POCKET GUIDE TO

# Micronutrient Management

Editors

**Kristen M. Roberts**
PhD, RDN, LD, CNSC, FASPEN, FAND

**Holly Estes-Doetsch**
MS, RDN, LD

**Marcia Nahikian-Nelms**
PhD, RDN, FAND

*Academy of Nutrition and Dietetics*
*Chicago, IL*

**.eat right.** Academy of Nutrition and Dietetics

Academy of Nutrition and Dietetics
120 S. Riverside Plaza, Suite 2190
Chicago, IL 60606

*Academy of Nutrition and Dietetics Pocket Guide to Micronutrient Management*

ISBN 978-0-88091-233-4 (print)
ISBN 978-0-88091-234-1 (eBook)
Catalog Number 233425 (print)
Catalog Number 233425e (eBook)

The views expressed in this publication are those of the authors and do not necessarily reflect policies and/or official positions of the Academy of Nutrition and Dietetics. Mention of product names in this publication does not constitute endorsement by the authors or the Academy of Nutrition and Dietetics. The Academy of Nutrition and Dietetics disclaims responsibility for the application of the information contained herein.

10    9    8    7    6    5    4    3    2    1

For more information on the Academy of Nutrition and Dietetics, visit www.eatright.org.

Library of Congress Cataloging-in-Publication Data

Names: Roberts, Kristen M., editor. | Estes-Doetsch, Holly, editor. |
  Nahikian-Nelms, Marcia, editor. | Academy of Nutrition and Dietetics,
  issuing body.
Title: Pocket guide to micronutrient management / [edited by] Kristen M.
  Roberts, Holly Estes-Doetsch, Marcia Nahikian-Nelms.
Description: Chicago, IL : Academy of Nutrition and Dietetics, [2024] |
  Includes bibliographical references and index.
Identifiers: LCCN 2024022368 (print) | LCCN 2024022369 (ebook) | ISBN
  9780880912334 (spiral bound) | ISBN 9780880912341 (ebook)
Subjects: MESH: Micronutrients--deficiency | Deficiency Diseases--therapy |
  Dietary Supplements | Nutrition Therapy
Classification: LCC RM216 (print) | LCC RM216 (ebook) | NLM QU 145.5 |
  DDC 615.8/54--dc23/eng/20240703
LC record available at https://lccn.loc.gov/2024022368
LC ebook record available at https://lccn.loc.gov/2024022369

Printed in Canada

# Contents

# List of Boxes, Tables, and Figures

## Boxes

# Tables

# Figures

# Contributors

## Editors

Kristen M. Roberts, PhD, RDN, LD, CNSC, FASPEN, FAND
Associate Professor, Gastroenterology, Hepatology, and Nutrition at
The Ohio State University Wexner Medical Center
Columbus, OH

Holly Estes-Doetsch, MS, RDN, LD
Clinical Instructor, Gastroenterology, Hepatology, and Nutrition at
The Ohio State University Wexner Medical Center
Columbus, OH

Marcia Nahikian-Nelms, PhD, RDN, FAND
Professor, Emeritus, College of Medicine, The Ohio State University
Columbus, OH

## Contributors

Mette M. Berger, MD, PhD
Professor Emeritus, Faculty of Biology and Medicine, Lausanne
University
Lausanne, Switzerland

Renée Blaauw, PhD, RD(SA)
Professor, Division of Human Nutrition, Faculty of Medicine and
Health Sciences, Stellenbosch University
Stellenbosch, South Africa

Leopoldo C. Cancio, MD, FACS, FCCM
Director, US Army Institute of Surgical Research Burn Center
Fort Sam Houston, TX

Emanuele Cereda, MD, PhD
Physician and Research Scientist, Fondazione IRCCS Policlinico San
Matteo
Pavia, Italy

Lingtak-Neander Chan, PharmD, BCNSP, FCCP, FASPEN
Professor of Pharmacy, Interdisciplinary Faculty in Nutritional
Sciences, University of Washington, Schools of
Pharmacy and Public Health
Seattle, WA

Mary Petrea Cober, PharmD, BCNSP, BCPPS, FASPEN
Professor, Pharmacy Practice, Northeast Ohio Medical University
Rootstown, OH

Osman Mohamed Elfadil, MBBS
Assistant Professor of Medicine, Mayo Clinic
Rochester, MN

David C. Evans, MD, FACS, FCCM, FASPEN
Adjunct Clinical Professor of Surgery, Ohio University
Medical Director, OhioHealth Nutrition Support Team, OhioHealth
Grant Medical Center
Columbus, OH

Kyle Hampson, PharmD, MPH, BCNSP, BCPPS, CNSC, FASPEN
Long Island University
Brooklyn, NY

Michelle L. Kozeniecki Schneider, MS, RDN, CNSC, CCTD, FASPEN
Lead Clinical Dietitian, Froedtert Hospital
Milwaukee, WI

Lance Kruger, PharmD, RPh
Senior Medical Science Liaison, Fresenius Medical Care
Avon, IN

Melissa Mroz-Planells, DCN, RDN
Kidney Nutrition Specialists
Seattle, WA

Manpreet S. Mundi, MD
Professor of Medicine, Mayo Clinic
Rochester, MN

Nancy Munoz, DCN, MHA, RDN, FAND
Chief, Nutrition and Food Service, VA Southern
Nevada Healthcare System
Las Vegas, NV

Gretchen Murray, RD, LD, CNSC
The Ohio State University Wexner Medical Center
Columbus, OH

Megan Nordlund, MS, RD, CSG
Clinical Dietitian, Harborview Medical Center
Seattle, WA

Julie Parrot, MS, RDN
Temple University Health System
Philadelphia, PA
Faculty of Health Sciences and Wellbeing, University of Sunderland
Visiting Research Fellow and PhD candidate
Sunderland, UK

Avani Patel, PharmD, MDN, RDN, LD
Pharmacist, Registered Dietitian Nutritionist
Plain City, OH

Jayshil J. Patel, MD
Associate Professor of Medicine, Medical College of Wisconsin
Milwaukee, WI

Kaitlin A. Pruskowski, PharmD, BCPS, BCCCP, FCCM
Clinical Pharmacist, Burn Critical Care,
US Army Institute of Surgical Research
JBSA Fort Sam Houston, TX

Beth A. Shields, MS, RDN, LD, CNSC
Chief of Nutritional Medicine & Metabolism,
US Army Institute of Surgical Research
Fort Sam Houston, TX

Nancy Storms Walsh, RDN
Dietitian, Retired
Rosebun, SD

Jane Ziegler, DCN, RDN, LDN
Professor and Interim Chair, Department of Clinical
and Preventive Nutrition, Rutgers University
Newark, NJ

# Reviewers

Mette M. Berger, MD, PhD
Professor Emeritus, Faculty of Biology and Medicine,
Lausanne University
Lausanne, Switzerland

Renée Blaauw, PhD, RD(SA)
Professor, Division of Human Nutrition, Faculty of Medicine and
Health Sciences, Stellenbosch University
Stellenbosch, South Africa

Laura Byham-Gray, PhD, RD
Professor, Department of Clinical and Preventative Nutritional
Sciences, School of Health Professions, Rutgers University
Newark, NJ

Lingtak-Neander Chan, PharmD, BCNSP, FCCP, FASPEN
Professor of Pharmacy and Interdisciplinary Faculty of
Nutritional Sciences, University of Washington
Seattle, WA

Kathleen Logan Coughlin, MS, RDN
Advanced Practice II Dietitian, Cleveland Clinic
Cleveland, OH

Olivia Gladys Funk, PharmD
Pharmacy Resident, Advent Health Orlando
Orlando, FL

Amanda E. Jacobson-Kelly, MD, MSc
Assistant Professor of Pediatrics, Division of Hematology/Oncology,
Nationwide Children's Hospital
Columbus, OH

Jennifer Kerner, MS, RDN, LD, CDCES
Clinical Dietitian, Advanced Practice,
University Hospitals of Cleveland
Westlake, OH

Mark Klang, MS, RPh, BCNSP, PhD, FASPEN
Core Manager, Research Pharmacy,
Memorial Sloan Kettering Cancer Center
New York, NY

Vanessa J. Kumpf, PharmD, BCNSP, FASPEN
Clinical Pharmacist Specialist, Nutrition Support,
Vanderbilt University Medical Center
Nashville, TN

Catherine M. McDonald, PhD, RDN, CSP
Clinical Dietitian, Primary Children's Hospital
Salt Lake City, UT

Kelly O'Donnell, MS, RDN, CNSC
Nutrition Support Specialist, University of Virginia Health System
Charlottesville, VA

Emma J. Osland, AdvAPD
Advanced Dietitian, Royal Brisbane and Women's Hospital
Herston, Australia

Neha Parekh, MS, RD, LD
Clinical Intake Coordinator, Cleveland Clinic
Cleveland, OH

Rebecca Romero, MHA, RD, LD, CLC
Clinical Manager, Nationwide Children's Hospital
Columbus, OH

Haley Schmidt, RD, CNSC
Neonatal Clinical Dietitian, Medical University of
South Carolina Shawn Jenkins Children's Hospital
Charleston, SC

# Foreword

Micronutrient health is a fundamental component of medical and nutrition therapies but has suffered from a lack of published and usable guidelines for practitioners. With the *Academy of Nutrition and Dietetics Pocket Guide to Micronutrient Management*, the editors—Kristen M. Roberts, PhD, RDN, LD, CNSC, FASPEN, FAND; Holly Estes-Doetsch, MS, RDN, LD; and Marcia Nahikian-Nelms, PhD, RDN, FAND—have brought the top subject-matter experts together to provide an evidence-based review of micronutrient physiology, deficiencies, and treatment in a practical handbook. This pocket guide takes an interprofessional approach, which is critical in health care today. This text fills a void in the published guidance for the treatment of both hospitalized and outpatient populations.

I have been practicing internationally as a registered dietitian nutritionist for the past decade. In that time, I have seen firsthand the impact of micronutrient deficiencies on the health of individuals worldwide. From rampant iron deficiency in women and children, to neural tube defects related to folate deficiency during pregnancy, to vitamin C deficiency in patients with burns, to blindness caused by vitamin A deficiency in children—micronutrient deficiencies are more common than we think. Furthermore, they are not limited solely to developing countries, existing in developed countries as well. The registered dietitian nutritionist has the skill set to assess, identify, and treat micronutrient deficiencies through a combination of the nutrition focused physical exam, diet history, and biochemical data. This book brings together the relevant micronutrient information and enables clinicians to strengthen their deficiency-assessment skills, create treatment plans, and enhance their practices, resulting in positive impacts on patient outcomes.

Lauri Wright, PhD, RDN, LD/N, FAND
Associate Professor and Director of Nutrition Programs,
University of South Florida
2023-2024 Academy of Nutrition and Dietetics President

# Acknowledgments

The editors give special thanks to the Academy of Nutrition and Dietetics, especially Stacey Zettle, MS, RDN, and Betsy Hornick, MS, RDN, for their ongoing support with planning, implementing, and editing this book. Thank you!

Thank you to my colleagues, specifically the nurse practitioners and gastroenterologists, for their support in making nutrition and micronutrient assessment a standard of care for all patients seen within the Division of Gastroenterology, Hepatology, and Nutrition at The Ohio State University. I also thank the students in the School of Health and Rehabilitation Sciences who continue to motivate me to be a better educator. Most importantly, I thank my family. Bryan, I could not be successful without your confidence in me and unconditional support for my career. Finally, to the "little people" in my life, Benjamin, Simon, and Anna—without you, this book would have been completed a year earlier.

*Kristen M. Roberts, PhD, RDN, LD, CNSC, FASPEN, FAND*

I extend a special thank-you to the students and faculty in the Master of Dietetics and Nutrition Program and the Division of Gastroenterology, Hepatology, and Nutrition at The Ohio State University for their support. I also wish to acknowledge the faculty in the Doctor of Clinical Nutrition program at Rutgers University for their mentorship and my family for their support.

*Holly Estes-Doetsch, MS, RDN, LD*

I gratefully acknowledge the ongoing support of the faculty, practitioners, and students in the School of Health and Rehabilitation Sciences in the College of Medicine at The Ohio State University.

*Marcia Nahikian-Nelms, PhD, RDN, FAND*

# About the Editors

**Kristen M. Roberts, PhD, RDN, LD, CNSC, FASPEN, FAND,** has formal training as a clinical and translational scientist with a specialization designated from the Center for Clinical and Translational Science at The Ohio State University. She has been a practicing clinical registered dietitian nutritionist for nearly 20 years and has expert knowledge in the management of intestinal failure, enteral and parenteral nutrition, and gastrointestinal diseases. In addition, she has attended the National Institutes of Health training program on dietary supplements and runs an active laboratory focusing on the development of micronutrient treatment strategies through the use of physical and biochemical assessment. Roberts has authored several peer-reviewed publications and speaks nationally on micronutrient assessment, fluid and electrolyte status, and acid-base balance. Her joint appointment is in the Division of Gastroenterology, Hepatology, and Nutrition and the School of Health and Rehabilitation Sciences, both at The Ohio State University. In clinical practice, she comanages a micronutrient assessment and treatment service. Roberts serves as a deputy editor for the journal *Nutrition in Clinical Practice* and is a fellow of the American Society for Parenteral and Enteral Nutrition (ASPEN) and the Academy of Nutrition and Dietetics. Most recently, she received the Distinguished Practice Award from the Dietitians in Nutrition Support dietetic practice group of the Academy of Nutrition and Dietetics, as well as the Distinguished Nutrition Support Dietitian, Advanced Clinical Practice Award from ASPEN.

**Holly Estes-Doetsch, MS, RDN, LD,** has been a registered dietitian nutritionist since 2006 and holds dual master of science degrees, one in nutrition and the other in exercise and sport science, from the University of Utah. She serves on the faculty of the School of Health and Rehabilitation Sciences at The Ohio State University, where she has taught medical nutrition therapy courses for graduate and undergraduate dietetics students since 2013. She has more than

10 years of clinical practice experience in acute care and outpatient settings and has worked with both pediatric and adult populations. Estes-Doetsch has presented on micronutrient management at the Academy of Nutrition and Dietetics Food & Nutrition Conference & Expo (FNCE) and comanages a micronutrient assessment and treatment service in the Division of Gastroenterology, Hepatology, and Nutrition at The Ohio State University. She codeveloped a case-based student training experience on micronutrient management during the COVID-19 pandemic as an opportunity for students to acquire supervised practice hours. In 2018, she and her coauthors received the Innovations in Nutrition and Dietetics Practice and Education poster session award from the Academy of Nutrition and Dietetics Council on Future Practice for research highlighting the value of using patient simulation to teach assessment of malnutrition, as presented at FNCE. In 2022, she received the Outstanding Dietetics Educator award from the Ohio Academy of Nutrition and Dietetics.

**Marcia Nahikian-Nelms, PhD, RDN, FAND,** is a professor of clinical health and rehabilitation sciences, the Assistant Dean for Academic Affairs in the School of Health and Rehabilitation Sciences, and the Director of Teaching and Learning for Faculty Advancement, Mentoring, and Engagement in the College of Medicine at The Ohio State University. She has practiced as a registered dietitian nutritionist and public health nutritionist for more than 45 years. She is the lead author of several textbooks, including *Nutrition Therapy and Pathophysiology* (now in its fourth edition) and *Medical Nutrition Therapy: A Case Study Approach* (now in its seventh edition), and has authored peer-reviewed journal articles and chapters for other texts. Her clinical expertise focuses on the development and practice of evidence-based nutrition therapy for both pediatric and adult populations. Nahikian-Nelms serves as one of the leads for interprofessional education and has contributed to simulation development within the seven health science colleges at The Ohio State University. She has received the university's Alumni Award for Distinguished Teaching, the Governor's Award for Outstanding Teaching for the

State of Missouri, the Outstanding Dietetic Educator in Missouri and Ohio award, the Outstanding Teacher in Health and Rehabilitation Sciences award, and the Provost's Research, Instruction and Development for Excellence Award from Southeast Missouri State University in recognition of her teaching.

CHAPTER 1

# Introduction and the Role of Interprofessional Care

Marcia Nahikian-Nelms, PhD, RDN, FAND

## Introduction

Micronutrient deficiencies are often viewed as either a historical medical issue that has been resolved with improved food supplies, enrichment, and fortification or a problem of extreme malnutrition occurring primarily in countries experiencing issues with food supply. As nutrition research has evolved, we have expanded our understanding of the role of micronutrients in acute and chronic disease, the impact of disease and treatments on micronutrient status, and the potential role of micronutrients in enhancing recovery from disease through complementation, repletion, supplementation, or treatment.[1] To support patient health outcomes, micronutrients must be considered as part of the assessment and treatment plan of individual patients.

Many patient populations under the care of specialized care teams are at risk for or present with micronutrient deficiencies. These include patients with renal disease, burns, wounds, and intestinal diseases, as well as those undergoing bariatric surgery or in critical care. A resource that captures this diversity of patients is needed to increase the identification and treatment of micronutrient concerns and subsequently improve patient outcomes. Published, disease-specific clinical guidelines for addressing micronutrient deficiencies when developing patient care plans are lacking, yet micronutrient deficiencies are present in a large percentage of inpatients and outpatients. This book is meant to serve as a reference for clinicians treating micronutrient deficiencies (not toxicities), and it approaches micronutrient management from an interprofessional perspective. Authors from various health disciplines have collaborated so that each chapter adequately reflects multidisciplinary perspectives of care. It was essential to have a *team* of health care professionals contribute to a publication of this importance, as micronutrient assessment and treatment are best achieved through an interprofessional approach.[2,3]

This book generally does not cover micronutrient management in specialized nutrition support, as these guidelines have been published elsewhere.[4,5] Conventional units are presented throughout this pocket guide to support the units most commonly seen by practicing clinicians. The international system of units (or SI units) can be accessed elsewhere.[6] Within this book, cut-off levels may vary based on the references cited within the chapter and the indications for treatment. This book does not address pediatric nutrition (other than neonates). Lastly, due to the paucity of research on micronutrient repletion, the guidelines within this handbook are suggested based on current practice. More research is needed to formalize disease-specific guidelines.

# Current Status of Micronutrient Management

The European Society for Clinical Nutrition and Metabolism (ESPEN) has clarified language for micronutrient management by defining the terminology for micronutrient assessment, monitoring, and prescription. This language is adopted in this text, and Box 1.1 on page 4 outlines the definitions.[1] These new definitions may represent a shift from the way clinicians previously spoke about micronutrient management. For example, in the ESPEN terminology, giving a patient a dosage of a micronutrient to restore its level in the body to what is physiologically normal is called *repletion*, whereas previously it was referred to as *supplementation*. In the new terminology, *supplementation* refers to giving dosages higher than standard amounts (ie, greater than Dietary Reference Intakes or Recommended Dietary Allowances). Of note, Chapter 14 (Metabolic and Bariatric Surgery) does not employ the ESPEN terminology, as this area of nutrition therapy uses practice guidelines from the American Society for Metabolic and Bariatric Surgery, in which supplementation, assay cut-off levels, and repletion amounts are typically different from those for patients who have not had bariatric surgery.

Screening and assessment for micronutrient complementation, repletion, supplementation, or pharmacological dosing takes into consideration what we know from the field of population health, the requirements to support normal growth and development, the typical contributions from dietary patterns, and increased needs during disease states. The most common micronutrients at risk for deficiency in the United States include calcium, iron, magnesium, potassium, choline, folate, and vitamins A, C, D, and E. These potential deficiencies are highlighted in the *Dietary Guidelines for Americans, 2020–2025* and multiple studies assessing nutritional intake that stem from the National Health and Nutrition Examination Survey (NHANES) program.[7-9] In addition, food-insecure households in the United States are at higher risk for inadequate dietary intakes of zinc and vitamins B6, B12, and K.[7] An examination of NHANES data from 2001-2016 further identifies pediatric risk to include iron, calcium, B6, choline, and potassium.[9] Another examination of NHANES dietary data, from 2005-2016, focused on specific nutrients known to support immune health. This analysis found that common inadequacies included zinc and vitamins A, C, D, and E.[10] The translation of population-based assessment to individual risk does not necessarily mean that a physiologic deficiency exists based on laboratory and clinical indices, but it does provide a framework for the clinician to

**BOX 1.1  European Society for Clinical Nutrition and Metabolism (ESPEN) Definitions of Micronutrient Prescriptions[1]**

## Complementation

| | |
|---|---|
| Oxford definition | The act of adding to something in a way that improves it or makes it more attractive, complete |
| ESPEN definition | The delivery of micronutrients to cover basal needs (eg, to complete enteral feeds or parenteral nutrition [PN]) |
| Comment | This action is typically needed to cover basal needs in case of progressive or insufficient enteral nutrition (EN). |
| Example | Provision of a multivitamin for a patient receiving EN (ie, a clinically stable patient with low body weight) when the pre-scribed EN volume meets energy and protein requirements but does not meet micronutrient requirements |

## Repletion

| | |
|---|---|
| Oxford definition | The act of making something full again by replacing what has been used |
| ESPEN definition | The delivery of micronutrients with the aim of restoring a normal status when the deficit is known; sometimes called supplementation, but this should be avoided |
| Comment | Repletion is employed when deficiencies or losses are identi-fied or presumed; it aims to restore a normal status. |
| Example | Provision of additional copper to a patient receiving long-term jejunal feeding who is identified as copper deficient, with the intent of reversing symptoms and restoring serum levels |

## Supplementation

| | |
|---|---|
| Oxford definition | The act of adding something to something else to improve or complete it |

| BOX 1.1 | European Society for Clinical Nutrition and Metabolism (ESPEN) Definitions of Micronutrient Prescriptions[1] (cont.) |
|---|---|
| ESPEN definition | The delivery of higher than standard doses (ie, superior to Dietary Reference Intake or PN recommendation); does not include pharmaconutrition but designates doses higher than basal requirements delivered in an attempt to correct depletion or deficiency |
| Comment | This term is applied without differentiation of amount whenever a micronutrient is prescribed. |
| Example | Addition of vitamin D and calcium for an individual at risk for osteoporosis |

### Pharmacologic dosing

| | |
|---|---|
| Oxford definition | Relating to the scientific study of drugs and their use in medicine |
| ESPEN definition | The delivery of a specific micronutrient to improve host defenses or any other biologic end point associated with good clinical evolution and to improve the outcome of patients who are critically ill |
| Comment | Generally, only one micronutrient is prescribed. The administration route is not determined. This is not a nutritional effect but rather a pharmacologic action. |
| Example | Therapeutic use of a high intravenous dose of vitamin C and thiamin in the intensive care unit as an adjunctive treatment for sepsis |

Adapted under CC BY NC ND from Berger MM, Shenkin A, Schweinlin A, et al. ESPEN micronutrient guideline. *Clin Nutr.* 2022;41(6):1357-1424. doi:10.1016/j.clnu.2022.02.015.1

realize the potential risk. During times of increased growth and need, such as infancy, adolescence, pregnancy, or lactation, micronutrient needs are higher. These additional requirements are accounted for in any screening or assessment and are reflected in the standard guidelines, Recommended Dietary Allowances, and nutrition support guidelines.[1,11]

Micronutrient deficiencies are logically associated with decreased dietary intake and with inferior-quality dietary intake. However, the recognition of malnutrition in the United States and in other countries has risen in importance. Patients who are hospitalized or of advanced age, those with chronic disease, and those who are experiencing acute inflammatory conditions are at substantial risk for malnutrition and micronutrient concerns.[12-15] The role of micronutrients in public health is also of the highest priority when creating evidence-based care guidelines as a component of disease prevention and treatment.[16-18]

Throughout this text, our clinicians draw from the literature to provide expert guidance for addressing micronutrient requirements influenced by acute disease and their subsequent treatments. Chapter 2 reviews regulatory standards for micronutrient formulations and discusses bioavailability, labeling, and third-party verification of content. Chapter 3 focuses on differences in product formulations and routes of micronutrient delivery, the awareness of which will aid clinical decision-making. Chapter 4 provides an overview of the impact of inflammation on micronutrient status and management, and Chapter 13 addresses the impact of critical illness on micronutrient status and the potential role of micronutrients in the treatment of critical illness. In acute-care crises, such as sepsis or traumatic brain injury, micronutrients are essential to support the metabolic pathways induced during inflammatory responses. Without replenishing stores or meeting increased requirements, health outcomes may be negatively affected. For example, during the COVID-19 pandemic, both vitamin C and D deficiencies were reported in patients hospitalized with the disease.[19] Chapters 5 through 8 outline the specifics of fat-soluble, water-soluble, iron, and trace mineral deficiencies. The remaining chapters review micronutrient deficiencies and treatment as related to various populations, including patients with gastrointestinal disease, renal disease, bariatric surgery, wounds, burns, and neonatal patients.

# Role of the Interprofessional Team

This text seeks to approach micronutrient management through an interprofessional lens. The physician (medical doctor or doctor of osteopathic medicine), registered dietitian nutritionist (RDN), registered nurse or nurse practitioner, and pharmacist (doctor of pharmacy or registered pharmacist) all bring unique knowledge, skills, and training to patient care, as described in Box 1.2.[20-23]

The RDN has extensive knowledge of each of the micronutrients and its role in normal physiology and disease pathophysiology. RDNs are trained to assess dietary adequacy and perform biochemical and physical

| BOX 1.2 | American Society for Parenteral and Enteral Nutrition (ASPEN) Standards of Professional Performance[20-23] |
|---------|-----------------------------------------------------------------------------------------------------------|
| Physician | The nutrition-support physician should know the patient's macronutrient, micronutrient, electrolyte, and fluid requirements, summarize and document these requirements in the medical record, and communicate them to the patient's primary health care team.[23] |
| Pharmacist | In collaboration with other health care professionals, the nutrition-support pharmacist should participate in the routine assessment of the patient's energy, protein, vitamin, mineral, fluid, and electrolyte requirements according to the patient's age, disease states, clinical conditions, and pharmacotherapy.[21] |
| Registered dietitian nutritionist (RDN) | The RDN should evaluate nutrition screening results, conduct a nutrition assessment using a nutrition focused physical exam, confer with interprofessional team members, determine a plan of care, and provide ongoing monitoring and adjustments to the plan of care.[20] |
| Registered nurse or nurse practitioner | The nursing professional should analyze data to determine the patient's nutritional status, as well as the energy, nutrient, and fluid requirements of the patient relevant to the impact of the clinical situation on nutrient requirements.[22] |

assessments using a nutrition focused physical exam to help determine micronutrient status. The 2017 Academy of Nutrition and Dietetics scope of practice for RDNs states that they may also "initiate, implement, and adjust protocol- or physician-order-driven nutrition-related medication orders and pharmacotherapy plans in accordance with established policy or protocols consistent with organizational policy and procedure."[24] The standards of professional performance for RDNs in nutrition support state that the individual scope of practice depends on the level of education and training (competent, proficient, and expert) and the competence level translates to the ability to make the appropriate decisions for assessment and treatment.[20] Federal regulations allow for RDNs to write orders without having to be appointed to the medical staff.[25]

The pharmacist is uniquely trained to determine the route and the type of formulation for micronutrients. The standards of practice for the nutrition-support pharmacist state that "in collaboration with other healthcare professionals, the [nutrition support professional] shall participate in the routine assessment of the patient's energy, protein, vitamin, mineral, fluid, and electrolyte requirements."[21] The registered nurse or nurse practitioner brings additional skills of physical assessment and clinical interviewing to the team, collaborates with other health care providers to assess nutritional requirements, and assists with the management of nutrition support devices, such as feeding tubes or vascular access devices.[22] The physician ultimately provides the medical governance over the patient's plan of care, informs other team members of the broader medical plan, and places the micronutrient treatment within that context.[23] Communication among these professionals promotes a complete plan for assessment, treatment, and monitoring.

Accreditation and licensing standards for all professions emphasize interprofessional collaboration. For example, pharmacy standards of practice require that pharmacists collaborate with other health care providers to ensure care coordination that will lead to positive patient outcomes.[26] The Accreditation Council for Graduate Medical Education expects medical residents to work within interprofessional teams to ensure patient safety and optimal patient outcomes.[27] Nursing practice standards also require collaboration with interprofessional teams to ensure positive outcomes.[28] Similarly, the standards of practice for RDNs encompass competencies of collaboration and team-based decision-making, not only in training but also in entry-level practice.[29] In 2021, the National Collaborative for Improving the Clinical Learning Environment published the first guidelines to create educational and treatment pathways for interprofessional learning.[30] Micronutrient management is an excellent model for bridging the classroom and clinical environments and, thereby, for demonstrating interprofessional practice and competence while ultimately improving patient outcomes.

Micronutrient management is uniquely suited to interprofessional collaboration. Evidence-based guidelines for many of the recommendations needed in complex management are lacking, and thus extensive critical thinking and clinical decision-making are required, necessitating a team-based approach. The *Pocket Guide to Micronutrient Management* models this collaborative clinical decision-making within each chapter as it guides the clinician through the existing literature and its application for care as it relates to each micronutrient and patient population. As each patient is unique, clinicians are encouraged to combine this information with their own clinical judgment for the best patient outcomes.

# References

1.  Berger MM, Shenkin A, Schweinlin A, et al. ESPEN micronutrient guideline. *Clin Nutr.* 2022;41(6):1357-1424. doi:10.1016/j.clnu.2022.02.015
2.  Jacob VS, Chattopadhyay SK, Thota AB, et al. Economics of team-based care in controlling blood pressure: a community guide systematic review. *Am J Prev Med.* 2015;49:772-783. doi:10.1016/j.amepre.2015.04.003
3.  Wang SM, Kung PT, Wang WH, Huang KH, Tsai WC. Effects of multidisciplinary team care on utilization of emergency care for patients with lung cancer. *Am J Manag Care.* 2014;20(8):e353-e364.
4.  Malone A, Carney LN, Carrera AL, Mays A, eds. *ASPEN Enteral Nutrition Handbook.* 2nd ed. American Society for Parenteral and Enteral Nutrition; 2019.
5.  Ayers P, Bobo ES, Hurt RT, Mays AA, Worthington PH, eds. *ASPEN Parenteral Nutrition Handbook.* 3rd ed. American Society for Parenteral and Enteral Nutrition; 2020.
6.  Adeli K, Higgins V, Bohn MK. Reference information for the clinical laboratory. In: Rafai N, Rossa WK, Young I, et al. eds. *Tietz Textbook of Laboratory Medicine.* 7th ed. Elsevier, 2023.

7.    US Department of Agriculture, US Department of Health and Human Services. *Dietary Guidelines for Americans, 2020-2025.* 9th ed. US Department of Agriculture and US Department of Health and Human Services; 2020. Accessed September 8, 2023. www.dietaryguidelines.gov /resources/2020-2025-dietary-guidelines-online-materials

8.    Cowan AE, Jun S, Tooze JA, et al. Total usual micronutrient intakes compared to the dietary reference intakes among US adults by food security status. *Nutrients.* 2020;12(1):38-49. doi:10.3390/nu12010038

9.    Bailey ADL, Fulgoni VL, Shah N, et al. Nutrient intake adequacy from food and beverage intake of US children aged 1-6 years from NHANES 2001-2016. *Nutrients.* 2021;13:827-840. doi:10.3390/nu13030827

10.   Reider CA, Chung RY, Devarshi PP, Grant RW, Mitmesser SH. Inadequacy of immune health nutrients: intakes in US adults, the 2005–2016 NHANES. *Nutrients.* 2020;12:1735-1751. doi:10.3390/nu12061735

11.   Institute of Medicine. *Dietary Reference Intakes: The Essential Guide to Nutrient Requirements.* National Academies Press; 2006.

12.   Berger MM, Ben-Harmouda N. Trace element and vitamin deficiency: quantum medicine or essential prescription? *Curr Opin Crit Care.* 2020;26:355-362. doi:10.1097/MCC.0000000000000737

13.   Lewis MJ. Alcoholism and nutrition: a review of vitamin supplementation and treatment. *Curr Opin Clin Nutr Metab Care.* 2020;23(2):138-144. doi:10.1097/MCO.0000000000000622

14.   Lee KS, Moser DK, Park JH, Lennie TA. The association of deficiencies of water-soluble vitamin intake with health-related quality of life and prognosis in patients with heart failure. *Qual Life Res.* 2021;30(4):1183-1190. doi:10.1007/s11136-020-02725-w

15.   Sauer AC, Goates S, Malone A, et al. Prevalence of malnutrition risk and the impact of nutrition risk on hospital outcomes: results from nutritionDay in the U.S. *JPEN J Parenter Enteral Nutr.* 2019;43(7):918-926. doi:10.1002/jpen.1499

16.   Mazidi M, Ofori-Asenso R, George ES, et al. Association between nutrient patterns and hypertension among adults in the United States: a population-based survey. *High Blood Press Cardiovasc Prev.* 2020;27(2):133-138. doi:10.1007/s40292-020-00364-3

17.   Epidemiology of Osteoporosis and Fragility Fractures. International Osteoporosis Foundation. Accessed October 26, 2021. www.osteoporosis .foundation/facts-statistics/epidemiology-of-osteoporosis-and-fragility -fractures

18.   DASH eating plan. National Heart, Lung, and Blood Institute. Accessed November 21, 2021. www.nhlbi.nih.gov/health-topics/dash-eating-plan

19.   Tomasa-Irriguible TM, Bielsa-Berrocal L. COVID-19: up to 82% critically ill patients had low vitamin C values. *BMC.* 2021;20(1):65-68. doi:10.1186 /s12937-021-00727-z

20. Corrigan ML, Bobo E, Rollins C, Mogensen KM. Academy of Nutrition and Dietetics and American Society for Parenteral and Enteral Nutrition: revised 2021 standards of practice and standards of professional performance for registered dietitian nutritionists (competent, proficient, and expert) in nutrition support. *Nutr Clin Pract.* 2021;36(6):1126-1143. doi:10.1002/ncp.10774

21. Tucker A, Ybarra J, Bingham A, et al. American Society for Parenteral and Enteral Nutrition (A.S.P.E.N.) standards of practice for nutrition support pharmacists. *Nutr Clin Pract.* 2015;30:139-146. doi:10.1177/0884533614550318

22. DiMaria-Ghalili RA, Gilbert K, Lord L, et al. Standards of nutrition care practice and professional performance for nutrition support and generalist nurses. *Nutr Clin Pract.* 2016;31(4):527-547. doi:10.1177/0884533616653835

23. Mascarenhas MR, August DA, DeLegge MH, et al. Standards of practice for nutrition support physicians. *Nutr Clin Pract.* 2012;27(2):295-299. doi:10.1177/0884533612438286

24. 2024 Scope and Standards of Practice for the RDN. Commission on Dietetic Registration; 2024. Accessed April 20, 2024. https://cdrnet.org/scope

25. Medicare and Medicaid Programs; regulatory provisions to promote program efficiency, transparency, and burden reduction; part II. *Fed Regist.* 2014;79(91):27106-27157. Codified as 42 CFR Parts 413, 416, 440, 442, 482, 483, 485, 486, 488, 491, and 493. Accessed August 9, 2021. www.gpo.gov/fdsys/pkg/FR-2014-05-12/pdf/2014-10687.pdf

26. Accreditation Council for Pharmacy Education. *Accreditation Standards and Key Elements for the Professional Program in Pharmacy Leading to the Doctor of Pharmacy Degree.* Draft Standards 2025. Accreditation Council for Pharmacy Education; 2024. Accessed April 21, 2024. www.acpe-accredit.org

27. Accreditation Council for Graduate Medical Education. *Common Program Requirements.* Accreditation Council for Graduate Medical Education; 2023.

28. Dickerson PS, Durkin GJ. Nursing Professional Development Standards of Practice: Standards 1–6. *J Nurses Prof Dev.* 2022;38(4):248-250. doi:10.1097/NND.0000000000000900

29. Commission on Dietetic Registration. *Essential Practice Competencies for the Commission on Dietetic Registration's Credentialed Nutrition and Dietetics Practitioners.* Academy of Nutrition and Dietetics; 2023.

30. National Collaborative for Improving the Clinical Learning Environment. *NCICLE Pathways to Excellence: Expectations for an Optimal Clinical Learning Environment to Achieve Safe and High-Quality Patient Care, 2021.* NCICLE; 2021. doi:10.33385/NCICLE.0003

CHAPTER 2

# Regulation of Dietary Supplements

Avani Patel, PharmD, MDN, RDN, LD

## Introduction

Micronutrient supplements are available in the form of dietary supplements (eg, over-the-counter oral supplements) or pharmaceutical products (eg, injectable trace elements and vitamins). As most consumers and health facilities use micronutrient supplements in the form of dietary supplements, it is important for health care providers to understand the quality and safety considerations associated with these products. This chapter covers how dietary supplements are regulated in the United States, third-party certification programs, and evidence-based professional resources for dietary supplements, including micronutrient products.

## Dietary Supplement Legislation

The US Food and Drug Administration (FDA) is the agency responsible for regulating dietary supplements in the United States.[1] Dietary supplements are regulated differently from prescription and over-the-counter medications. Three key pieces of legislation were instrumental in providing the regulatory framework for dietary supplements: the Dietary Supplement Health and Education Act of 1994 (DSHEA), the Dietary Supplement and Nonprescription Drug Consumer Protection Act of 2006, and the FDA Food Safety Modernization Act of 2010.

DSHEA is the principal legislation for dietary supplements in the United States.[2,3] It was passed as an amendment to the Federal Food, Drug, and Cosmetic Act of 1938.[1] Before DSHEA, dietary supplements were regulated as foods under the Food, Drug, and Cosmetic Act. DSHEA provided key definitions, outlined how dietary supplements would be regulated by the FDA, established labeling requirements, and created the Office of Dietary Supplements at the National Institutes of Health.

DSHEA defined the terms *dietary supplement*, *dietary ingredient*, and *new dietary ingredient*. *Dietary supplement* is defined in Box 2.1.[3]

---

**BOX 2.1  Definition of a Dietary Supplement[3]**

According to the Dietary Supplement Health and Education Act of 1994, a dietary supplement is a substance that:

- is taken by mouth as a pill, powder, tablet, or liquid;
- is intended to supplement the diet;
- contains one or more dietary ingredient(s); and
- is identified on the front panel of the product's label as being a dietary supplement.

---

Under DSHEA, *dietary ingredients* include but are not limited to substances such as vitamins, minerals, herbs and other botanicals, amino acids, and any dietary substances used to supplement the diet by increasing the total dietary intake.[3] The list also includes any concentrate, metabolite, constituent, extract, or combination of these substances.

A *new dietary ingredient* is an ingredient in a dietary supplement that was not sold in the United States before October 15, 1994.[3] Ingredients on the market before this date are "grandfathered" ingredients and are considered safe based on their historical record. It is the responsibility of the manufacturer to ensure the safety of grandfathered ingredients before selling them on the market. Dietary supplements containing new dietary ingredients require a 75-day notification to the FDA by the manufacturer before being marketed, as well as a premarket safety notification.[4] The premarket safety notification includes the information used by the manufacturer to determine that the new dietary ingredient is safe if used for the recommended conditions and according to directions on the label.

DSHEA established that the FDA would regulate dietary supplements as a separate subcategory of foods, not as new drugs or food additives.[3] Dietary supplements may not be sold as conventional food items, nor as the sole item constituting a meal or a diet. They do not require premarket approval from the FDA unless they contain a new dietary ingredient. Manufacturers of dietary supplements do not need to demonstrate proof of safety and efficacy before marketing their products, as is required of manufacturers of drugs (both prescription and nonprescription). Under DSHEA, dietary supplement manufacturers are responsible for ensuring the safety of their products, not the FDA. In the event of safety concerns, the FDA must prove that a dietary supplement is unsafe before it can limit the sale of the product or remove it from the market. Dietary supplements are not allowed to have an indication for use, which means efficacy cannot be measured. Instead of submitting data to support the efficacy and safety of a product, manufacturers are only required to submit the statement that will appear on the product label to the FDA within 30 days of marketing the product.

The Dietary Supplement and Nonprescription Drug Consumer Protection Act of 2006 was passed as an amendment to the Food, Drug, and Cosmetic Act. It established requirements for the reporting and recordkeeping of adverse events by responsible parties—namely, the manufacturers, packers, and distributors of dietary supplements.[5] The act stipulates that the label of a dietary supplement marketed in the United States must include a domestic address or domestic telephone number to which adverse effects can be reported. The responsible party must report any serious adverse event associated with the use of its product in the United States to the FDA. The submission of an adverse event report does not necessarily imply that the dietary supplement product caused the adverse event. The responsible party must maintain records of reported adverse events for 6 years, and these records are subject to inspection by an authorized representative of the Department of Health and Human Services.

The most recent legislation to affect the regulation of dietary supplements is the FDA Food Safety Modernization Act, which was enacted in 2010.[6] This act granted the FDA mandatory recall authority over adulterated and (some) misbranded food products—including dietary supplements. This provision allows the FDA to remove dietary supplements with safety concerns more quickly from the market. The act also required the FDA to publish guidance clarifying what constitutes a *new dietary ingredient*.

# Current Good Manufacturing Practices

DSHEA empowered the FDA to establish current good manufacturing practice (CGMP) requirements for dietary supplements.[7] CGMP regulations apply to any individual or entity that manufactures, packages, labels, or holds dietary supplements,[7] and they outline the minimum requirements for carrying out these activities. CGMP regulations must be followed by domestic and foreign companies that manufacture or distribute dietary supplements in areas where the FDA has authority.[4] Such companies must develop standards of practice that ensure quality and reproducibility in manufacturing. An example of a CGMP requirement is the written master manufacturing record; such a record must be created and used for each individual supplement formulation and for every batch size to guarantee consistency and homogeneity among batches of supplements. Other examples include the establishment of laboratory control processes and specifications for product-testing methods and the creation of protocols for holding reserve samples of products in conditions that prevent contamination or deterioration.

# Dietary Supplement Labeling

Manufacturers of dietary supplements are permitted to display claims about a supplement's effects on general wellness, bodily structure or function,[8] and nutritional deficiency disease on their product labels. Examples of claims about effects on bodily structure or function include, "calcium builds strong bones" or "fiber maintains bowel regularity."[9] If a label bears such a claim, it must also include the following FDA disclaimer: *This claim has not been evaluated by the Food and Drug Administration. This product is not intended to diagnose, treat, cure, or prevent any disease.*[8] The disclaimer is intended to distinguish structure or function claims from health claims, which are evaluated and approved by the FDA. It also distinguishes structure or function claims from drug claims, which are intended for the prevention or treatment of disease.[2] Claims regarding nutrient deficiency disease may describe the value of the product as it relates to a disease of nutrient deficiency; however, the claim must also indicate how widespread the disease is in the United States.[8]

Manufacturers of products with labels containing one or more of the aforementioned types of claims must notify the FDA of the claim within 30 days of marketing the product.[10] The FDA will evaluate the scientific evidence, including evidence-based research pertaining to the claim, and may request additional evidence from the manufacturer to substantiate the claim.

Further dietary supplement labeling requirements are outlined in the US Code of Federal Regulations (21 CFR 101.36).[11-13] Key requirements include the following:

- statement of identity (product name) and a statement that the product is a dietary supplement
- Supplement Facts panel
- list of any ingredients that do not appear on the Supplement Facts panel
- name and address of the manufacturer, packager, or distributor
- net quantity of contents

# Adulterated and Misbranded Products

The Food, Drug, and Cosmetic Act empowers the FDA to take action against any adulterated or misbranded dietary supplement.[14,15] The FDA may only take such action after the product is on the market, and the burden of proof falls on the FDA. A dietary supplement is considered misbranded if the label is false or misleading.[15] Box 2.2 provides more information on adulterated dietary supplements.[14]

---

**BOX 2.2  Adulterated Dietary Supplements[14]**

A dietary supplement is considered adulterated if any of the following is true:

- It is "injurious to health" or "presents a significant or unreasonable risk of illness or injury under conditions of use recommended or suggested in labeling" or "under normal conditions of use."
- It contains a new dietary ingredient for which there is insufficient safety information with regard to risk of illness or injury.
- It contains an ingredient that poses an "imminent hazard" to health.

---

# Regulation of Dietary Supplement Advertisements

Advertisements for dietary supplements are regulated by the Federal Trade Commission (FTC).[16] The FTC oversees print and broadcast advertising, infomercials, internet advertisements, catalogs, and other materials that directly market dietary supplements. This differs from the FDA's purview, which includes product labels, package inserts, and any point-of-sale promotional materials. The FTC often collaborates with the FDA to evaluate claims made by manufacturers of dietary supplements in their advertising. Advertisements sent via mail may also be regulated by the US Postal Inspection Service.

# Dietary Supplement Additives

The Food Additives Amendment of 1958 helped establish a framework for how additives are regulated. Additives are substances added to foods or dietary supplements to alter certain characteristics of the final product; they may, for example, improve a product's texture or appearance, or increase its shelf life.[17] For dietary supplements, the main dietary ingredients used in the product are not considered additives. Ingredients such as binders, excipients, and fillers *are* considered food additives by the FDA and are regulated as such. The FDA maintains a list of two groups of additives that are exempt from the regulatory process[17]:

- *prior-sanctioned substances*—additives that the FDA or US Department of Agriculture established as safe before the passing of the Food Additives Amendment

- substances *"generally recognized as safe" (GRAS)*—additives that are considered safe because of a long history of safety data or published scientific evidence supporting their safety (eg, salt, sugar, and spices)

If a new food additive is neither prior-sanctioned nor GRAS, the manufacturer must prove its safety to the FDA.

## Concern for Allergens

There are concerns that allergens may make their way into the formulations of dietary supplements as additives. How often additives result in a clinically significant adverse reaction is difficult to determine, though the possibility cannot be ruled out. Because over-the-counter dietary supplements are regulated as food products, the FDA requires that the presence of any of the nine major food allergens be indicated on the product label, along with the source of the allergen (sesame, fish, shellfish, tree nuts, soy, milk, wheat, peanuts, egg).[18] The name of the allergen can appear in two ways:

- in parentheses immediately after the ingredient within the ingredient list, as in "lecithin (soy)"

- in a separate "contains" statement located either next to, after, or under the list of ingredients, as in "Contains: soy"

These labeling requirements do *not* extend to prescription and nonprescription medications.

In addition, allergens other than the nine major food allergens do not need to be labeled and can be difficult to identify. For example, gluten (found in wheat, barley, or rye) is sometimes used as a binding or filler agent in food and pharmaceutical products.[19] Although wheat is one of the top nine allergens and must be listed on product labels, barley and rye are not. The amount of gluten present in food product can be problematic for patients with gluten intolerance or celiac disease. It is important to seek out dietary supplements (such as multivitamin/mineral products) that are labeled gluten-free for these patients. The FDA has clear rules defining the term *gluten-free* and when it can be used on a label. A product must contain less than 20 parts per million of gluten to be labeled *gluten-free, no gluten, free of gluten*, or *without gluten*.[20] Because of the variability in dietary supplement quality, the risk of gluten contamination in dietary supplements cannot be excluded.[21]

# Quality and Safety Concerns

Although DSHEA provided the framework for the regulation of dietary supplements, concerns for safety and efficacy remain, as premarketing safety and efficacy determinations are not required.[2] Self-regulation of the dietary supplement industry has resulted in a market full of products of varying quality. The FDA's ability to regulate dietary supplements is challenged by the vast number of products. Lack of verified analytical methods for every active ingredient used in supplements makes this task even more challenging.[22] Misbranding, adulteration, and contamination remain ongoing challenges for regulation.

# Third-Party Certification of Dietary Supplements

A number of independent organizations provide third-party certifications of dietary supplements. As third-party entities, these organizations are not involved in the manufacturing or sale of the products. The process of certifying dietary supplements may include independent testing for quality, evaluation of claims made on labels, or assessing compliance with CGMP requirements. Quality factors of products, such as identity, ingredient quality, purity, potency, composition, and performance characteristics (eg, dissolution and disintegration), may be assessed.[23] Products must meet acceptable limits for contaminants such as pesticides, heavy metals, microbes, and toxic botanical species. Because neither DSHEA requirements nor CGMP regulations identify specific testing or quality standards for dietary supplements, institutions such as the United States Pharmacopeia (USP) and NSF have set their own standards for quality and safety.[24,25] Manufacturer participation in third-party certification programs is voluntary. Products that meet the standards can display the certification logo of the organization that verified the product. Although third-party certifications can ensure certain quality characteristics of dietary supplement products, they cannot confirm efficacy or safety.

## United States Pharmacopeia

USP is a science-based nonprofit organization established in 1820.[24] It sets standards of identity, strength, quality, and purity for drug products, drug substances, excipients, dietary supplements, and food ingredients.[26] USP standards have been acknowledged in the Federal Food, Drug and Cosmetic Act since its enactment in 1938. Although USP standards are referenced in US legislation, USP is an independent organization from the government. USP collaborates with volunteer scientific experts, academic institutions, practitioner groups, volunteers from industry, and federal agencies to establish standards for dietary supplements. It launched its Dietary Supplement Verification Program in 2001. Although USP plays a role in setting standards of quality for dietary supplements, the enforcement of standards and provisions falls on the FDA or other

US government agencies.[23] Meeting USP standards is voluntary for manufacturers of dietary supplements.

## NSF

NSF is an independent global organization that develops standards and certification programs for various aspects of public health, including food, water, consumer products, and the environment.[27] NSF was established in 1944 (as the "National Sanitation Foundation") to help develop standards for public health and safety in the United States. It subsequently expanded into the global market, changing its name to NSF International in 1990, and in 2022 simplified its name to NSF. Accredited by the American National Standards Institute (ANSI), it uses NSF/ANSI 173 as the standard for testing and certifying dietary supplements.[25] Input from federal agencies, industry representatives, and consumer representatives was used to establish the NSF/ANSI 173 standards.

In addition to setting standards, NSF performs tests and audits, and offers services such as certification programs, training, education, risk management, and consultation. NSF offers three types of certifications: *Contents Tested and Certified*, *Certified for Sport*, and *GMP Registered*. Certified for Sport certifies supplements marketed to athletes. Products are tested for substances banned by most major athletic organizations, as well as undeclared ingredients such as steroids, narcotics, and stimulants.[28] Products meeting standard criteria may display the *Contents Tested and Certified* or the *Certified for Sport* seal on product packaging. Manufacturers that meet the standards for the *GMP Registered* mark may display it on promotional materials, but it is not intended for product packaging.

## ConsumerLab.com

ConsumerLab.com, a private organization established in 1999, was the first third-party certification program for dietary supplements in the United States.[29] It provides consumers and health care professionals with independent test results and information on products such as dietary supplements, prescription medications, sports and energy products, functional foods, foods and beverages, and personal care products. Unlike USP and NSF, ConsumerLab.com does not establish its own standards for quality; it uses standards based on international research and recommendations from organizations and resources such as USP, the World Health Organization, and California Proposition 65.[23] One service it provides is product reviews, which evaluate multiple brands of products that claim to have the same primary ingredient. The reviewers purchase samples directly at the retail level at various times during the year to avoid sampling bias, and they typically buy a mix of popular and smaller brands.

The third-party certification programs are summarized in Box 2.3.[29-32]

---

### BOX 2.3  Third-Party Certification Programs[29-32]

**United States Pharmacopeia (USP)[30]**

Not-for-profit

**Services**

Product quality control and manufacturing process evaluation

Laboratory testing of product samples to check for adherence to standards of quality found in USP-National Formulary or applicable manufacturer specifications

Annual off-the-shelf testing of products that have received USP verification to ensure products continue to meet quality standards

Facility audits to ensure adherence to good manufacturing practice standards

**What the certification or verification mark means**

Product contains the ingredients declared on the label in the correct quantity

Product does not contain certain contaminants above acceptable limits

Product has met performance standards for dissolution and distribution in the body

Product was produced according to US Food and Drug Administration current good manufacturing practices

**NSF[31]**

Not-for-profit

**Services**

Label claim review to ensure product contains the ingredients declared on the label in the correct quantity

---

### BOX 2.3  Third-Party Certification Programs[29-32] (cont.)

**Services (cont.)**

Toxicology review

Ensure product does not contain certain contaminants above acceptable limits or any undeclared contaminants

**What the certification or verification mark means**

Product contains the ingredients declared on the label in the correct quantity

Product does not contain certain contaminants above acceptable limits; includes checking for over 200 substances banned by most major athletic organizations (Certified for Sports mark)

Product has met performance standards for dissolution and distribution in the body

 *ConsumerLab.com[29,32]*
For profit

## Services

Quality checks for individual products, or multilabel testing program for manufacturers of private label and multibrand products

Raw material and private label certification program for entities that supply ingredients to manufacturers

Custom analysis and consulting services for special purpose testing, analysis, and other consulting services

Publication of testing methods and quality standards used for testing of products

Product reviews, conducted every 24-36 months

**What the certification or verification mark means**

Products meets recognized standards of identity and level of quality indicated on label

Product does not contain certain contaminants above specific limits

Product disintegrates in a manner that is accessible to the body

Product is tested for quality criteria annually; sample is obtained from products in the open market

## Reporting Adverse Events

Manufacturers of dietary supplements, including many micronutrient products, do not have to prove product safety or efficacy before selling their products on the US market. For this reason, the reporting of adverse events by health professionals, consumers, and patients is essential in helping the FDA identify supplements that pose a health risk to the public. The FDA may use adverse-event reporting to restrict or ban the sale of products, as in the case of ephedra-containing products.[33] Ephedra was sold in the United States as an herbal supplement and was marketed for its energy-boosting and weight-loss effects. The FDA received more than 18,000 adverse-event reports related to ephedra-containing products and used these reports as grounds for banning the sale of such products, which it successfully did in 2004.[34]

Adverse events related to dietary supplements and micronutrient pharmaceutical products can be reported to MedWatch, which is the FDA's safety information and adverse-event reporting program (www.fda.gov/safety/medwatch-fda-safety-information-and-adverse-event-reporting-program), or to the Safety Reporting Portal of the US Department of Health and Human Services (www.safetyreporting.hhs.gov). MedWatch receives reports of adverse events for regulated products, including dietary supplements, biologics, cosmetics, drug products, foods and beverages, medical devices, and radiation-emitting products.[35] The Safety Reporting Portal streamlines adverse-event reporting among federal agencies, including the FDA, Centers for Disease Control and Prevention, Agency for Healthcare Research and Quality, Office for Human Research Protections, Department of Defense, and Department of Veterans Affairs.[36] Health professionals, researchers, public health officials, and consumers may also submit adverse events to the Safety Reporting Portal.

## Additional Resources

Box 2.4 provides additional professional resources for information on dietary supplements.

**BOX 2.4  Professional Resources for Information on Micronutrients and Dietary Supplements**

## US Food and Drug Administration

Current information on dietary supplements (www.fda.gov/food/dietary -supplements)

Adverse-event reporting for dietary supplements via MedWatch (www.fda .gov/safety/medwatch-fda-safety-information-and-adverse-event-reporting -program)

Information on regulation of dietary supplements, including guidelines for label-ing and structure or function claims (www.fda.gov/food/dietary-supplements -guidance-documents-regulatory-information/dietary-supplement-labeling -guide)

Safety alerts and warnings for dietary supplements (www.fda.gov/safety/recalls -market-withdrawals-safety-alerts)

Patient education materials (www.fda.gov/food/information-consumers-using -dietary-supplements/supplement-your-knowledge)

## Micronutrient Information Center at the Linus Pauling Institute, Oregon State University

Information on the impact of vitamins, minerals, phytochemicals, and other dietary factors on health and disease (https://lpi.oregonstate.edu/mic)

## US Department of Agriculture

National Agricultural Library (www.nal.usda.gov)

Information on dietary supplements via Nutrition.gov (www.nutrition.gov /topics/dietary-supplements)

## United States Pharmacopeia (USP)

Establishes standards of identity, strength, quality, and purity packaging, and labeling for dietary supplements (www.usp.org/dietary-supplements-herbal -medicines)

Newsletters, updates, safety data sheets, and a dedicated website (www.quality -supplements.org) that identifies manufacturers and individual dietary supple-ment products that have obtained the USP Verified mark

*Continued on next page*

---

**BOX 2.4  Professional Resources for Information on Micronutrients and Dietary Supplements (cont.)**

### Office of Dietary Supplements (ODS), National Institutes of Health (NIH)

Newsletters (https://ods.od.nih.gov/News/ODS_Update.aspx), fact sheets for individual vitamins and minerals (https://ods.od.nih.gov/factsheets/list-all/), and ODS- and NIH-funding grants, contracts, and other funding opportunities (https://ods.od.nih.gov/Funding/grantsandfunding.aspx)

Access to ODS Population Studies Program (https://ods.od.nih.gov/Research/populationstudies.aspx), which evaluates dietary supplement use and assesses supplement use in specific populations and in relation to lifestyle, overall health status, and disease risk

Access to federally funded research on dietary supplements (https://ods.od.nih.gov/Research/CARDS_Database.aspx)

### TRC Healthcare NatMed Pro Database

Comprehensive, subscription-based natural medicines database of dietary supplements, herbal medicines, and complementary and integrative therapies; contains over 1,400 monographs plus safety and efficacy information; updated daily (https://trchealthcare.com/about-us/products/natural-medicines)

Includes an interaction checker and the Natural Medicines Brand Evidence-Based Rating (NMBER) system, which uses scientific evidence to rate products on safety, effectiveness, and quality

Includes continuing education for clinical management of disease states using natural or alternative medicines

---

# References

1.   Federal Food, Drug, and Cosmetic Act, 21 USC, ch. 9. Accessed March 19, 2022. https://uscode.house.gov/view.xhtml?path=/prelim@title21/chapter9&edition=prelim

2.   Dickinson A. History and overview of DSHEA. *Fitoterapia*. 2011;82(1):5-10. doi:10.1016/j.fitote.2010.09.001

3.   Dietary Supplement Health and Education Act of 1994, Pub L No. 103-417, 108 Stat 4325 (1994). Accessed February 16, 2022. www.congress.gov/bill/103rd-congress/senate-bill/784/text

4.	Frankos VH, Street DA, O'Neill RK. FDA regulation of dietary supplements and requirements regarding adverse event reporting. *Clin Pharmacol Ther.* 2010;87(2):239-244. doi:10.1038/clpt.2009.263

5.	Dietary Supplement and Nonprescription Drug Consumer Protection Act, Pub L No. 109-462, 120 Stat 3469 (2006). Accessed March 19, 2022. www.govinfo.gov/app/details/STATUTE-120/STATUTE-120-Pg3469

6.	Full text of the Food Safety Modernization Act (FSMA) [2010]. US Food and Drug Administration. Updated December 13, 2017. Accessed March 18, 2022. www.fda.gov/food/food-safety-modernization-act-fsma/full -text-food-safety-modernization-act-fsma

7.	Current good manufacturing practice in manufacturing, packaging, labeling, or holding operations for dietary supplements; final rule. *Fed Regist.* 2007;72(121):34752-34958. Codified as 21 CFR Part 111. Accessed February 23, 2022. www.govinfo.gov/content/pkg/FR-2007-06-25/html /07-3039.htm

8.	Certain Types of Statements for Dietary Supplements. 21 CFR §101.93. Accessed February 23, 2022. www.ecfr.gov/current/title-21/chapter-I /subchapter-B/part-101/subpart-F/section-101.93

9.	Label claims for conventional foods and dietary supplements. US Food and Drug Administration. March 7, 2022. Accessed March 19, 2022. www .fda.gov/food/food-labeling-nutrition/label-claims-conventional-foods -and-dietary-supplements

10.	Guidance for industry: substantiation for dietary supplement claims made under section 403(r) (6) of the Federal Food, Drug, and Cosmetic Act. US Food and Drug Administration. January 2009. Current as of September 20, 2018. Accessed February 23, 2022. www.fda.gov /regulatory-information/search-fda-guidance-documents/guidance -industry-substantiation-dietary-supplement-claims-made-under -section-403r-6-federal-food

11.	Nutrition labeling of dietary supplements. 21 CFR §101.36 (2012). Accessed March 18, 2022. www.govinfo.gov/app/details/CFR-2012 -title21-vol2/CFR-2012-title21-vol2-sec101-36

12.	Food; designation of ingredients. 21 CFR §101.4 (2011). Accessed August 8, 2022. www.govinfo.gov/app/details/CFR-2011-title21-vol2 /CFR-2011-title21-vol2-sec101-4

13.	Food; name and place of business of manufacturer, packer, or distributor. 21 CFR §101.5 (2011). Accessed August 8, 2022. www.accessdata .fda.gov/scripts/cdrh/cfdocs/cfcfr/cfrsearch.cfm?cfrpart=101

14.	Adulterated food, 21 USC §342 (2011). Accessed March 18, 2022. www .govinfo.gov/app/details/USCODE-2011-title21/USCODE-2011-title21 -chap9-subchapIV-sec342

15. Dietary supplement labeling exemptions, 21 USC §343-2 (2011). Accessed March 18, 2022. www.govinfo.gov/app/details/USCODE-2011-title21 /USCODE-2011-title21-chap9-subchapIV-sec343-2

16. Federal Trade Commission. Health Products Compliance Guidance. December 20, 2022. Accessed February 6, 2024. www.ftc.gov/business -guidance/resources/health-products-compliance-guidance

17. Overview of food ingredients, additives, and colors. US Food and Drug Administration. February 20, 2020. Accessed November 21, 2021. www.fda.gov/food/food-ingredients-packaging/overview-food -ingredients-additives-colors

18. Food allergies. US Food and Drug Administration. August 18, 2021. Accessed November 21, 2021. www.fda.gov/food/food-labeling-nutrition /food-allergies

19. Gluten in medications. Beyond Celiac. Accessed August 9, 2022. www.beyondceliac.org/living-with-celiac-disease/gluten-in-medication

20. Gluten and food labeling. US Food and Drug Administration. January 10, 2022. Accessed August 14, 2022. www.fda.gov/food/nutrition-education -resources-materials/gluten-and-food-labeling

21. For healthcare practitioners. USP [United States Pharmacopeia] Quality Supplements website. June 3, 2016. Accessed March 15, 2022. www.quality-supplements.org/healthcare-practitioners

22. Bailey RL. Current regulatory guidelines and resources to support research of dietary supplements in the United States. *Crit Rev Food Sci Nutr.* 2020;60(2):298-309. doi:10.1080/10408398.2018.1524364

23. Akabas SR, Vannice G, Atwater JB, Cooperman T, Cotter R, Thomas L. Quality certification programs for dietary supplements. *J Acad Nutr Diet.* 2016;116(9):1370-1379. doi:10.1016/j.jand.2015.11.003

24. Public standards promote and protect public health. USP [United States Pharmacopeia] *Quality Matters* blog. March 17, 2015. Accessed March 17, 2022. https://qualitymatters.usp.org/public-standards-promote-and -protect-public-health

25. Standards development. NSF. Accessed March 17, 2022. www.nsf.org /standards-development

26. Recognition of USP compounding standards. USP. Accessed March 15, 2022. www.usp.org/compounding/legal-considerations

27. About NSF. NSF. Accessed March 15, 2022. www.nsf.org/about-nsf

28. What our mark means. Certified for Sport, NSF. Accessed March 16, 2022. www.nsfsport.com/our-mark.php

29. About ConsumerLab.com. ConsumerLab.com. Accessed March 16, 2022. www.consumerlab.com/about

30. Verification services. USP [United States Pharmacopeia]. Accessed March 15, 2022. www.usp.org/services/verification-services

31. Supplement and vitamin certification. NSF. Accessed June 30, 2021. www.nsf.org/knowledge-library/supplement-vitamin-certification

32. Quality Certification Program. ConsumerLab.com. Accessed March 16, 2022. www.consumerlab.com/quality-certification-program

33. Final rule declaring dietary supplements containing ephedrine alkaloids adulterated because they present an unreasonable risk. *Fed Regist*. 2004;69(28):6788-6854. Accessed August 13, 2022. www .federalregister.gov/documents/2004/02/11/04-2912/final-rule -declaring-dietary-supplements-containing-ephedrine-alkaloids -adulterated-because-they

34. Zell-Kanter M, Quigley MA, Leikin JB. Reduction in ephedra poisonings after FDA ban. *N Engl J Med*. 2015;372(22):2172-2174. doi:10.1056 /NEJMc1502505

35. MedWatch: the FDA safety information and adverse event reporting program. US Food and Drug Administration. December 16, 2021. Accessed March 17, 2022. www.fda.gov/safety/medwatch-fda-safety -information-and-adverse-event-reporting-program

36. History [of the Safety Reporting Portal]. Safety Reporting Portal. Accessed March 17, 2022. www.safetyreporting.hhs.gov/SRP2/en/About.aspx

# CHAPTER 3

# Product Formulations

Avani Patel, PharmD, MDN, RDN, LD

## Introduction

The appropriate selection of a micronutrient product for supplementation or repletion is an essential component of micronutrient management. Understanding the concepts of pharmacokinetics, including bioavailability, can prove valuable when comparing different routes of administration. Bioavailability considerations for specific micronutrients can guide the selection of an optimal micronutrient product. The benefits and limitations of different dosage forms should be considered, especially with regard to individual patient characteristics. Once a product is selected, providing a complete nutrition prescription is essential. This chapter defines pharmacokinetics, bioavailability, and the components of the nutrition prescription. The concepts discussed within this chapter are applied to specific micronutrients discussed in section 2 of this pocket guide. Of note, enteral and parenteral delivery of micronutrients are covered in other resources.[1,2]

## Pharmacokinetics Overview

Pharmacokinetics is the study of how the body interacts with foreign chemicals (eg, a drug or nutrient) over the time of exposure.[3] Principles of pharmacokinetics are used in pharmacology to deliver drug therapy safely and effectively. Understanding these principles can assist health care providers with prescribing, adjusting, and monitoring drug or nutrient therapy. This section provides an overview of pharmacokinetics in the context of drug administration; however, concepts of pharmacokinetics can also be applied to nutrient products.

The pharmacokinetic profile of a drug is determined by measuring its absorption, distribution, metabolism, and elimination from the body.[4] Generally speaking, *absorption* is the means by which a drug moves from the site of administration into the bloodstream or systemic circulation. Solubility, dissolution, and accompanying excipients are factors that may affect absorption. One way to categorize the extent to which a drug is absorbed after administration is in terms of bioavailability. *Bioavailability* is the proportion of a drug that is able to enter the systemic circulation and exert a biological effect at the site of action.[5] *Distribution* is the process by which the drug travels through the bloodstream. *Metabolism* is the sum of the body's enzymatic actions that alter the drug to facilitate elimination from the body. *Elimination* is how the drug is removed from the body, typically via urine, feces, exhalation, or sweat. Depending on the characteristics of the compound, elimination can be affected by the perfusion rate to the organ that metabolizes or clears the drug from the body.[4] Underlying organ function can also be a factor, as is the case with decreased renal clearance of drugs when renal function is compromised.

# Bioavailability

Bioavailability is typically expressed as a percentage or fraction of the drug absorbed. It is noted as $F$ and can be represented in a graph by displaying the concentration-time curve of the active ingredient after administration. The same active ingredient administered through different routes will have different bioavailabilities and pharmacokinetic profiles. Thus, it is critical to consider differences in bioavailability when determining the optimal dose of a micronutrient product to be prescribed and administered in order to optimize efficacy and prevent toxicity.

Variables that affect bioavailability include dissolution (the extent to which a solid dosage form dissolves), intestinal absorption, and presystemic (first-pass) metabolism.[6] Other factors that may affect bioavailability include gastric and intestinal pH, which is especially important for certain formulations or compounds that are stable in specific pH; bile flow, which is important, for example, when administering fat-soluble vitamins; and permeability of the compound.[7,8] Not all administration routes are affected by these factors to the same degree. For example, the intravenous route of administration is considered to have 100% bioavailability, because it is administered directly into the circulation.

## Presystemic (First-Pass) Metabolism

Presystemic metabolism is the metabolism of the active ingredient before it reaches the systemic circulation. The liver and gastrointestinal (GI) tract are the two largest contributors to presystemic metabolism, with the liver contributing to a greater extent. Presystemic metabolism can also occur in the vasculature, lungs, or other tissues. Factors that influence metabolism in the liver and intestinal wall include enzymatic activity, plasma protein, and GI motility. Because metabolism of the active ingredient alters its structure and function, drugs or nutrients that undergo extensive presystemic metabolism have lower bioavailability. The presystemic effect varies due to individual differences such as age, sex, disease state, and genetic factors that could influence the rate of enzyme induction and inhibition.[9] Disease factors that restrict the flow of blood to organs such as the liver and kidneys can also influence presystemic metabolism. For example, patients with cirrhosis have reduced activity of select cytochrome P450 (CYP) enzymes that normally function to metabolize drugs and other substances in the body.[10] Once the drug is metabolized, the subsequent metabolites can be classified as pharmacologically active or inactive. If the metabolites are pharmacologically active, the dose needs to be adjusted in accordance with the biological activity of the metabolite.[5] If the drug is metabolized to a great extent to inactive metabolites, a higher dose is needed to achieve the same therapeutic activity.

## Bioavailability and Routes of Administration

To increase bioavailability, pharmaceutical manufacturers have developed products that can be administered via alternative routes, such as intravenous, intramuscular, and sublingual. Bioavailability of the product changes with different routes of administration, thus the dose and frequency of administration should be adjusted accordingly.[5] Box 3.1 illustrates this using vitamin B12 as an example.[5,11-13]

> **BOX 3.1  Example of Vitamin B12 Dosing Differences Based on Bioavailability and Route of Administration**[5,11-13]
>
> ### Vitamin B12 maintenance dosing recommendation
>
> The recommended maintenance dose of cyanocobalamin given orally to treat vitamin B12 deficiency is 1,000 mcg once per day (following an appropriate loading dose).
>
> Intranasal administration of cyanocobalamin requires a lower maintenance dose, usually 500 mcg once per week.[11]
>
> ### Explanation
>
> Oral vitamin B12 requires a higher dose due to saturable active absorption through cubilin-mediated intrinsic factor–cobalamin transport in the ileum.[12,13]
>
> Absorption via passive diffusion is limited due to the highly polar properties of vitamin B12.[12] Nasal administration bypasses these limitations of intestinal absorption and allows for entry into systemic absorption via the nasal mucosa.[5]
>
> Nasal administration requires a lower dose and frequency than oral administration does to achieve the same therapeutic effect.

# Bioavailability Considerations for Micronutrient Supplements

When developing the Dietary Reference Intakes (DRIs), the Food and Nutrition Board of the Institute of Medicine recognized the following factors that affect nutrient bioavailability[14]:

- concentration of the nutrient
- dietary factors
- chemical form of the nutrient
- supplements taken separately from meals
- nutrition and health of the individual
- excretory losses
- nutrient-nutrient interactions

As mentioned earlier, the concepts of bioavailability can be applied to micronutrient products. However, it is important to consider that the bioavailability of nutrients is influenced by a number of factors that set it apart from the bioavailability of drugs.

Nutrient bioavailability is complicated by the fact that absorption and utilization depend on the individual's nutritional and physiological status. Iron absorption can be used as an example. There is no known mechanism for active excretion of iron from the body; therefore, iron absorption is the primary manner in which the body regulates iron levels. Generally, absorption increases when the body's requirement for iron is high and decreases when requirement is low. The body senses the demand through several regulatory pathways, including iron supply to the erythroid marrow, increases in erythropoietic rate, and the amount of total iron stores in the body. This effect is seen until high doses of iron are administered, at which point the body's normal feedback regulation is disrupted and absorption is increased. When compared to dose-response curves of drug products, dose-response curves exhibited by nutritional supplements are harder to predict and are also confounded by other variables, such as concurrent illnesses.[15]

The plasma reference ranges for many micronutrients were determined based on average intake in healthy people. It is unclear whether those ranges apply to individuals experiencing different disease states. In addition, the plasma concentration of a micronutrient may not accurately represent the total body pool of the nutrient.

Because of the lack of standardization of specific formulations among manufacturers of over-the-counter nutrient supplements, other ingredients may be added to individual products that can affect bioavailability.[16] In addition, nutritional supplements exert biological effects and affect health in a manner that is difficult to quantify.[14] Box 3.2 summarizes the special considerations for nutrient supplements and bioavailability.[17-19]

**BOX 3.2  Special Considerations for Micronutrient Supplements and Bioavailability[17-19]**

Bioavailability can vary between different dosage forms and routes of administration for the same micronutrient.

Bioavailability data for over-the-counter micronutrient supplements may be limited and less applicable compared to data for standard pharmaceutical products.

Because of differences in formulations, differences in manufacturing practices, and limited research on over-the-counter micronutrient supplements, determining exact pharmacokinetic and bioavailability data for individual products is difficult. Generally, route of administration has the largest impact on bioavailability; drug and nutrient products with the same dosage forms generally have comparable bioavailability.

Meal composition may affect the bioavailability of certain oral products. For example, iron is most efficiently absorbed on an empty stomach, whereas absorption of calcium is improved with meals.[17,18]

Absorption of oral supplements is dependent on individual digestive and absorptive capabilities of the gastrointestinal (GI) tract. (Consider alterations in GI anatomy—eg, bariatric surgery or short bowel syndrome.) For example, a patient who has undergone terminal ileum resection would benefit from the intranasal, intramuscular, or subcutaneous route of administration of vitamin B12. Vitamin B12 is normally absorbed in the terminal ileum, so traditional oral preparations would result in little or no absorption.

Malabsorptive disorders (eg, celiac disease, chronic diarrhea, exocrine pancreatic insufficiency) affect absorption. For example, a patient with exocrine pancreatic insufficiency would have limited absorption of fat-soluble vitamins in food or supplements without concomitant supplementation of pancreatic enzyme replacement therapy.[19]

Food-nutrient and nutrient-nutrient interactions must be considered. For example, foods that contain phytates, tannins, calcium, soy, or egg protein may decrease absorption of iron. Vitamin C improves nonheme iron absorption from food by reducing iron from ferric to the ferrous state throughout the GI tract.[18]

# Route of Administration

Route of administration is the way in which a drug or micronutrient is delivered into the body. When choosing a route of administration, consider the following:

- Is the intended effect of the micronutrient product local or systemic? Most micronutrient treatment is intended for systemic circulation and subsequent transport to the site of action.[5]

- What is the desired onset of action? This is measured from time of administration to when the therapeutic effects of the micronutrient product can first be observed.[5]

- What is the intended duration of action? This is measured as the length of time over which the therapeutic effects of the micronutrient product can be observed. This can be expressed in terms of *half-life*—the amount of time it takes for half of the product to be cleared from the body. Oral, subcutaneous, and intramuscular routes of administration may have longer durations of action.[5]

- What is the intended duration of treatment? This is the length of time micronutrient treatment is needed for acute, subchronic, or chronic therapy.[20]

-  What are the individual patient preferences or relevant characteristics of the patient?

  o The oral route may not be appropriate for patients who cannot swallow, are experiencing vomiting, or have limited GI absorption capabilities.

  o In-office administration of a longer-acting micronutrient formulation may be appropriate if patient adherence to a daily-use regimen is a concern. For example, vitamin B12 can be administered via the intramuscular or subcutaneous route.

  o Age can influence which route of administration is most appropriate. Flavored solution, suspension, or syrup may be more suitable than tablet or capsule forms for children.

- Are there concerns regarding product availability or expense?
  - Product availability can be a factor when there are shortages, back orders, or recalls.
  - Expense is an important consideration, as the cost of micronutrient products can vary considerably among routes of administration. Solid oral dosage forms, such as tablets and capsules, are generally lower in cost. Intravenous, intramuscular, and subcutaneous formulations are more expensive.

# Oral Administration

Micronutrients intended for the oral route of administration come in a variety of dosage forms. Tablet, capsule, oral liquid, effervescent, and chewable forms are intended to be swallowed, absorbed at a designated site in the GI tract, introduced into systemic circulation, and transported to the target site.[5] Because these dosage forms pass through the GI tract, they may be affected by the presence and quantity of food in the gut at the time of administration. Food-nutrient interactions and nutrient-nutrient interactions are also concerns with oral administration.

Sublingual formulations are intended to be placed under the tongue for absorption via mucosa in the oral cavity. Similarly, buccal formulations are placed in the cheek for absorption via mucosa in the oral cavity. The target for a sublingual or buccal formulation can be local or systemic. Box 3.3 on page 38 provides a summary of oral formulations.[5,20-23]

# Intravenous Administration

Micronutrients can be formulated for direct administration into a vein. The intravenous route is ideal for micronutrients that have a high degree of presystemic metabolism or have poor absorption in the GI tract.[5] Micronutrients administered intravenously should be done so at a rate that is both efficacious and safe. Box 3.4 on page 41 provides a summary of intravenous formulations.[5]

## BOX 3.3  Oral Micronutrient Forms and Considerations[5,20-23]

### Tablets and capsules

Tablet          Solid dosage forms made by compression and molding tech-
                niques; may or may not contain additives such as diluents,
                coatings, or coloring agents[21]

Capsule         Solid dosage forms prepared by enclosing active ingredient (with
                or without additives) in a hard or soft shell[22]

**Advantages**

Generally safe, convenient, and
cost-effective

Prolonged shelf life

**Disadvantages**

Subject to presystemic metabolism,
though the extent depends on the
specific nutrient

### Extended-release, delayed-release, or enteric-coated tablets and capsules

Solid dosage forms made with delayed-release technology; formulated to
remain unchanged as they pass through the stomach and release active ingredient in the intestine for absorption[21]

**Advantages**

Enhanced absorption for micronutrients that normally are rendered
inactive in the stomach

May improve tolerability of micronutrients that cause stomach upset
or irritate the stomach lining

Longer duration of action than immediate-release tablets or
capsules, facilitating less frequent
administration

Prolonged shelf life

**Disadvantages**

Higher cost than immediate-release
tablets or capsules

Subject to presystemic metabolism,
though the extent depends on the
specific nutrient

Slower onset of action

Not ideal for feeding tubes, as most
extended-release or delayed-
release tablets or capsules should not
be crushed

### Chewable tablets

Solid tablets that quickly disintegrate when chewed; usually flavored and colored[21]

Should be chewed completely and then swallowed

**BOX 3.3 Oral Micronutrient Forms and Considerations[5,20-23] (cont.)**

## Chewable tablets (cont.)

### Advantages

May be ideal for children and adults who cannot or prefer not to swallow tablets or capsules

Easier to carry and more convenient to administer than solutions

May be better absorbed than tablets or capsules in patients with malabsorption or ostomies

### Disadvantages

Unpleasant taste or aftertaste

Due to coloring and appearance, may look like candy; precautions should be taken to keep out of reach of children

Subject to presystemic metabolism, though the extent depends on the specific nutrient

## Effervescent tablets

Solid tablets that easily dissolve and contain effervescent salts that release gas when mixed with water[21]

### Advantages

May be ideal for children and adults who cannot or prefer not to swallow tablets or capsules

Are mixed with water before administration, resulting in quicker dissolution than other solid dosage forms

May be better absorbed than tablets or capsules in patients with malabsorption or ostomies

### Disadvantages

Unpleasant taste or aftertaste

More expensive than solid tablets or capsules

Subject to presystemic metabolism, though the extent depends on the specific nutrient

May contain high levels of sodium or potassium, which can be a concern for patients in certain disease states

## Solutions, syrups, and suspensions

| | |
|---|---|
| Solution | Liquid dosage forms in which active ingredient is dissolved in an aqueous solution[5] |
| Syrup | Solutions containing sucrose; thicker consistency than non-syrup solutions[5] |
| Suspension | Liquid dosage forms in which active ingredient is in the form of a fine powder mixed in a fluid vehicle; active ingredient is insoluble in the liquid, and suspension must be shaken before administration[5] |

*Continued on next page*

## BOX 3.3  Oral Micronutrient Forms and Considerations[5,20-23] (cont.)

### Solutions, syrups, and suspensions (cont.)

| Advantages | Disadvantages |
|---|---|
| Generally safe, convenient, and cost-effective | Subject to presystemic metabolism, though the extent depends on the specific nutrient |
| Suitable for children and adults who cannot or prefer not to swallow solid dosage forms | Suspension forms must be shaken before administration |
| Generally dissolve and absorb faster than solid forms | May have limited shelf life once multidose packages are opened |
| May be better absorbed than tablets or capsules in patients with malabsorption or ostomies | May use sweeteners such as sorbitol, mannitol, or similar sugar alcohols[23] that are partially digested in the small intestine and then proceed to the large intestine, where they are broken down and fermented by bacteria, potentially causing gastrointestinal symptoms such as bloating, gas, or osmotic diarrhea |
| Liquid formulations preferred when administering via a feeding tube | |

### Sublingual (under the tongue) or buccal (between the gum and cheek) formulations

Solid tablets, such as troches, lozenges, or liquid drops

Sublingual route has more rapid absorption than buccal[20]

| Advantages | Disadvantage |
|---|---|
| Easy to administer | May cause irritation in the oral cavity |
| Bypass presystemic metabolism | Salivary clearance (substances removed from the oral cavity because of the flow of saliva or motions associated with swallowing) |
| Ideal for micronutrients that are destroyed by gastric juice or have poor gastrointestinal absorption | Permeability may be selective |
| | Patient education needed to ensure proper technique is followed |

---

**BOX 3.4  Intravenous Micronutrient Forms and Considerations[5]**

### Intravenous (IV) formulations

Can be a single injection (for lower volume) or an IV drip infusion (for larger volume)[5]

| Advantages | Disadvantages |
|---|---|
| Rapid onset of action, as administration is directly into circulation | Requires IV access |
| 100% bioavailability due to bypassing presystemic metabolism | Limited time to treat or prevent toxicity, due to rapid absorption |
| | Strict sterile protocols for administration |
| Suitable for patients who are unconscious or patients unwilling or unable to take drugs via oral route | Prolonged infusion time to achieve desired effect |
| | Pain or discomfort related to IV site |
| | More expensive than oral dosage forms |
| | Requires administration by trained health care personnel, as well as proper medical equipment |

---

# Subcutaneous Administration

Subcutaneous formulations are administered by an injection beneath the skin, generally in the forearm, upper arm, thigh, or buttocks. Once injected, the active ingredient enters local blood capillaries by diffusion or filtration, and subsequently enters systemic circulation. Box 3.5 on page 42 provides a summary of subcutaneous formulations.[5]

# Intramuscular Administration

Intramuscular formulations are injected into the skeletal muscle. The gluteal, deltoid, and lumbar muscles are common sites of administration.[5] Because intramuscular injections penetrate deeper than subcutaneous injections, clinicians must take care to avoid any major nerves or blood vessels when selecting points of injection. Box 3.6 on page 43 provides a summary of intramuscular formulations.[5]

---

**BOX 3.5  Subcutaneous Micronutrient Forms and Considerations[5]**

### Subcutaneous injection

Aqueous solution or suspension intended for injection beneath the skin, which can deliver volumes of 2 mL or less

| Advantages | Disadvantages |
|---|---|
| Preferred route if prolonged duration of action is desired, as absorption is slower | Can deliver only small volumes (usually 2 mL or less) |
| Self-administration possible with proper training | Not appropriate if rapid absorption is desired |
| | Potential for local irritation; rotation of injection sites recommended with repeated injections |
| | Absorption rates potentially altered by physical activity, due to increased blood circulation |
| | Pain related to injection |
| | Limited shelf life once multidose packages are opened |

---

# Intranasal Administration

Intranasal formulations are administered to the mucosa in the nasal cavity.[5] They may be formulated for local effects or for systemic circulation. Systemic effects are achieved through drug absorption by microvilli, which run along the highly vascularized nasal mucosa. Systemic absorption via nasal route bypasses presystemic metabolism; however, the active ingredient may be metabolized to some extent by local enzymes in the nasal mucosa. Box 3.7 on page 44 provides a summary of intranasal formulations.[20]

> **BOX 3.6 Intramuscular Micronutrient Forms and Considerations[5]**
>
> ### Intramuscular injection
> Aqueous or oleaginous (oil-based) solutions or suspensions that can deliver volumes of up to 5 mL[5]
>
> | Advantages | Disadvantages |
> |---|---|
> | Faster onset of action than subcutaneous route | Strict sterile protocols for administration |
> | Preferred route if a prolonged duration of action is desired, as active ingredient is released over time | More expensive than oral dosage forms |
> | | Pain related to administration of injection |
> | Alternative route for drugs that cause irritation when administered in subcutaneous tissue | Potential for local irritation; rotation of injection sites recommended with repeated injections |
> | Can deliver larger volumes than subcutaneous administration (but smaller volumes than intravenous) | Limited shelf life once multidose packages are opened |
> | | Requires administration by trained health care personnel, or training and education of patient |

# The Micronutrient Nutrition Prescription

When making recommendations for micronutrient supplementation or repletion strategies, clinicians should indicate all of the necessary elements in a written nutrition prescription. Even if the product is to be purchased over the counter, the nutrition prescription should give the patient clear and direct instructions. A complete prescription includes the following:

- date of issue
- patient name
- patient date of birth
- provider name and address
- name of the vitamin or mineral

- dosage strength
- dosage form
- delivery route
- dose frequency
- relevant directions for administration (eg, with or without meals)
- quantity to be initially filled by the pharmacist or purchased by the patient (if over the counter)
- number of refills (if filled at a pharmacy) or duration of treatment (if over the counter)
- prescriber signature

---

### BOX 3.7  Intranasal Micronutrient Forms and Considerations[20]

#### *Intranasal*

Solutions, sprays, inhalants, ointments, or gels[20]

| Advantages | Disadvantages |
|---|---|
| Bypasses presystemic metabolism | Potential for local irritation |
| Alternative to oral dosage form | Unpleasant taste after administration |
| | Requires training of patient in proper application technique |
| | Limited products available because few micronutrients can be absorbed intranasally |
| | Products not shareable; use is limited to one person |
| | Actual dose absorbed may vary with administration technique |
| | Potential for absorption may be negatively affected by concurrent respiratory illness |
| | Limited shelf life once multidose packages are opened |

Although not part of the nutrition prescription itself, instructions regarding laboratory tests should be communicated to the patient if such testing will be needed to assess the efficacy of the treatment or supplementation. Patients should be counseled to inform their pharmacists of any micronutrient treatments they are receiving in a prescriber's office or taking over the counter.

# References

1.  Malone A, Carney LN, Carrera AL, Mays A, eds. *ASPEN Enteral Nutrition Handbook*. 2nd ed. American Society for Parenteral and Enteral Nutrition; 2019.

2.  Ayers P, Bobo ES, Hurt RT, Mays AA, Worthington PH, eds. *ASPEN Parenteral Nutrition Handbook*. 3rd ed. American Society for Parenteral and Enteral Nutrition; 2020.

3.  Grogan S, Preuss CV. Pharmacokinetics. In: *StatPearls (online)*. StatPearls Publishing; 2022. NCBI Bookshelf. Accessed August 17, 2022. www.ncbi.nlm.nih.gov/books/NBK557744

4.  Bauer LA. Clinical pharmacokinetics and pharmacodynamics. In: DiPiro JT, Yee GC, Posey L, Haines ST, Nolin TD, Ellingrod V, eds. *Pharmacotherapy: A Pathophysiologic Approach*. 11th ed. McGraw-Hill; 2020:15.

5.  Allen LV Jr. Dosage form design: biopharmaceutical and pharmacokinetic considerations. In: *Ansel's Pharmaceutical Dosage Forms and Drug Delivery Systems*. 11th ed. Wolters Kluwer; 2018:127-161.

6.  Pond SM, Tozer TN. First-pass: elimination basic concepts and clinical consequences. *Clin Pharmacokinet*. 1984;9(1):1-25. doi:10.2165/00003088-198409010-00001

7.  Vraníková B, Gajdziok J. Biologická dostupnost léčiva a možnosti jejího ovlivňování [Bioavailability and factors influencing its rate]. *Ceska Slov Farm*. 2015;64(1-2):7-13.

8.  Grossmann RE, Tangpricha V. Evaluation of vehicle substances on vitamin D bioavailability: a systematic review. *Mol Nutr Food Res*. 2010;54(8):1055-1061. doi:10.1002/mnfr.200900578

9.  Tam YK. Individual variation in first-pass metabolism. *Clin Pharmacokinet*. 1993;25(4):300-328. doi:10.2165/00003088-199325040-00005

10. Elbekai RH, Korashy HM, El-Kadi AOS. The effect of liver cirrhosis on the regulation and expression of drug metabolizing enzymes. *Curr Drug Metab*. 2004;5(2):157-167. doi:10.2174/1389200043489054

11. Cyanocobalamin (vitamin B12): drug information. UpToDate. Accessed July 29, 2021. www-uptodate-com.proxy.lib.ohio-state.edu/contents /cyanocobalamin-vitamin-b12-drug-information

12. Seetharam B, Yammani RR. Cobalamin transport proteins and their cell-surface receptors. *Expert Rev Mol Med*. 2003;5(18):1-18. doi:10.1017 /S1462399403006422

13. Allen LH. Bioavailability of vitamin B12. *Int J Vitam Nutr Res*. 2010;80( 4-5):330-335. doi:10.1024/0300-9831/a000041

14. Hambidge KM. Micronutrient bioavailability: Dietary Reference Intakes and a future perspective. *Am J Clin Nutr*. 2010;91(5):1430S-1432S. doi:10 .3945/ajcn.2010.28674B

15. Srinivasan VS. Bioavailability of nutrients: a practical approach to in vitro demonstration of the availability of nutrients in multivitamin-mineral combination products. *J Nutr*. 2001;131(4):1349S-1350S. doi:10 .1093/jn/131.4.1349S

16. Heaney RP. Factors influencing the measurement of bioavailability, taking calcium as a model. *J Nutr*. 2001;131(4):1344S-1348S. doi:10.1093/jn /131.4.1344S

17. Calcium carbonate: drug information. UpToDate. Accessed July 29, 2021. www-uptodate-com.proxy.lib.ohio-state.edu/contents/calcium -carbonate-drug-information

18. Teucher B, Olivares M, Cori H. Enhancers of iron absorption: ascorbic acid and other organic acids. *Int J Vitam Nutr Res*. 2004;74(6):403-419. doi:10.1024/0300-9831.74.6.403

19. Dominguez-Muñoz JE. Management of pancreatic exocrine insufficiency. *Curr Opin Gastroenterol*. 2019;35(5):455-459. doi:10.1097 /MOG.0000000000000562

20. Mathias NR, Hussain MA. Non-invasive systemic drug delivery: developability considerations for alternate routes of administration. *J Pharm Sci*. 2010;99(1):1-20. doi:10.1002/jps.21793

21. Allen LV Jr. Tablets. In: *Ansel's Pharmaceutical Dosage Forms and Drug Delivery Systems*. 11th ed. Wolters Kluwer; 2018:203-229.

22. Allen LV Jr. Capsules. In: *Ansel's Pharmaceutical Dosage Forms and Drug Delivery Systems*. 11th ed. Wolters Kluwer; 2018:186-202.

23. Interactive Nutrition Facts label: sugar alcohols. US Food and Drug Administration. October 2021. Accessed July 29, 2022. www.accessdata .fda.gov/scripts/interactivenutritionfactslabel/assets/InteractiveNFL_ SugarAlcohols_October2021.pdf

CHAPTER 4

# The Impact of Inflammation

Mette M. Berger, MD, PhD, and
Renée Blaauw, PhD, RD(SA)

## Introduction

Whether acute or chronic, inflammation affects nutritional and micro-nutrient status directly, as it is the main trigger of catabolism. Because micronutrients are key components for the normal functioning and metabolism of cells in the body, deficiencies may have serious implications, and clinicians must be able to diagnose them with fair certitude: the short-term and long-term consequences of micronutrient deficiencies are profound.[1] As blood levels for most micronutrients drop in the presence of inflammation,[2] the low values should always be interpreted with an indicator of the inflammatory status, such as C-reactive protein (CRP), $\alpha$1-acid glycoprotein (AGP), or interleukin-6 (IL-6), to distinguish a true deficiency from inflammation-induced redistribution.[3,4] Micronutrients are a cornerstone of the immune response,[5] but their role in the inflammatory response and its resolution varies.[6]

This chapter addresses the pathophysiology of inflammation and discusses the impact of the inflammatory process on markers of micronutrient status. Recommendations on the assessment of micronutrient status, along with indications on how results could be interpreted in acute and chronic settings, are provided. Lastly, management and monitoring action steps are proposed.

# Pathophysiology of Inflammation

Inflammation is a standardized response to external injury (eg, a burn, trauma, surgery) or internal injury (eg, infection, cancer). It is a universal, complex process that involves innate and adaptive immunity aimed at healing.[7] It can remain an acute response or evolve into a chronic process. Inflammation is initiated by resident immune cells already present in the involved tissue, mainly macrophages, histiocytes, Kupffer cells, and mast cells.[2] These cells possess surface receptors known as pattern recognition receptors (PRRs), which recognize (ie, bind) two subclasses of molecules: pathogen-associated molecular patterns (PAMPs) and damage-associated molecular patterns (DAMPs). These undergo activation and release inflammatory mediators responsible for the clinical signs of inflammation—namely, vasodilation and increased blood flow (causing redness and heat), as well as increased vascular permeability resulting in exudation (leakage) of plasma proteins and fluid into the tissues, causing edema (interstitial) and swelling (intracellular).

In parallel, inflammation results in the synthesis of acute-phase proteins, such as CRP, AGP, ferritin, serum amyloid A and P, ceruloplasmin, and fibrinogen.[8] There is a mirror decrease of "negative acute-phase proteins," such as albumin, transferrin, retinol-binding protein (RBP), and prealbumin (Figure 4.1).[9] Several negative acute-phase proteins are carriers of trace elements and vitamins; therefore, these changes affect the circulating concentrations of micronutrients. The alterations in protein metabolism by injury in various forms and changes in the plasma and tissue protein concentrations were first described by J. A. Owen in 1967.[10]

Inflammation leads to a redistribution of most micronutrients from the circulating compartment to other organs, resulting in low circulating levels for most of them.[11] For this reason, low levels do not necessarily indicate deficiency or even depletion. Table 4.1 on page 50 summarizes the changes in micronutrient levels in the blood compartment during inflammation.[11-13] Additional laboratory measurements to help differentiate the inflammatory effect, as well as the extent of the expected

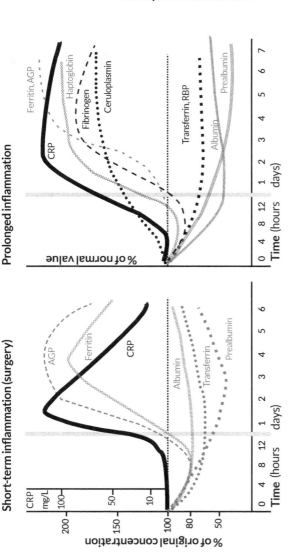

FIGURE 4.1 Evolution of acute-phase proteins and micronutrient carriers in short-lived and prolonged inflammation[a,9]

Abbreviations: AGP, α1-acid glycoprotein; CRP, C-reactive protein; RBP, retinol-binding protein.
[a] In the absence of preexisting micronutrient deficiencies.

49

**TABLE 4.1  Direction of Change in Micronutrient Levels in the Blood Compartment During Inflammation[a,11-13]**

| Micronutrient | Direction change due to inflammation[b] |
|---|---|
| *Trace element and other laboratory measurements to consider (when relevant)* | |
| Chromium | Variable |
| Copper | ↑↑ |
| • Ceruloplasmin | ↑↑ |
| Iron | ↓↓ |
| • Ferritin | ↑↑ |
| • Hepcidin | ↑ |
| • Soluble transferrin receptor | Ø |
| Manganese | Ø - ↑ |
| Molybdenum | Ø |
| Selenium | ↓↓↓ |
| • Plasma glutathione peroxidase 3 | Ø - ↓ |
| Zinc | ↓↓ |
| *Vitamin and other laboratory measurements to consider (when relevant)* | |
| Thiamin (vitamin B1) | Ø - ↑[c] |
| Riboflavin (vitamin B2) | ↓ - ↓↓[c] |
| Niacin (vitamin B3) | Ø |
| Vitamin B6 (pyridoxine) | Ø - ↓[c] |
| Biotin (vitamin B7) | Ø |
| Folate (vitamin B9) | Ø |
| Vitamin B12 (cobalamin) | Ø - ↑ |
| Vitamin A | ↓ |
| • Retinol-binding protein | ↓ |
| Vitamin C | ↓↓↓ |
| Vitamin D | ↓↓ |
| Vitamin E | ↓ |
| Vitamin K | ↓ |

[a] Refer to Chapters 5-8 for a review of the assays used in micronutrient determinations.

[b] Number of arrows indicates the intensity of the change; Ø = no change due to inflammation

[c] Results dependent on methodology. Erythrocyte measurements are less affected by inflammation than are whole-blood measurements.

changes, are indicated. The unreliability of blood levels in determining micronutrient status has been emphasized by many.[3] Observational studies have shown in otherwise healthy individuals with no deficiency that within 12 to 24 hours of minor elective surgery, plasma concentrations of several trace elements and vitamins fall markedly, without any change in whole-body micronutrient status.[14] Low micronutrient levels in the blood may persist for weeks in people with severe conditions, including those with a chronic illness. Although some low blood levels may be explained by the redistribution of micronutrients from the circulating compartment to other organs, true deficiency may be present: the difficulty lies in untangling the two components. Indeed, some micronutrients may be directly "consumed" in antioxidation (eg, vitamin C),[15,16] resulting in an absolute acute deficiency.

Inflammation is a component of most acute and chronic diseases. Patients who are critically ill nearly always present with an inflammatory response, often quite massive, similar to that seen in surgery, burns, and wound healing.[12] Other conditions associated with an inflammatory response (acute or chronic) include inflammatory bowel disease, arthritis, obesity, metabolic syndrome, diabetes mellitus, cardiovascular disease, cancer, pancreatitis, acute respiratory distress syndrome and chronic obstructive pulmonary disease, chronic kidney disease, autoimmune diseases, and neurodegenerative diseases such as Parkinson disease, Alzheimer disease, and epilepsy.[17] Older adults are also often affected, as aging is associated with developing a low-level, systemic, chronic inflammation.[18] Due to the underlying inflammatory nature of all of these conditions, micronutrient status should always be interpreted along with an inflammatory parameter.

# Grading of Inflammation

For most micronutrients, circulating blood concentrations are the only clinically available indicator of status. It is important to differentiate a true deficiency from a drop in circulating levels due to redistribution associated with the inflammatory response. An awareness of the extent of inflammation is of utmost importance to accurately assess micronutrient status and decide on appropriate action, particularly when there are economic, laboratory availability, or micronutrient shortage issues.

While blood tests are the most common way to measure micronutrients, they can also be measured in different matrixes, such as in the intracellular compartment (red blood cells, leukocytes) or tissues (ie, hair, nails, organs). The tissues will be less affected by inflammation, and some tests are more invasive. Taking into consideration the difficulty in interpretating blood levels, various attempts for adjustments have been proposed, but none are entirely satisfactory. There is an additional risk of error associated with some scientists/clinicians expressing their results as a percentage of their local reference ranges, which differ between continents and complicate interpretation. This emphasizes the role of the protein carriers and micronutrient-related enzymes providing additional functional information about the micronutrients.

The principal markers of inflammation are CRP, high sensitivity CRP (hs-CRP), AGP, and IL-6, with testing for the latter two being unavailable in many health care centers. Most studies dealing with alterations of blood levels associated with inflammation have used CRP as the marker. The use of CRP to grade inflammation is recommended as follows[11]:

- CRP level of 1.0 to 2.0 mg/dL: mild inflammation
- CRP level of 2.1 to 8.0 mg/dL: moderate inflammation
- CRP level of 8.1 mg/dL or higher: severe inflammation

The micronutrients most sensitive to inflammation are iron, selenium, riboflavin, vitamin B6, vitamin C, and vitamin D, which begin to show a modest decrease when CRP levels exceed 1.0 mg/dL.[19,20] The impact of inflammation becomes substantial when CRP levels rise above 2.0 mg/dL, with a graded decrease of micronutrient concentrations associated with increasing CRP levels. Because most micronutrient levels decrease as soon as CRP exceeds 2.0 mg/dL, hs-CRP, which aims at detecting mild inflammation, is not sensitive enough to diagnose micronutrient variations in most cases, except with vitamins C and B6, where a true reflection of the status can only be made if CRP is less than 0.5 mg/dL.[11,14]

The Biomarkers Reflecting Inflammation and Nutritional Determinants of Anemia (BRINDA) project was designed to improve the interpretation of nutrient biomarkers in settings of inflammation and to generate context-specific estimates of risk factors for anemia. Although its focus is anemia (a worldwide public health issue), BRINDA has provided important insights regarding the interpretation of laboratory results. Using data from a series of studies conducted in the context of malaria and HIV, the project was able to provide guidance on how to adjust biomarkers for several micronutrients using the inflammation markers AGP and CRP in several countries. In 2021, BRINDA developed an open-source, all-in-one, R-package statistical programming extension for inflammation adjustment for RBP, serum retinol, ferritin, soluble transferrin receptor (sTfR), and zinc using the two inflammation indicators (AGP and CRP) for various population groups.[21]

# Biomarkers to Assist in Interpreting Laboratory Results in Inflammation

The impact of "pure" inflammation on micronutrient blood levels has been investigated in healthy volunteers. The investigations show that additional biomarkers are required. One such study, conducted in 52 healthy individuals exposed to norovirus, examined the relationships between CRP, AGP, and micronutrient biomarkers from 0 to 35 days following virus exposure. The norovirus infection resulted in mild inflammation (median CRP level of 1.6 mg/dL). Significant alterations from baseline were observed for ferritin (elevated on day 3), hepcidin (elevated on days 2 and 3), serum iron (depressed on days 2–4), transferrin saturation (depressed on days 2–4), and retinol (depressed on days 3, 4, and 7).[22] This section reviews the most commonly available biomarkers of the effect of inflammation on micronutrient status, followed by a case study that demonstrates how to best interpret and act on the laboratory results for these biomarkers.

## Albumin Status

Albumin is a marker of disease severity and a negative acute-phase reactant, but by no means is it a nutritional marker in the presence of inflammation.[23] Because albumin carries variable proportions of numerous circulating micronutrients (eg, vitamin A, zinc, vitamin B6, vitamin C, selenium), decreased plasma albumin will decrease the micronutrient concentrations in the blood.[11] One large study has shown that the impact of the systemic inflammatory response may be adjusted based on albumin concentrations. For example, in the cohort of 743 patients, plasma zinc level was associated with both CRP and albumin, and the adjustment for albumin was useful. But for selenium, although its level was associated with both CRP and albumin, the adjustment for albumin did not work, likely because changes in albumin have numerous causes different from those influencing selenium status: the authors recommended determination of plasma glutathione peroxidase 3 (GPX3) or intracellular measurements.[24] This example shows that adjustment based on albumin concentrations does not apply to all micronutrients.

# Iron Status

Iron deficiency is a worldwide public health issue, and anemia indicates severe deficiency. The strong impact of inflammation can result in substantial changes in iron metabolism. Iron levels in the blood during a state of inflammation will always be low, potentially causing a state of functional iron deficiency. On one hand, too much iron is deleterious, so hypoferremia has been considered a positive attribute in the short term, as it reduces the amount of circulating iron accessible to invading microbes. However, iron deficiency with the development of anemia of chronic disease due to prolonged shunting of iron from important processes (ie, functional unavailability) can ultimately have multiple negative effects on cognitive, cardiopulmonary, and neuromuscular functions.[25] Because inflammation decreases circulating iron concentrations, the correct diagnosis of true deficiency is essential and must be supported by measures of additional proteins—namely, ferritin, transferrin, and hepcidin.

## Ferritin

A true iron deficiency is indicated by reduced ferritin (iron storage protein) levels in the absence of inflammation. Unfortunately, ferritin is an acute-phase reactant and is upregulated in proportion to the inflammatory insult: iron stores will increase as circulating iron is shunted from circulation.[25] Faced with the unreliability of ferritin to reflect iron deficiency in the presence of inflammation, one group of researchers attempted to improve the diagnosis of deficiency by testing two additional acute-phase markers, CRP and AGP,[26] and found that this combination could be useful in interpreting the ferritin level.

## Transferrin and Related Markers

Although not available everywhere, transferrin is used to determine potential iron overload in patients for whom intravenous iron therapy may pose increased risks. High transferrin saturation values have been associated with adverse outcomes (eg, in critically ill patients).[25] Transferrin saturation is of less value for diagnosing functional iron deficiency; soluble transferrin receptor (sTfR) is a more precise alternative.[21,25] The sTfR is the cleaved extracellular portion of transferrin receptor 1 that is released into serum. It is not an acute-phase reactant, and its concentration is a reliable marker of iron depletion, enabling the prediction of iron stores in the bone marrow.[27]

## Hepcidin

Hepcidin, a peptide hormone produced by the hepatocytes, regulates intestinal iron absorption, distribution, and liver storage and is considered the "master regulator" of iron. It has become the marker of choice for monitoring iron status in cases of acute inflammation. It is considered a better marker than transferrin but is not yet widely available.[28] Although the immediate changes in ferritin and transferrin are initiated directly by cytokines, hepcidin determines the severity and duration of an iron-restricted state. Hepcidin acts by binding to and degrading ferroportin, a cellular iron exporter found in duodenal cells, macrophages, and hepatocytes. It is upregulated in the presence of inflammation.[25]

In a randomized study of 133 critically ill patients with anemia, serum hepcidin concentration—but not ferritin or transferrin saturation—was able to identify patients in whom intravenous iron therapy effectively reduced red blood cell transfusion requirements.[29] Another randomized study, which included 399 patients, assessed whether hepcidin levels could accurately guide the treatment of iron deficiency in critically ill patients with anemia. The results showed that hepcidin-guided iron repletion was associated with a significant reduction in mortality at 90 days after discharge from intensive care and with an improved 1-year survival rate.[28]

# Copper Status

Because copper is one of the few micronutrients that increases with inflammation, a low serum copper value with an elevated CRP level always reflects deficiency.[12] The best way to confirm copper status is by its simultaneous determination with levels of CRP and the copper-transporter ceruloplasmin, a positive acute-phase reactant. A normal ceruloplasmin level or a normal serum copper level, or both, together with an elevated CRP indicates that copper status is suboptimal (although perhaps not yet deficient). A low ceruloplasmin level with high CRP will confirm a true copper deficiency.

# Selenium Status

The plasma enzyme GPX3 indicates short-term changes in selenium status, whereas GPX1 measures status across the erythrocyte life span and is, therefore, a better indicator of long-term status.[12] These seleno-proteins are dependent on an adequate blood selenium level of greater than 90 mcg/L.[30] Decreased GPX3 activity is a good indicator of selenium inadequacy.[12]

Plasma selenium levels fall in proportion to the inflammatory insult. Therefore, the simultaneous determination of an inflammatory marker such as CRP is essential. Practitioners should consider low plasma selenium levels with suspicion in the presence of a CRP level exceeding 2.0 mg/dL.[11] Whatever the grade of inflammation, a plasma selenium level of less than 32 mcg/L should be considered indicative of a severe deficiency and prompt selenium administration.[12]

# Vitamin A Status

RBP is the carrier protein of vitamin A and is a negative acute-phase protein. RBP levels drop rapidly with inflammation, thus affecting the body's circulating vitamin A status.[12] Serum vitamin A levels should be assessed through RBP and the acute-phase markers CRP, which rises quickly following infection, and AGP, which rises more slowly over a longer period of time. The BRINDA project studied vitamin A deficiency diagnosis, using RBP levels of less than 20 mcg/dL (0.7 mcmol/L) as a cutoff for deficiency, and showed that the adjustment differed among demographic groups. Although there was a linear relationship between inflammation (CRP, AGP) and vitamin A deficiency in preschool children, there was no significant impact in women.* The combination of these variables facilitates assessment of the severity of the impact of the inflammation and takes into consideration the duration of the inflammation (differentiating between early and late convalescence). The BRINDA authors concluded that, in settings where inflammation or malaria is present, the burden of vitamin A deficiency may be overestimated.[31] This is critical in contexts where vitamin A intervention programs are implemented, as concerns have arisen about the potential for excessive vitamin A exposure.

The case study at the end of this chapter illustrates how to use biomarkers to determine micronutrient status and therapy.

# Proposed Actions and Monitoring

Taking an isolated blood micronutrient measurement is of limited value. Repeated determinations are required when the aim is diagnosis of deficiency or when monitoring response to treatment. For short-term inflammation, such as in a patient suffering from the flu or recovering from elective surgery, it is best to wait for the CRP level to return to normal before making any determination of micronutrient status. However, clinicians often have no choice as to timing when a reasonable clinical suspicion of deficit exists. If the clinical indicators imply a micronutrient deficiency, serum levels can be determined, and repletion can commence while waiting for laboratory results. A second determination should then be done to confirm or monitor repletion.

If a patient is at potential long-term risk for deficiency (eg, if receiving long-term parenteral nutrition or recovering from gastrointestinal surgery), it is important to establish a baseline value and then follow up at 6- or 12-month intervals. Table 4.2 on page 58 proposes monitoring routines for various micronutrients and biomarkers indicated in different clinical scenarios.[12,32-38]

The Impact of Inflammation

---

* Study participants were described as women. Gender was not further specified.

**TABLE 4.2 Proposed Micronutrient Monitoring Routines for Various Conditions[a,12,32-38]**

| Clinical condition | Anemia | IBD and exclusive jejunal feeding[36,37] | High-output intestinal fistulas[36] | Obesity and post-bariatric surgery | Chronic dialysis[34] | CRRT[38] | Major burns[39] | Long-term PN in short bowel conditions | Liver failure (acute and chronic) |
|---|---|---|---|---|---|---|---|---|---|
| Proposed monitoring frequency | Baseline then 1 mo after treatment | Baseline then every 6 mo | Baseline then every 1-3 mo | Baseline then every 6 mo | Baseline then every 6 mo | After first 2 wk then every 2 wk | Weekly | Baseline then every 6 mo | Baseline then every 6 mo |
| Copper | (x)[b] | × | × | × | (x)[b] | × | × | | × |
| Iron | × | × | | × | | × | × | | |
| Manganese | | | | | | | | × | × |
| Selenium | | × | × | × | | × | × | × | |
| Zinc | × | × | × | × | | × | × | × | × |
| Thiamin (vitamin B1) | × | × | | | | × | | | |
| Riboflavin (vitamin B2) | | × | | | | | | | |

| | | | | | | | |
|---|---|---|---|---|---|---|---|
| Vitamin B6 (pyridoxine) | × | | | | | × | × |
| Biotin (vitamin B7) | × | × | | | | | |
| Folate (vitamin B9) | × | | × | | | × | |
| Vitamin B12 (cobalamin) | × | × | × | | | | × |
| Vitamin C | | | × | × | | × | |
| Vitamin A | × | × | × | × | | × | × |
| Vitamin D | × | × | × | | × | | × |
| Vitamin E | × | × | × | × | | × | × |
| Vitamin K | × | × | × | | | | |
| CRP or AGP | × | × | × | × | × | × | × |
| Ferritin | × | × | | | | | |
| Hepcidin | × | (x)[b] | | | | | × |
| Ceruloplasmin | (x)[b] | × | × | × | | × | |

Abbreviations: AGP, 1-acid glycoprotein; CRP, C-reactive protein; CRRT, continuous renal replacement therapy; IBD, inflammatory bowel disease; PN, parenteral nutrition.

[a]Not all micronutrients and biomarkers are included, as they are only available in research protocols.

[b](x) = to be determined in second round of investigations.

Clinical and research experience indicate that micronutrient values that are 20% lower than the lowest reference value in the presence of inflammation are likely to signify a deficiency[39,40] and may improve with repletion. In addition, decreased values in the absence of inflammation should always be considered a deficiency.

# Case Study

The following case study illustrates the use of biomarkers in determining the presence or absence of micronutrient deficiencies.

A 68-year-old male patient (weight, 75 kg; BMI, 27) is transferred to the intensive care unit (ICU) for acute respiratory failure requiring intubation and mechanical ventilation 10 days after an extensive skin and muscle resection to both thighs in the context of toxic shock syndrome. Vacuum-assisted drains are draining 500 mL/d per leg, which is compensated by saline. He has gained 8 kg since hospital admission.

The patient was not malnourished prior to being admitted. Following the initial surgery and up to the time of transfer to the ICU, he was given only oral food, and the dietitian noted an intake of 25% at best. The dietitian recommended two oral nutritional supplements per day, but the patient did not take them. The patient is hemodynamically stable, having received two units of packed red blood cells. Enteral nutrition is started on ICU day 2. After an initial blood draw on admission to the ICU (day 1), a second blood draw is taken on day 2.

**Day 1 and day 2 blood results are provided. After interpretation, an additional blood draw is requested on day 3.**

| Laboratory value (units) | Reference range[a] | Day 1 | Day 2 | Interpretation | Day 3 |
|---|---|---|---|---|---|
| Potassium (mEq/L) | 3.5-4.5 | 3.7 | 3.1 | Further decrease on day 2 indicates refeeding syndrome | 3.5 |
| Phosphate (mg/dL) | 0.8-1.2 | 2.5 | 0.9 | Further decrease on day 2 reflects refeeding syndrome | 1.7 |
| Glucose (mg/dL) | 70-100 | 234 | 227 | Hyperglycemia due to insulin resistance—treat with insulin | 162 |
| Hemoglobin (g/dL) | 11-12 | 7.6 | 8.8 | Severe anemia | 8.9 |
| Albumin (g/dL) | 3.5-4.5 | 2.5 | 2.8 | Generally low with inflammation | 2.8 |
| CRP (mg/dL) | <1 | 28 | 25 | Major inflammation is present due to large wounds | 24 |
| 25-hydroxyvitamin D3 (ng/mL) | 12-40 | | 4.6 | Very low value likely indicates vitamin D deficiency | |
| Copper (mcg/dL) | 64-140 | 52 | | Deficiency is quasi-certain, but ask for ceruloplasmin level to confirm deficiency—start repletion | |
| Iron (mcg/dL) | 60-170 | 28 | | Possible deficiency (loss through surgery)—ask for ferritin and hepcidin levels | 34 |
| Selenium (mcg/L) | 65-110 | 31 | | Deficient—if available, ask for GPX3 level | |
| Zinc (mcg/dL) | 90-150 | 65 | | Likely not deficient | |
| Ceruloplasmin (mg/dL) | 14-40 | | | Low—confirms copper deficiency | 11 |
| Ferritin (ng/mL) | 12-300 | | | Elevated—positive acute-phase reactant | 750 |
| sTfR (mg/L) | 1.8-4.6 | | | Elevated in response to iron deficiency | 5.7 |
| Hepcidin[b] (ng/mL) | 17.2-91.2 | | | Low | 15 |

Abbreviations: CRP, C-reactive protein; GPX3, plasma glutathione peroxidase 3; sTfR, soluble transferrin receptor.

[a] Per hospital laboratory assay

[b] Hepcidin is not approved by the US Food and Drug Administration for the evaluation of iron deficiency; however, the European Society for Clinical Nutrition and Metabolism endorses this assessment with a Grade A recommendation.

The Impact of Inflammation

# Suggested Actions Based on Interpretation of Laboratory Results

Proceed cautiously with an increase in energy intake because of the presence of **refeeding syndrome**.[41,42]

For **vitamin D** deficiency, recommend a loading dose (1,250 mcg or 50,000 IU) and ensure a minimum of 50 mcg/d (2,000 IU/d) enterally.[12]

Low **copper** and **ceruloplasmin** levels, along with high CRP levels, indicate a copper deficiency—recommend 4 mg copper intravenously per day for 10 days,[12] then repeat sampling.

As no further markers for **selenium** are available, and the value indicates severe deficiency, recommend 100 mcg selenium intravenously for 7 to 10 days.[12]

Given the mildly low **zinc level**, recommend an adequate amount to meet the Dietary Reference Intake, and ask for a repeat measurement on day 10 (after 1 week).

The patient's **iron** deficiency is likely caused by bleeding from the wounds. Low stores are confirmed by a low hepcidin level and an elevated sTfR level (a high ferritin value only reflects inflammation): recommend transfusion, and consider administering 1 g iron as carboxymaltose as soon as the CRP level is below 1.0 mg/dL.[12]

# *References*

1.  Sriram K, Lonchyna VA. Micronutrient supplementation in adult nutrition therapy: practical considerations. *JPEN J Parenter Enteral Nutr.* 2009;33(5):548-562. doi:10.1177/0148607108328470

2.  McMillan DC, Maguire D, Talwar D. Relationship between nutritional status and the systemic inflammatory response: micronutrients. *Proc Nutr Soc.* 2019;78(1):56-67. doi:10.1017/S0029665118002501

3.  Thurnham DI, Northrop-Clewes CA. Inflammation and biomarkers of micronutrient status. *Curr Opin Clin Nutr Metab Care.* 2016;19(6):458-463. doi:10.1097/MCO.0000000000000323

4.  Namaste SM, Aaron GJ, Varadhan R, Peerson JM, Suchdev PS, BRINDA Working Group. Methodologic approach for the Biomarkers Reflecting Inflammation and Nutritional Determinants of Anemia (BRINDA) project. *Am J Clin Nutr.* 2017;106(suppl 1):333S-347S. doi:10.3945/ajcn.116.142273

5.  Gombart AF, Pierre A, Maggini S. A review of micronutrients and the immune system-working in harmony to reduce the risk of infection. *Nutrients.* 2020;12(1):236. doi:10.3390/nu12010236

6.  Sears B, Saha AK. Dietary control of inflammation and resolution. *Front Nutr.* 2021;8:709435. doi:10.3389/fnut.2021.709435

7.  Oishi Y, Manabe I. Macrophages in inflammation, repair and regeneration. *Int Immunol.* 2018;30(11):511-528. doi:10.1093/intimm/dxy054

8.  Kumar P, Shen Q, Pivetti CD, Lee ES, Wu MH, Yuan SY. Molecular mechanisms of endothelial hyperpermeability: implications in inflammation. *Expert Rev Mol Med.* 2009;11:e19. doi:10.1017/S1462399409001112

9.  Fleck A. Clinical and nutritional aspects of changes in acute-phase proteins during inflammation. *Proc Nutr Soc.* 1989;48(3):347-354. doi:10.1079/pns19890050

10. Owen JA. Effect of injury on plasma proteins. *Adv Clin Chem.* 1967;9:1-41. doi:10.1016/s0065-2423(08)60284-x

11. Duncan A, Talwar D, McMillan DC, Stefanowicz F, O'Reilly DS. Quantitative data on the magnitude of the systemic inflammatory response and its effect on micronutrient status based on plasma measurements. *Am J Clin Nutr.* 2012;95(1):64-71. doi:10.3945/ajcn.111.023812

12. Berger MM, Shenkin A, Schweinlin A, et al. ESPEN micronutrient guideline. *Clin Nutr.* 2022;41(6):1357-1424. doi:10.1016/j.clnu.2022.02.015

13. Ghashut RA, McMillan DC, Kinsella J, Talwar D. Erythrocyte concentrations of B1, B2, B6 but not plasma C and E are reliable indicators of nutrition status in the presence of systemic inflammation. *Clin Nutr ESPEN*. 2017;17:54-62. doi:10.1016/j.clnesp.2016.10.007

14. Salota R, Omar S, Sherwood RA, Raja K, Vincent RP. Clinical relevance of trace element measurement in patients on initiation of parenteral nutrition. *Ann Clin Biochem*. 2016;53(6):680-685. doi:10.1177/0004563216633489

15. Oudemans-van Straaten HM, Man A, de Waard MC. Vitamin C revisited. *Crit Care*. 2014;18(4):460. doi:10.1186/s13054-014-0460-x

16. Berger MM, Oudemans-van Straaten HM. Vitamin C supplementation in the critically ill patient. *Curr Opin Clin Nutr Metab Care*. 2015;18(2):193-201. doi:10.1097/MCO.0000000000000148

17. Chen L, Deng H, Cui H, et al. Inflammatory responses and inflammation-associated diseases in organs. *Oncotarget*. 2017;9(6):7204-7218. doi:10.18632/oncotarget.23208

18. Sendama W. The effect of ageing on the resolution of inflammation. *Ageing Res Rev*. 2020;57:101000. doi:10.1016/j.arr.2019.101000

19. Tuuminen T, Sorsa M, Tornudd M, Poussa T, Antila E, Jaakkola K. The association between high sensitivity C-reactive protein and micro-nutrient levels: a cross-sectional analysis based on a laboratory database. *Clin Nutr ESPEN*. 2019;33:283-289. doi:10.1016/j.clnesp.2019.06.011

20. Shenkin A, Talward D, Berger MM. Uses and abuses of micronutrient blood tests in assessing nutritional status. *Nutr Clin Pract*. 2022;38(1):56-69. doi:10.1002/ncp.10924

21. Luo H, Addo O, Jahan A. BRINDA: computation of BRINDA adjusted micronutrient biomarkers for inflammation. R package version 0.1.3. 2021. Accessed January 2022. https://cran.r-project.org/web/packages/BRINDA/index.html

22. Williams AM, Ladva CN, Leon JS, et al. Changes in micronutrient and inflammation serum biomarker concentrations after a norovirus human challenge. *Am J Clin Nutr*. 2019;110(6):1456-1464. doi:10.1093/ajcn/nqz201

23. Shenkin A. Serum prealbumin: is it a marker of nutritional status or of risk of malnutrition? *Clin Chem*. 2006;52(12):2177-2179. doi:10.1373/clinchem.2006.077412

24. Ghashut RA, McMillan DC, Kinsella J, Vasilaki AT, Talwar D, Duncan A. The effect of the systemic inflammatory response on plasma zinc and selenium adjusted for albumin. *Clin Nutr*. 2016;35(2):381-387. doi:10.1016/j.clnu.2015.02.010

25. Litton E, Lim J. Iron metabolism: an emerging therapeutic target in critical illness. *Crit Care*. 2019;23(1):81. doi:10.1186/s13054-019-2373-1

26. Thurnham DI, McCabe LD, Haldar S, Wieringa FT, Northrop-Clewes CA, McCabe GP. Adjusting plasma ferritin concentrations to remove the effects of subclinical inflammation in the assessment of iron deficiency: a meta-analysis. *Am J Clin Nutr.* 2010;92(3):546-555. doi:10.3945/ajcn.2010.29284

27. Baillie FJ, Morrison AE, Fergus I. Soluble transferrin receptor: a discriminating assay for iron deficiency. *Clin Lab Haematol.* 2003;25(6):353-357. doi:10.1046/j.0141-9854.2003.00548.x

28. Lasocki S, Asfar P, Jaber S, et al. Impact of treating iron deficiency, diagnosed according to hepcidin quantification, on outcomes after a prolonged ICU stay compared to standard care: a multicenter, randomized, single-blinded trial. *Crit Care.* 2021;25(1):62. doi:10.1186/s13054-020-03430-3

29. Litton E, Baker S, Erber W, et al. Hepcidin predicts response to IV iron therapy in patients admitted to the intensive care unit: a nested cohort study. *J Intensive Care.* 2018;6:60. doi:10.1186/s40560-018-0328-2

30. Hatanaka N, Nakaden H, Yamamoto Y, Matsuo S, Fujikawa T, Matsusue S. Selenium kinetics and changes in glutathione peroxidase activities in patients receiving long-term parenteral nutrition an effects of supplementation with selenite. *Nutrition.* 2000;16(1):22-26. doi:10.1016/s0899-9007(99)00183-5

31. Larson LM, Namaste SM, Williams AM, et al. Adjusting retinol-binding protein concentrations for inflammation: Biomarkers Reflecting Inflammation and Nutritional Determinants of Anemia (BRINDA) project. *Am J Clin Nutr.* 2017;106(suppl 1):390S-401S. doi:10.3945/ajcn.116.142166

32. Berger MM, Reintam-Blaser A, Calder PC, et al. Monitoring nutrition in the ICU. *Clin Nutr.* 2019;38(2):584-593. doi:10.1016/j.clnu.2018.07.009

33. Fiaccadori E, Sabatino A, Barazzoni R, et al. ESPEN guideline on clinical nutrition in hospitalized patients with acute or chronic kidney disease. *Clin Nutr.* 2021;40(4):1644-1668. doi:10.1016/j.clnu.2021.01.028

34. Goosen C, Baumgartner J, Mikulic N, et al. Examining associations of HIV and iron status with nutritional and inflammatory status, anemia, and dietary intake in South African schoolchildren. *Nutrients.* 2021;13(3):962. doi:10.3390/nu13030962

35. Couper C, Doriot A, Siddiqui MTR, Steiger E. Nutrition management of the high-output fistulae. *Nutr Clin Pract.* 2021;36(2):282-296. doi:10.1002/ncp.10608

36. Bischoff SC, Escher J, Hébuterne X, et al. ESPEN practical guideline: clinical nutrition in inflammatory bowel disease. *Clin Nutr.* 2020;39(3):632-653. doi:10.1016/j.clnu.2019.11.002

37. Berger MM, Broman M, Forni L, Ostermann M, De Waele E, Wischmeyer PE. Nutrients and micronutrients at risk during renal replacement therapy: a scoping review. *Curr Opin Crit Care*. 2021;27(4):367-377. doi:10.1097/MCC.0000000000000851

38. Rousseau AF, Losser MR, Ichai C, Berger MM. ESPEN endorsed recommendations: nutritional therapy in major burns. *Clin Nutr*. 2013;32(4):497-502. doi:10.1016/j.clnu.2013.02.012

39. Berger MM, Soguel L, Shenkin A, et al. Influence of early antioxidant supplements on clinical evolution and organ function in critically ill cardiac surgery, major trauma and subarachnoid hemorrhage patients. *Crit Care*. 2008;12(4):R101. doi:10.1186/cc6981

40. Berger MM, Baines M, Raffoul W, et al. Trace element supplements after major burns modulate antioxidant status and clinical course by way of increased tissue trace element concentration. *Am J Clin Nutr*. 2007;85(5):1293-1300. doi:10.1093/ajcn/85.5.1293

41. Doig GS, Simpson F, Heighes PT, et al. Restricted versus continued standard caloric intake during the management of refeeding syndrome in critically ill adults: a randomised, parallel-group, multicentre, single-blind controlled trial. *Lancet Respir Med*. 2015;3(12):943-952. doi:10.1016/S2213-2600(15)00418-X

42. da Silva JSV, Seres DS, Sabino K, et al. ASPEN consensus recommendations for refeeding syndrome. *Nutr Clin Pract*. 2020;35(2):178-195. doi:10.1002/ncp.10474

# CHAPTER 5

# Deficiencies in Fat-Soluble Vitamins

Kristen M. Roberts, PhD, RDN, LD, CNSC, FASPEN, FAND, and Lingtak-Neander Chan, PharmD, BCNSP, FCCP, FASPEN

## Introduction

This chapter addresses the role of fat-soluble vitamins (A, D, E, and K) in human physiology and the pathology that occurs when their concentrations in the body are inadequate. Although fat-soluble vitamins present a higher risk for toxicity than most of the water-soluble nutrients do, the focus of the chapter is on the assessment of inadequacies, not toxicities. Currently, no evidence-based guidelines exist that clearly identify a dosing strategy for fat-soluble vitamins based on particular laboratory values. Assessment for deficiency and the subsequent determination of a dosing strategy requires a complex evaluation of biochemical, physical, and clinical factors. Physical findings may not manifest until the later stages of deficiency; therefore, positive findings are not required to initiate treatment. Further research on protocols for supplementation and repletion in various disease states is needed to develop firm guidance. The chapter reviews the clinical assessment (in older children and adults) for determining a fat-soluble vitamin deficiency and the dosing strategies suggested for repletion. These findings should be coordinated with the clinical picture to optimize a treatment plan. Dietary Reference Intakes (DRIs) for the fat-soluble vitamins are provided in Table 5.1.[1-3]

| TABLE 5.1 Dietary Reference Intakes for Fat-Soluble Vitamins[1-3] | | | | |
|---|---|---|---|---|
| **Population (age)** | **Vitamin A[a] (RDA)** | **Vitamin D[b] (RDA)** | **Vitamin E (RDA)** | **Vitamin K (AI)** |
| Children (9-13 y) | M: 600 mcg F: 600 mcg | M: 15 mcg F: 15 mcg | M: 11 mg F: 11 mg | M: 60 mcg F: 60 mcg |
| Adults (>14 y) | M: 900 mcg F: 700 mcg | M: 15 mcg F: 15 mcg | M: 15 mg F: 15 mg | M: 75-120 mcg F: 75-90 mcg |
| Older adults (>70 y) | M: 900 mcg F: 700 mcg | M: 20 mcg F: 20 mcg | M: 15 mg F: 15 mg | M: 120 mcg F: 90 mcg |
| Pregnant | F: 750-770 mcg | F: 15 mcg | F: 15 mg | F: 75-90 mcg |
| Lactating | F: 1,200-1,300 mcg | F: 15 mcg | F: 19 mg | F: 75-90 mcg |

Abbreviations: AI, Adequate Intake; F, females; M, males; RDA, Recommended Dietary Allowance.

[a] As retinol activity equivalents

[b] 1 mcg cholecalciferol = 40 IU vitamin D

# Digestion, Absorption, and Metabolism of Fat-Soluble Vitamins

Fat-soluble vitamins are introduced into the human body through foods (refer to the Appendix on page 331 for food sources), medications (eg, lipid injectable emulsions), supplements, and biosynthesis from the intestinal microbiota (as seen with vitamin K). Fat-soluble vitamins in the diet are embedded within the food matrix. Mechanical and chemical emulsification in the mouth, stomach, and small intestine extract these essential micronutrients from foods by increasing the surface area for penetration by lingual, gastric, and pancreatic lipase.[4] The emulsification process facilitates absorption, rendering these nutrients bioavailable. As biliary secretions enter the small intestine through the common bile duct, micelle formation occurs, facilitating luminal entry into the epithelial cells. As fat-soluble vitamins and fatty acids enter the epithelial cells, chylomicrons are packaged and released through the central lacteals into the lymphatic system. The fat-soluble vitamins have a similar fate to dietary fat and, thus, circulate for immediate use.[4,5] When cellular demand diminishes, circulating vitamins return to the liver and adipose tissue for storage.[4]

# Pathophysiology of Deficiencies

Deficiencies in fat-soluble vitamins can occur with inadequate intake (oral, enteral, or parenteral), increased losses (eg, maldigestion, malabsorption, or drug-nutrient and nutrient-nutrient interactions), or increased physiological requirements (eg, burns or critical illness).[6,7] Few formal guidelines exist for dosing strategies to rectify suboptimal status.[8-11] Deficiencies in fat-soluble nutrients often co-occur with other nutrient deficiencies in most clinical scenarios,[7] but they have also been documented in isolation. Vitamin D deficiency is the most common isolated deficiency and is reported in populations with limited sun exposure (eg, institutionalized populations or those living at distances farther from the equator) and inadequate intake.[12,13]

When a fat-soluble vitamin deficiency is suspected, the clinician must consider the patient's micronutrient intake, the pathophysiology contributing to micronutrient deficiency risk, a biochemical assessment, and the clinical presentation (if positive findings are present) to improve the likelihood of identifying a true deficiency. In cases of hypoproteinemia, deficiencies may be more prevalent, as the transport of fat-soluble vitamins requires carrier proteins. Physical findings most often occur when the vitamin deficiency is severe or prolonged. Individuals at risk for deficiency will benefit from routine biochemical assessments. As with all micronutrient treatment regimens, there is concern for toxicity, so continued monitoring after treatment is essential to reevaluate whether further treatment is appropriate once homeostasis is achieved.

# Vitamin A

Vitamin A comes in two main forms: preformed retinoids and provitamin A carotenoids (eg, beta carotene), which are found in animal and plant sources, respectively. Vitamin A performs cellular functions essential to vision, growth, embryonic development, cellular differentiation, immune function, and reproductive health. Vitamin A deficiency is associated with night vision loss, infertility, impaired immune function, and growth abnormalities.[14] These abnormalities have been reported in individuals with alcohol-use disorder, chronic intestinal failure, inflammatory bowel disease, and liver disease, and in patients recovering from bariatric surgery (Chapter 14).[7] To determine whether an individual is getting enough vitamin A, the total vitamin A and carotenoid intake should be calculated and compared to the appropriate DRI (refer to Table 5.1). Historically, vitamin A was measured in International Units (IU), but in 2016 the US Food and Drug Administration revised the Nutrition Facts and Supplement Facts labels and began using retinol activity equivalents (RAE).[15] Vitamin A supplements are available in various salt forms of preformed vitamin A or provitamin A, including retinol, retinyl esters, beta carotene, α carotene, and β cryptoxanthin.

## Screening and Assessment

Vitamin A deficiency is a public health concern in many developing countries, with the main causes being parasitic infections, infection, and malabsorption. Deficiency in a healthy adult eating a typical diet in a developed country is rare, as the liver contains more than 90% of vitamin A stores, which is sufficient to maintain normal status for approximately 6 months.[5] Clinical suspicion of vitamin A deficiency warrants a nutrition focused physical exam (NFPE), a clinical interview that includes a diet history or food frequency questionnaire, and a biochemical assessment. Unfortunately, positive physical findings or changes in visual acuity are associated with a severe deficiency, thus physical findings are of limited use in identifying early signs of deficiency. A case study evaluated the association between follicular hyperkeratosis and micronutrient deficiencies and found severe malnutrition, not micronutrient deficiency (eg, vitamins E and A), to be the contributing factor in the development of follicular hyperkeratosis.[16] This case report highlights how physical findings pose challenges to interpretation, as manifestations can be multifactorial or unrelated to a specific vitamin or mineral deficiency. When physical findings are positively correlated with suboptimal serum retinol concentrations, repletion is necessary, and suggested dosing varies based on the patient's age and the severity of the physical finding. An expert review of vitamin A suggested up to 200,000 IU (60,000 mcg RAE) on days 1, 2, and 14 when corneal lesions are identified, with expected clinical improvement within 1 week of treatment.[5] Milder presentations (such as Bitot spots) warrant much lower dosages (eg, 10,000 IU or 3,000 mcg RAE per day), with expected improvements within a few weeks.[17] However, clinical trials are needed to confirm these suggested repletion doses in various disease states.

Zinc and iron play critical roles in the transport and mobilization of vitamin A from adipose tissue; therefore, deficiencies in these minerals can lead to vitamin A deficiency, especially when protein-energy malnutrition is present. Laboratory assessment of serum or plasma zinc levels, iron levels (serum iron, ferritin, and total iron-binding capacity), and an inflammatory marker (eg, CRP) should occur concomitantly with determination of serum or plasma retinol concentrations. Elevated levels of inflammatory biomarkers raise concerns about the potential for the inaccurate interpretation of zinc, iron, and vitamin A test results (refer to Chapter 4).[18]

# Vitamin D

Vitamin D is essential for maintaining calcium homeostasis and, therefore, contributes to bone metabolism and growth, suppression of inflammation, and the prevention of hypocalcemic tetany.[19] Worldwide, vitamin D deficiency has been reported in up to 90% of various populations.[20] Table 5.1 reviews the DRIs for vitamin D, which are based on its role in bone health and calcium regulation. The primary source of vitamin D is ultraviolet B rays through direct exposure of the skin to sunlight, but in many situations sun exposure alone does not produce enough endogenous previtamin D to meet physiological needs.

Thus, optimal dietary vitamin D intake is critical for preventing clinical deficiency. Few foods contain naturally occurring vitamin D, and fortified foods provide an essential source for those living in areas with minimal sunlight or at high latitudes. Regardless of the source, vitamin D must undergo two hydroxylation reactions to convert to the physiological active form of vitamin D (1,25-dihydroxyvitamin D, or calcitriol), with the first hydroxylation occurring in the liver and the second in the kidney.[19]

# Screening and Assessment

People with malabsorptive conditions, hepatic or renal diseases, liver failure, Whipple disease, celiac sprue, Crohn's disease, or inadequate vitamin D intake, as well as those experiencing drug-nutrient interactions, are at risk for vitamin D deficiency and require screening. Vitamin D is predominately stored in adipose tissue, so the total vitamin D pool is increased in most individuals who are obese. However, because vitamin D is sequestered into the adipocytes, obesity is associated with decreased plasma vitamin D concentrations. Rapid weight loss, such as that which occurs in the first few months following bariatric surgery, can transiently increase plasma vitamin D concentrations because of the redistribution of vitamin D from the fat depot.[21,22]

Biochemical assessment in conjunction with a review of the patient's medical, diet, dietary-supplement, and sun-exposure histories assist in correctly identifying a deficiency. A patient interview revealing muscle weakness, bone pain, or stool characteristics associated with steatorrhea should heighten suspicion for potential deficiency. The NFPE may reveal nonspecific growth abnormalities in children, but there is a lack of correlation with other physical findings in the adult population. Serum or plasma total 25-hydroxyvitamin D (calcidiol) concentration has a serum half-life of 15 days and reflects the total vitamin D reserve in the body. Serum 1,25-dihydroxyvitamin D (calcitriol), which is assessed mostly in patients with chronic kidney disease, should not be used for routine monitoring of vitamin D status.[23]

Although not all micronutrients are affected by inflammation, inclusion of an inflammatory marker such as CRP should be considered when assessing multiple micronutrient deficiencies, as vitamin D is a negative acute-phase reactant (refer to Chapter 4).

## Special Considerations

Ergocalciferol (vitamin D2) and cholecalciferol (vitamin D3) are appropriate for supplementation or repletion, even in people who cannot complete the final hydroxylation (ie, those with renal disease). The National Kidney Foundation Kidney Disease Outcomes Quality Initiative guideline confirms with an expert opinion that both vitamin D2 and vitamin D3 are sufficient for treatment of deficiency, yet additional research on outcomes in chronic kidney disease is needed (Chapter 10).[24]

# Vitamin E

Vitamin E—of which $\alpha$-tocopherol is the most biologically active form—is an important antioxidant that regulates immune function, protects neuronal cells, decreases lipid peroxidation, and supports the stability of the erythrocyte membranes. DRIs are established (Table 5.1). Unlike the other fat-soluble vitamins, vitamin E is stored in multiple sites, including adipose, heart, lung, muscle, liver, and brain tissues and the adrenal glands.[25] Optimal storage is likely responsible for the poor correlation between suboptimal dietary intake and $\alpha$-tocopherol status in the blood.

## Screening and Assessment

In the context of serum or plasma assessment, it is critical to evaluate the patient for hyperlipidemia, as this condition increases the concentrations of $\alpha$-tocopherol.[7,26] To calculate the effective serum vitamin E concentration, the $\alpha$-tocopherol level should be divided by a summation of total cholesterol (mg/dL) and triglycerides (mg/dL). In people with elevated lipid concentrations, a cholesterol and triglyceride–adjusted concentration is useful in the interpretation to prevent underestimating vitamin E status.

Vitamin E deficiency occurs in conjunction with other fat-soluble vitamin deficiencies in individuals with fat malabsorption, as occurs with chronic pancreatitis, cystic fibrosis, or cholestatic liver disease, and less frequently because of poor dietary intake.[27] Genetic conditions can increase the risk of developing vitamin E deficiency, as seen in ataxia with vitamin E deficiency and abetalipoproteinemia.[28]

The NFPE does not help identify vitamin E deficiency because there are no documented dermatological manifestations specific to vitamin E deficiency. However, in people with chronic anemia from immune-mediated hemolysis (eg, drug-induced hemolytic anemia, especially with glucose-6-phosphate dehydrogenase deficiency), pallor may be present on the NFPE. Also, individuals with neuromuscular dysfunction may have visual impairment, nystagmus, and ophthalmoplegia.[7,29]

Serum α-tocopherol concentrations are suggested to be affected by inflammation when the CRP level is greater than 8 mg/dL (refer to Chapter 4).[7]

# Special Considerations

Investigations have suggested that implementation of high-dose vitamin E (exceeding the DRI for age and sex) in various conditions, including nonalcoholic fatty liver disease, may be effective; however, inconclusive evidence or negative findings limit the ability to recommend this practice. In 2010, researchers investigated the impact of vitamin E vs pioglitazone vs placebo on fibrosis in biopsy-proven metabolic dysfunction-associated steatohepatitis without concomitant diabetes, and data suggested a benefit of vitamin E (800 IU/d).[30] This study was published in the *New England Journal of Medicine* and subsequently included in a 2020 review article in the *Journal of the American Medical Association*.[31] Both publications greatly increased the visibility of these findings. However, numerous conflicting reports of increased mortality in specific populations, and ensuing concerns, limit the applicability of this treatment to all clinical scenarios.[32-34]

# Vitamin K

Vitamin K (ie, phylloquinone and the menaquinones) has essential functions as a cofactor for proteins in bone metabolism and as a coenzyme for a vitamin K–dependent carboxylase involved in the blood clotting cascade.[35] It is transported via triglycerides, mainly as a component of very low-density lipoproteins.[36] Matrix Gla protein is a vitamin K–dependent protein that reduces calcifications; therefore, a vitamin K deficiency may lead to vascular calcifications and related comorbidities. However, people with vascular calcifications and heart disease may also be at an increased risk, due to the lack of vitamin K–dependent matrix-GLA-protein activity.[37,38] Dietary phylloquinone comes from leafy green vegetables, and consistent intake can minimize adverse drug events in patients taking warfarin. DRIs are established (refer to Table 5.1), yet it is critical to understand that most menaquinones are derived from intestinal microbes.[35]

## Screening and Assessment

Most vitamin K deficiencies are found in individuals with fat malabsorption, pancreatic or biliary dysfunction, or chronic antibiotic use. Vitamin K is rapidly metabolized, and serum concentrations are poor predictors of vitamin K status. However, there appears to be a strong correlation between serum vitamin K and triglyceride concentrations.[36,39] The NFPE may reveal reddish-purple spots or bone demineralization in the presence of clinical deficiency. Fat malabsorption or chronic antibiotic use, combined with a positive NFPE, warrants vitamin K assessment.

There is no direct biomarker of vitamin K body status. Plasma concentrations of total phylloquinone may be affected by inflammation when the CRP level exceeds 1 mg/dL.[7] Elevated prothrombin time or an international normalized ratio can be a reliable, indirect surrogate biomarker of the functional status of vitamin K but lacks sufficient sensitivity to identify a preclinical deficiency. Other possible biomarkers include undercarboxylated osteocalcin, which is a protein induced by vitamin K absence, and a vitamin K–to-triglyceride ratio.[36,39]

# Deficiency Assessment Strategies and Nutrient Interactions

Box 5.1 summarizes assessment strategies for determining fat-soluble vitamin status.[5,7,14,19,25,26,35,36,39-43] Box 5.2 on page 80 lists drug-nutrient and nutrient-nutrient interactions involving the fat-soluble vitamins.[44-45]

---

**BOX 5.1  Assessment Strategies for Determining Fat-Soluble Vitamin Status[5,7,14,19,25,26,35,36,39-43]**

### *Vitamin A*

**Pertinent biochemical tests**

Retinol, serum

Retinol-binding protein, serum

C-reactive protein, serum[a]

Iron studies, serum[b]

Complete blood count, serum

Zinc, serum or plasma

Carotene, plasma

**Clinical assessment of deficiency**

| | |
|---|---|
| *Physical findings* | Symmetrical follicular papules with keratin plugs present on extensor surfaces |
| | Hair casts (thin, cylindrical buildup that encompasses the hair shaft) |
| | Signs and symptoms associated with iron-deficiency anemia (eg, pallor, koilonychia, stomatitis, glossitis) |
| | Hyperkeratosis |
| | Bitot spots |
| *Clinical findings* | Decreased visual acuity |
| | Xerophthalmia |
| | Compromised immune function |

---

**BOX 5.1  Assessment Strategies for Determining Fat-Soluble Vitamin Status**[5,7,14,19,25,26,35,36,39-43] **(cont.)**

**Special considerations**

Optimize dosing of pancreatic exocrine replacement therapy (PERT) in patients with pancreatic insufficiency.

In patients with anemia associated with hypovitaminosis A and iron deficiency, treatment with vitamin A and iron is essential to improve hemoglobin concentration.

Inflammation causes a decline in serum retinol and retinol-binding protein concentrations.

Retinol conversion: 1 retinol activity equivalent (RAE) = 1 mcg retinol = 12 mcg dietary beta carotene.

## *Vitamin D*

**Pertinent biochemical tests**

25-hydroxyvitamin D, serum or plasma

Standard tests measure total (free and bound) 25-hydroxyvitamin D2 and 25-hydroxyvitamin D3

C-reactive protein, serum[a]

Parathyroid hormone

Total calcium, serum; *or* ionized calcium[c]

**Clinical assessment of deficiency**

| | |
|---|---|
| *Physical findings* | Growth abnormalities (in children) |
| *Clinical findings* | Bone pain |
| | Muscle weakness |
| | Steatorrhea |

**Special considerations**

Optimize dosing of PERT in patients with pancreatic insufficiency.

*Continued on next page*

---

**BOX 5.1  Assessment Strategies for Determining Fat-Soluble Vitamin Status[5,7,14,19,25,26,35,36,39-43] (cont.)**

## *Vitamin E*

### Pertinent biochemical tests

α-tocopherol concentration

C-reactive protein, serum[a]

Cholesterol, serum

Triglyceride, serum

### Clinical assessment of deficiency

| *Clinical findings* | Steatorrhea |
| --- | --- |
| | Neuromuscular dysfunction |
| | Decreased visual acuity |

### Special considerations

Optimize dosing of PERT in patients with pancreatic insufficiency.

In the setting of hyperlipidemia, α-tocopherol should be adjusted by the summation of serum cholesterol and triglyceride concentrations. A ratio of α-tocopherol (mg) to total lipids (g) of <0.8 indicates vitamin E inadequacy.[25,41,42]

Use caution in patients with concurrent fat malabsorption, as this condition may alter the ratio of α-tocopherol to total lipids by overestimating the presence of a deficiency.

Pay careful attention when treating vitamin E deficiency in patients taking warfarin, as they are at increased risk for hemorrhage.

## *Vitamin K*

### Pertinent biochemical tests

Prothrombin time

Vitamin K, serum

Triglyceride, serum

PIVKA-II (if available)

---

**BOX 5.1  Assessment Strategies for Determining Fat-Soluble Vitamin Status[5,7,14,19,25,26,35,36,39-43] (cont.)**

### Clinical assessment of deficiency

| *Clinical findings* | Bleeding |
| --- | --- |
| | Hemorrhage |
| | Bone demineralization |
| | Osteoporosis |

### Special considerations

Optimize dosing of PERT in patients with pancreatic insufficiency.

Chronic use of antibiotics may cause vitamin K deficiency.

Serum vitamin K is a biomarker of recent intake due to vitamin K's rapid clearance from blood, but it is unsuitable for monitoring vitamin K status.

Triglyceride and plasma phylloquinone concentrations are correlated, and it is suggested to calculate a phylloquinone-to-triglyceride ratio to determine the risk of deficiency.[35,38] The reference range for the ratio is 0.20-2.20. Results below the reference range should be considered a possible vitamin K deficiency.[35]

[a] Refer to Chapter 4 for assessment information on the use of C-reactive protein.
[b] Iron studies include serum iron, serum ferritin, total iron-binding capacity, and transferrin saturation.
[c] Serum calcium and ionized calcium concentrations cannot be used in isolation to assess the need for calcium repletion or supplementation strategies. The clinician must assess nutritional intake and bone density to determine calcium requirements.

*Deficiencies in Fat-Soluble Vitamins*

## BOX 5.2 Drug-Nutrient and Nutrient-Nutrient Interactions for Fat-Soluble Vitamins[44,45]

| Interacting substance (drug or other nutrient) | Mechanism for vitamin interference |
|---|---|
| **Vitamin A** | |
| Retinoic acid and ethanol | Chronic ethanol consumption induces cytochrome P450 (CYP)3A4 enzymes that increase retinoic acid degradation. |
| Isotretinoin (13-cis-retinoic acid) | Isotretinoin increases plasma total all-trans-retinoic acid concentration and may increase the risk of vitamin A toxicity. |
| Iron and zinc supplementation | Iron and zinc have the same absorption site, leading to competitive binding. Iron is required to mobilize vitamin A stores. Zinc is needed to synthesize retinol-binding protein, which is essential for vitamin A transport. |
| Orlistat | Orlistat reduces vitamin A absorption into the enterocyte in a dose-dependent manner. |
| **Vitamin D** | |
| Drugs that induce CYP3A4 enzymes (eg, phenytoin, carbamazepine, rifampin, dexamethasone) | These drugs increase the catabolism of calcidiol through the induction of CYP3A4. |
| **Vitamin E** | |
| Anticoagulants (eg, warfarin) | Vitamin E can have a potential antithrombotic effect at high doses (>1,000 IU) and may increase bleeding or bruising if taken concurrently with anticoagulant therapy. |

---

**BOX 5.2  Drug-Nutrient and Nutrient-Nutrient Interactions for Fat-Soluble Vitamins[44,45] (cont.)**

**Vitamin K**

| | |
|---|---|
| Warfarin | Warfarin antagonizes the activity of vitamin K. |
| Antibiotics | Antibiotics deplete vitamin K–producing intestinal microbes and may inhibit vitamin K mechanisms. |

**All fat-soluble vitamins**

| | |
|---|---|
| Bile acid sequestrants (eg, cholestyramine, colestipol) | These drugs prevent the reabsorption of bile salts and thus deplete bile salt pools, leading to increased risk of fat malabsorption. |

---

# Treatment, Monitoring, and Evaluation

Box 5.3 on page 82 summarizes the various treatment forms and regimens for addressing abnormalities in fat-soluble vitamin status.[44-47] Box 5.4 on page 85 provides the appropriate monitoring and evaluation plans associated with each micronutrient deficiency.[48-51] Because there is heterogeneity among the many published dosing strategies, these suggestions do not preclude the use of clinical judgment by health care providers.

> **BOX 5.3  Available Treatment Forms and Suggested Regimens for Treating Fat-Soluble Vitamin Deficiencies[44-47]**

## Vitamin A

### Treatment forms

| | |
|---|---|
| Oral | Various salt forms, ranging from preformed vitamin A (commonly as retinol esters [eg, retinyl acetate and retinyl palmitate], beta carotene, or a combination of both) to tablets and capsules in strengths ranging from 1,000-50,000 IU (300-15,000 mcg retinol activity equivalents [RAE]) |
| Injection | Solution of water-miscible vitamin A palmitate for intramuscular (IM) use (50,000 IU/mL or 15,000 mcg RAE/mL) (prescription product) |

### Treatment regimens[a,b]

*Hypovitaminosis A (in patients aged 8 years and older)*

| | |
|---|---|
| By mouth (PO) | 100,000 IU/d (30,000 mcg RAE/d) for 3 days, followed by 50,000 IU/d (15,000 mcg RAE/d) for 2 weeks |
| | Follow-up therapy: 10,000-20,000 IU/d (3,000–6,000 mcg RAE/d) for 2 months |
| IM injection | 100,000 IU/d (30,000 mcg RAE/d) for 3 days, followed by 50,000 IU/d (15,000 mcg RAE/d), IM (or PO), for 2 weeks |
| | Follow-up therapy: 10,000 to 20,000 IU/d (3,000–6,000 mcg RAE/d), PO, for 2 months |

*Xerophthalmia (in patients aged 1 year and older):*

200,000 IU (60,000 mcg RAE), PO, for 1 dose; repeat the next day and again in 2 to 3 weeks for total of 3 doses

*Night blindness or Bitot spots in females of reproductive age*

5,000 to 10,000 IU/d (1,500–3,000 mcg RAE/d), PO; 10,000 IU/d (3,000 RAE/d) maximum or 25,000 IU (7,500 mcg RAE) once weekly for no more than 4 weeks

*Malabsorption (eg, cholestasis, biliary atresia)*

5,000-15,000 IU/d (1,500-4,500 mcg RAE/d), PO, using water-miscible product

**BOX 5.3   Available Treatment Forms and Suggested Regimens for Treating Fat-Soluble Vitamin Deficiencies[44-47](cont.)**

## Vitamin D

### Treatment forms

| | |
|---|---|
| Oral | Ergocalciferol (vitamin D2) and cholecalciferol (vitamin D3) as tablets, capsules, or solutions of various strengths over the counter (OTC) |
| | Ergocalciferol, 1,250 mcg (50,000 IU) (prescription product) |
| Injection[c] | Not available (neither cholecalciferol nor ergocalciferol) as a standalone injectable product in the United States. Replacement therapy should be via the oral route. |

### Treatment regimens[a]

*Hypovitaminosis D (in adults)*

1,250 mcg (50,000 IU) once weekly for 8 to 12 weeks. For every 25 mcg (1,000 IU) increase in oral vitamin D intake, the corresponding increase in plasma 25-hydroxyvitamin D is estimated to be ~7 ng/mL in 3 to 4 months.

Increase daily maintenance dose for patients with malabsorption, intestinal resection, Roux-en-Y gastric bypass, obesity, or concurrent use of cytochrome P450 (CYP3A4) enzyme–inducing drugs to prevent redeveloping deficiency. As much as 150 to 250 mcg/d (6,000-10,000 IU/d) may be required. Closely monitor 25-hydroxyvitamin D concentrations.

## Vitamin E

### Treatment forms

| | |
|---|---|
| Oral | Available OTC in many forms, including RRR-▢-tocopherol, dl-▢-tocopherol, tocotrienol, and tocopherol polyethylene glycol succinate (a water-soluble form) |
| Injection | Not available as a standalone parenteral product in the United States, except as part of an injectable multiple-vitamin complex |

### Treatment regimens[a]

*Hypovitaminosis E*

15-25 IU per kilogram of body weight daily for documented clinical deficiency. Dose requirements are higher in patients with fat malabsorption, chronic pancreatitis, cholestatic hepatobiliary diseases, or intestinal resection.

*Deficiencies in Fat-Soluble Vitamins*

*Continued on next page*

---

**BOX 5.3  Available Treatment Forms and Suggested Regimens for Treating Fat-Soluble Vitamin Deficiencies[44-47] (cont.)**

## Vitamin K

### Treatment forms

Oral        Available OTC in many forms as phylloquinone, phytonadione, menaquinone-4, menaquinone-7

               Phytonadione is the only available prescription form in the United States

Injection     Phytonadione solution

               IM: Not recommended because of the risk of hematoma

               Subcutaneous (SC): An acceptable approach, although absorption may vary

               Intravenous (IV): Dilute dose in a minimum of 50 mL of a compatible IV solution; administer slowly using an infusion pump over 10 to 20 min. Infusion rate should not exceed 1 mg/min.

### Treatment regimens[a]

*Prevention of hypovitaminosis K*

    Typical regimen: up to 1 mg/d, PO, or 5 mg once weekly

*Hypovitaminosis K*

    1 to 5 mg/d, SC or PO

    10 mg once, IV

    In patients with severe malabsorption or who are unable to take oral medications, consider SC and IV administration.

---

[a] Based on published literature; not all regimens are approved by the US Food and Drug Administration.

[b] Contraceptive measures are necessary during vitamin A repletion in females of reproductive age. Careful monitoring of vitamin A concentrations is needed if repletion is occurring during pregnancy, especially in the first trimester.

[c] Calcitriol is available as an injectable product, as well as an oral capsule and solution, but calcitriol is not used to treat vitamin D deficiency. Its primary indications include secondary hyperparathyroidism in patients with chronic kidney disease, or hypocalcemia associated with hypoparathyroidism or pseudohypoparathyroidism.

**BOX 5.4  Recommendations for Monitoring Fat-Soluble Vitamin Deficiencies[48-51]**

## Vitamin A

### Monitoring recommendations

The target retinol concentration is 30 mcg/dL or higher.

Recheck serum retinol concentration every 3 months until vitamin A status normalizes.

In patients with elevated C-reactive protein (CRP) levels at initial assessment, recheck CRP at the time of serum retinol recheck.

In patients with iron-deficiency anemia at initial assessment or who are being treated for anemia, redo iron studies and do a complete blood count (CBC) at the time of serum retinol recheck.

In patients with zinc deficiency at initial assessment, recheck serum or plasma zinc values at the time of serum retinol recheck.

Corneal lesions may resolve in 2 weeks with high doses of vitamin A. Bitot spots may resolve within 4 weeks with lower doses.

### Other considerations

Dosing is in retinol activity equivalents (RAE) or mcg (1:1).

Patients should take oral supplements with food to improve bioavailability.

Recommend a water-miscible formulation in patients with fat malabsorption (eg, chronic pancreatitis, cholecystectomy).

Enteral nutrition dosing is similar to oral dosing.

## Vitamin D

### Monitoring recommendations

The target total plasma 25-hydroxyvitamin D concentration is 20 ng/mL or higher.

If 1,250 mcg (50,000 IU) once weekly does not substantially increase plasma 25-hydroxyvitamin D concentration, consider increasing the regimen to 1,250 mcg (50,000 IU) twice or three times weekly for 8 weeks.

Recheck 25-hydroxyvitamin D concentration every 3 months until normalization of vitamin D status.

In patients with an elevated CRP level at initial assessment, recheck CRP at the time of serum 25-hydroxyvitamin D recheck.

*Continued on next page*

*Deficiencies in Fat-Soluble Vitamins*

## BOX 5.4 Recommendations for Monitoring Fat-Soluble Vitamin Deficiencies[48-51] (cont.)

### Vitamin D (cont.)

#### Other considerations

Patients should take oral supplements with food to improve bioavailability.

The dose requirement is increased in patients with small bowel resection or cholecystectomy because they may have decreased absorption.

A single dose of more than 1,250 mcg (>50,000 IU) is not recommended, as it may be associated with increased fall risk in older adults.

Calcitriol is primarily used in patients with chronic kidney disease to prevent metabolic bone disease.

### Vitamin E

#### Monitoring recommendations

Repletion of 100 mg/d is necessary when ⍺-tocopherol concentrations are less than 5 mcg/mL or the ratio of ⍺-tocopherol (g) to lipids (g) is less than 0.8.

#### Other considerations

Patients should take oral supplements with food to improve bioavailability.

Tocopherol polyethylene glycol succinate is an inhibitor of intestinal P-glycoprotein, which can cause major drug interactions. Use with caution.

### Vitamin K

#### Monitoring recommendations

With vitamin K treatment, prothrombin time should normalize in patients with a confirmed deficiency.

#### Other considerations

Only 30% to 40% of an oral dose is retained and will have a maximum impact on serum concentrations after 24 hours.

# References

1. Food and Nutrition Board, Institute of Medicine. *Dietary Reference Intakes for Thiamin, Riboflavin, Niacin, Vitamin B6, Folate, Vitamin B12, Pantothenic Acid, Biotin, and Choline.* National Academies Press; 1998.

2. Food and Nutrition Board, Institute of Medicine. *Dietary Reference Intakes for Vitamin C, Vitamin E, Selenium, and Carotenoids.* National Academies Press; 2000.

3. Food and Nutrition Board, Institute of Medicine. *Dietary Reference Intakes for Calcium and Vitamin D.* National Academies Press; 2011.

4. Zhang Y, Zhang T, Liang Y, Jiang L, Sui X. Dietary bioactive lipids: a review on absorption, metabolism, and health properties. *J Agric Food Chem.* 2021;69(32):8929-8943. doi:10.1021/acs.jafc.1c01369

5. Tanumihardjo SA, Russell RM, Stephensen CB, et al. Biomarkers of Nutrition for Development (BOND)—vitamin A review. *J Nutr.* 2016;146(9):1816S-1848S. doi:10.3945/jn.115.229708

6. Nosewicz J, Sparks A, Hart PA, et al. The evaluation and management of macronutrient deficiency dermatoses. *J Am Acad Dermatol.* 2022;87(3):640-647. doi:10.1016/j.jaad.2022.04.007

7. Berger MM, Shenkin A, Schweinlin A, et al. ESPEN micronutrient guideline. *Clin Nutr.* 2022;41(6):1357-1424. doi:10.1016/j.clnu.2022.02.015

8. Arvanitakis M, Ockenga J, Bezmarevic M, et al. ESPEN guideline on clinical nutrition in acute and chronic pancreatitis. *Clin Nutr.* 2020;39(3):612-631. doi:10.1016/j.clnu.2020.01.004

9. Bischoff SC, Escher J, Hébuterne X, et al. ESPEN practical guideline: clinical nutrition in inflammatory bowel disease. *Clin Nutr.* 2020;39(3):632-653. doi:10.1016/j.clnu.2019.11.002

10. Rubio-Tapia A, Hill ID, Kelly CP, Calderwood AH, Murray JA; American College of Gastroenterology. ACG clinical guidelines: diagnosis and management of celiac disease. *Am J Gastroenterol.* 2013;108(5):656-677. doi:10.1038/ajg.2013.79

11. Turck D, Braegger CP, Colombo C, et al. ESPEN-ESPGHAN-ECFS guidelines on nutrition care for infants, children, and adults with cystic fibrosis. *Clin Nutr.* 2016;35(3):557-577. doi:10.1016/j.clnu.2016.03.004

12. Alia E, Kerr PE. Vitamin D: skin, sunshine, and beyond. *Clin Dermatol.* 2021;39(5):840-846. doi:10.1016/j.clindermatol.2021.05.025

13. Jaworeck S, Kriwy P. It's sunny, be healthy? An international comparison of the influence of sun exposure and latitude lines on self-rated health. *Int J Environ Res Public Health.* 2021;18(8):4101. doi:10.3390/ijerph18084101

14.  Vitamin A and carotenoids: fact sheet for health professionals. Office of Dietary Supplements, National Institutes of Health. Updated June 15, 2022. Accessed July 5, 2023. https://ods.od.nih.gov/factsheets/VitaminA -HealthProfessional

15.  Food labeling: revision of the Nutrition and Supplement Facts labels. Final rule. *Fed Regist*. 2016;81(103):33741-33999.

16.  Maronn M, Allen DM, Esterly NB. Phrynoderma: a manifestation of vitamin A deficiency? . . . The rest of the story. *Pediatr Dermatol*. 2005;22(1):60-63. doi:10.1111/j.1525-1470.2005.22113.x

17.  Ross DA. Recommendations for vitamin A supplementation. *J Nutr*. 2002;132(9 suppl):2902S-2906S. doi:10.1093/jn/132.9.2902S

18.  Sheftel J, Tanumihardjo SA. Systematic review and meta-analysis of the relative dose-response tests to assess vitamin A status. *Adv Nutr*. 2021;12(3):904-941. doi:10.1093/advances/nmaa136

19.  Vitamin D: fact sheet for health professionals. Office of Dietary Supplements, National Institutes of Health. Updated August 12, 2022. Accessed July 5, 2023. https://ods.od.nih.gov/factsheets/VitaminD -HealthProfessional

20.  Kamboj P, Dwivedi S, Toteja GS. Prevalence of hypovitaminosis D in India and way forward. *Indian J Med Res*. 2018;148(5):548-556. doi:10.4103 /ijmr.IJMR_1807_18

21.  Hajhashemy Z, Shahdadian F, Ziaei R, Saneei P. Serum vitamin D levels in relation to abdominal obesity: a systematic review and dose-response meta-analysis of epidemiologic studies. *Obes Rev*. 2021;22(2):e13134. doi:10.1111/obr.13134

22.  Carrelli A, Bucovsky M, Horst R, et al. Vitamin D storage in adipose tissue of obese and normal weight women. *J Bone Miner Res*. 2017;32(2):237-242. doi:10.1002/jbmr.2979

23.  Holick MF. Vitamin D status: measurement, interpretation, and clinical application. *Ann Epidemiol*. 2009;19(2):73-78. doi:10.1016/j.annepidem .2007.12.001

24.  Ikizler TA, Burrowes JD, Byham-Gray LD, et al. KDOQI clinical practice guideline for nutrition in CKD: 2020 update. *Am J Kidney Dis*. 2020;76 (3 suppl 1):S1-S107. doi:10.1053/j.ajkd.2020.05.006

25.  Vitamin E: fact sheet for health professionals. Office of Dietary Supplements, National Institutes of Health. Updated March 26, 2021. Accessed July 5, 2023. https://ods.od.nih.gov/factsheets/VitaminE -HealthProfessional

26.  Traber MG, Jialal I. Measurement of lipid-soluble vitamins—further adjustment needed? *Lancet*. 2000;355(9220):2013-2014. doi:10.1016 /S0140-6736(00)02345-X

27. Food and Nutrition Board, Institute of Medicine. *Dietary Reference Intakes for Vitamin C, Vitamin E, Selenium, and Carotenoids.* National Academies Press; 2000.

28. Jayaram S, Soman A, Tarvade S, Londhe V. Cerebellar ataxia due to isolated vitamin E deficiency. *Indian J Med Sci.* 2005;59(1):20-23.

29. Satya-Murti S, Howard L, Krohel G, Wolf B. The spectrum of neurologic disorder from vitamin E deficiency. *Neurology.* 1986;36(7):917-921. doi:10.1212/wnl.36.7.917

30. Sanyal AJ, Chalasani N, Kowdley KV, et al. Pioglitazone, vitamin E, or placebo for nonalcoholic steatohepatitis. *N Engl J Med.* 2010;362(18):1675-1685. doi:10.1056/NEJMoa0907929

31. Sheka AC, Adeyi O, Thompson J, Hameed B, Crawford PA, Ikramuddin S. Nonalcoholic steatohepatitis: a review. *JAMA.* 2020;323(12):1175-1183. doi:10.1001/jama.2020.2298

32. Abner EL, Schmitt FA, Mendiondo MS, Marcum JL, Kryscio RJ. Vitamin E and all-cause mortality: a meta-analysis. *Curr Aging Sci.* 2011;4(2):158-170. doi:10.2174/1874609811104020158

33. Ballon-Landa E, Parsons JK. Nutrition, physical activity, and lifestyle factors in prostate cancer prevention. *Curr Opin Urol.* 2018;28(1):55-61. doi:10.1097/MOU.0000000000000460

34. Schürks M, Glynn RJ, Rist PM, Tzourio C, Kurth T. Effects of vitamin E on stroke subtypes: meta-analysis of randomised controlled trials. *BMJ.* 2010;341:c5702. doi:10.1136/bmj.c5702

35. Vitamin K: fact sheet for health professionals. Office of Dietary Supplements, National Institutes of Health. Updated March 29, 2021. Accessed July 5, 2023. https://ods.od.nih.gov/factsheets/VitaminK-HealthProfessional/

36. Azharuddin MK, O'Reilly DS, Gray A, Talwar D. HPLC method for plasma vitamin K1: effect of plasma triglyceride and acute-phase response on circulating concentrations. *Clin Chem.* 2007;53(9):1706-1713. doi:10.1373/clinchem.2007.086280

37. Barrett H, O'Keeffe M, Kavanagh E, Walsh M, O'Connor EM. Is matrix Gla protein associated with vascular calcification? A systematic review. *Nutrients.* 2018;10(4):415. doi:10.3390/nu10040415

38. Schurgers LJ, Cranenburg EC, Vermeer C. Matrix Gla-protein: the calcification inhibitor in need of vitamin K. *Thromb Haemost.* 2008;100(4):593-603.

39. Zhang Y, Bala V, Mao Z, Chhonker YS, Murry DJ. A concise review of quantification methods for determination of vitamin K in various biological matrices. *J Pharm Biomed Anal.* 2019;169:133-141. doi:10.1016/j.jpba.2019.03.006

40.  Nosewicz J, Spaccarelli N, Roberts KM, et al. The epidemiology, impact, and diagnosis of micronutrient nutritional dermatoses part 1: zinc, selenium, copper, vitamin A, and vitamin C. *J Am Acad Dermatol*. 2022;86(2):267-278. doi:10.1016/j.jaad.2021.07.079

41.  Zimmerman L, McKeon B. Osteomalacia. In: *StatPearls (online)*. StatPearls Publishing; 2022. NCBI Bookshelf. Accessed December 13, 2023. www.ncbi.nlm.nih.gov/books/NBK551616

42.  Horwitt MK, Harvey CC, Dahm CH Jr, Searcy MT. Relationship between tocopherol and serum lipid levels for determination of nutritional adequacy. *Ann N Y Acad Sci*. 1972;203:223-236. doi:10.1111/j.1749-6632 .1972.tb27878.x

43.  Thurnham DI, Davies JA, Crump BJ, Situnayake RD, Davis M. The use of different lipids to express serum tocopherol: lipid ratios for the measurement of vitamin E status. *Ann Clin Biochem*. 1986;23(pt 5):514-520. doi:10.1177/000456328602300505

44.  Micromedex (database). Merative. 2023. Accessed July 5, 2023. www.micromedexsolutions.com

45.  Facts and Comparisons: drug referential resource. Wolters Kluwer. 2023. Accessed July 5, 2023. www.wolterskluwer.com/en/solutions/lexicomp /facts-and-comparisons

46.  Drugs@FDA: FDA-approved drugs. US Food and Drug Administration. Accessed July 5, 2023. www.accessdata.fda.gov/scripts/cder/daf/index.cfm

47.  DailyMed. National Library of Medicine. Accessed July 5, 2023. www.dailymed.nlm.nih.gov/dailymed/index.cfm

48.  Pazirandeh S, Burns D. Overview of vitamin A. UpToDate. August 22, 2022. Accessed July 6, 2023. www.uptodate.com/contents/overview-of -vitamin-a

49.  Dawson-Hughes B. Vitamin D deficiency in adults: definition, clinical manifestations, and treatment. UpToDate. May 23, 2023. Accessed July 6, 2023. www.uptodate.com/contents/vitamin-d-deficiency-in-adults -definition-clinical-manifestations-and-treatment

50.  Pazirandeh S, Burns D. Overview of vitamin E. UpToDate. July 12, 2022. Accessed July 6, 2023. www.uptodate.com/contents/overview-of -vitamin-e

51.  Pazirandeh S, Burns D. Overview of vitamin K. UpToDate. March 16, 2023. Accessed July 6, 2023. www.uptodate.com/contents/overview-of -vitamin-k

# Deficiencies in Water-Soluble Vitamins

Holly Estes-Doetsch, MS, RDN, LD, and
Lingtak-Neander Chan, PharmD, BCNSP, FCCP, FASPEN

## Introduction

The nine water-soluble vitamins—eight B vitamins plus vitamin C—are listed in Box 6.1 on page 92. Water-soluble vitamins (with the exception of vitamin B12) are absorbed primarily via the duodenum or proximal jejunum enterocytes. Whereas hepatic storage of vitamin B12 may delay deficiency for several years, the storage capacity for other water-soluble vitamins is limited, and these undergo renal excretion with excessive intake.[1] For some water-soluble vitamins, such as thiamin, depletion may occur in as little as 3 to 4 weeks if physiological requirements are not met.[1,2] The biological roles of the B vitamins are vast, but many serve as cofactors or coenzymes for metabolic reactions, play roles in the synthesis of neurotransmitters and nucleic acids, combat oxidative stress, and support erythropoiesis. The Dietary Reference Intakes (DRIs) for the water-soluble vitamins are listed in Table 6.1 on page 94.[3] Food sources can be found in the Appendix.

*Deficiencies Water-Soluble Vitamins*

> **BOX 6.1  Water-Soluble Vitamins**
>
> Thiamin (vitamin B1)
> Riboflavin (vitamin B2)
> Niacin (vitamin B3; nicotinic acid)
> Pantothenic acid (vitamin B5)
> Vitamin B6 (pyridoxine, pyridoxal, pyridoxamine)
> Biotin (vitamin B7)
> Folate (vitamin B9)
> Vitamin B12 (cobalamin)
> Vitamin C (ascorbic acid)

# Pathophysiology of Deficiencies

Several of the B vitamins—namely riboflavin, niacin, pantothenic acid, vitamin B6, and biotin—rarely develop into isolated deficiencies, but deficiencies in these vitamins may occur in conjunction with other deficiencies. Isolated deficiencies are most likely to occur in patients with inborn errors of metabolism, which affect the body's utilization of certain nutrients. Aside from poor dietary intake of water-soluble vitamins, other risk factors for concurrent deficiencies are excessive nutrient losses via wounds, the gastrointestinal tract, urinary system, or renal replacement therapy. In addition, chronic alcohol consumption can affect water-soluble vitamin status by (1) impairing absorption, (2) altering metabolism if liver cirrhosis is present, or (3) compromising dietary intake if alcohol is replacing foods in the diet.[4] Many drug-nutrient interactions may also cause altered absorption or metabolism of water-soluble vitamins, and ultimately deficiency, and are reviewed in this chapter.

# Overview of Physical and Biochemical Assessments

Patients with suspected water-soluble vitamin deficiency should have their hair, eyes, lips, oral cavity, skin, and nails examined for the following signs:

- neurological manifestations (eg, polyneuropathy, numbness, ataxia, loss of gait abnormality, paresthesia, and new-onset memory loss), which may be particularly associated with thiamin, folate, and vitamin B12 deficiencies

- hair loss and brittle nails, which may be related to biotin deficiency[5]

- pallor of the skin and conjunctiva, which may present with folate, vitamin B6, or vitamin B12 depletion if anemia is present

- seborrheic dermatitis, which has been reported in severe cases of riboflavin, vitamin B6, and biotin deficiency[5]

- pellagrous dermatitis (characterized by inflamed, hyperpigmented patches of sun-exposed skin), which is consistent with niacin deficiency[5,6]

The biochemical assessment of water-soluble vitamin status can be challenging, as serum levels often reflect recent dietary intake but not tissue stores. Although inflammation does not seem to influence serum or plasma concentrations of many water-soluble vitamins, there is evidence that transient decreases in serum or plasma riboflavin, vitamin B6, and vitamin C levels can occur (see Chapter 4).[7] Vitamins B6 and C appear to be particularly sensitive to changes in inflammation.[8]

# Thiamin

Thiamin supports the structure and function of the central nervous system and serves as a cofactor for enzymatic reactions in glycolysis, the Krebs cycle, and the pentose phosphate pathway.[2,9] Depletion causes metabolic alterations, impairing production of adenosine triphosphate and possibly leading to acute acidemia as a result of lactic acidosis and

TABLE 6.1 Dietary Reference Intakes for Water-Soluble Vitamins[3]

| Population | Thiamin[a] (mg/d) | Riboflavin[a] (mg/d) | Niacin[a] (mg/d) | Pantothenic acid[b] (mg/d) | Vitamin B6[a] (mg/d) | Biotin[b] (mcg/d) | Folate[a] (mcg/d) | Vitamin B12[a] (mcg/d) | Vitamin C[a,c] (mg/d) |
|---|---|---|---|---|---|---|---|---|---|
| *Males* | | | | | | | | | |
| 9-13y | 0.9 | 0.9 | 12 | 4 | 1.0 | 20 | 300 | 1.8 | 45 |
| 14-18y | 1.2 | 1.3 | 16 | 5 | 1.3 | 25 | 400 | 2.4 | 75 |
| 19-30y | 1.2 | 1.3 | 16 | 5 | 1.3 | 30 | 400 | 2.4 | 90 |
| 31-50y | 1.2 | 1.3 | 16 | 5 | 1.3 | 30 | 400 | 2.4 | 90 |
| 51-70y | 1.2 | 1.3 | 16 | 5 | 1.7 | 30 | 400 | 2.4 | 90 |
| >70y | 1.2 | 1.3 | 16 | 5 | 1.7 | 30 | 400 | 2.4 | 90 |
| *Females* | | | | | | | | | |
| 9-13y | 0.9 | 0.9 | 12 | 4 | 1.0 | 20 | 300 | 1.8 | 45 |
| 14-18y | 1.0 | 1.0 | 14 | 5 | 1.2 | 25 | 400 | 2.4 | 65 |
| 19-30y | 1.1 | 1.1 | 14 | 5 | 1.3 | 30 | 400 | 2.4 | 75 |
| 31-50y | 1.1 | 1.1 | 14 | 5 | 1.3 | 30 | 400 | 2.4 | 75 |
| 51-70y | 1.1 | 1.1 | 14 | 5 | 1.5 | 30 | 400 | 2.4 | 75 |
| >70y | 1.1 | 1.1 | 14 | 5 | 1.5 | 30 | 400 | 2.4 | 75 |

**Pregnant**

| | | | | | | | | | |
|---|---|---|---|---|---|---|---|---|---|
| ≤18y | 1.4 | 1.4 | 18 | 6 | 1.9 | 30 | 600 | 2.6 | 80 |
| 19-30y | 1.4 | 1.4 | 18 | 6 | 1.9 | 30 | 600 | 2.6 | 85 |
| 31-50y | 1.4 | 1.4 | 18 | 6 | 1.9 | 30 | 600 | 2.6 | 85 |

**Lactating**

| | | | | | | | | | |
|---|---|---|---|---|---|---|---|---|---|
| ≤18y | 1.4 | 1.6 | 17 | 7 | 2.0 | 35 | 500 | 2.8 | 115 |
| 19-30y | 1.4 | 1.6 | 17 | 7 | 2.0 | 35 | 500 | 2.8 | 120 |
| 31-50y | 1.4 | 1.6 | 17 | 7 | 2.0 | 35 | 500 | 2.8 | 120 |

[a] Recommended Dietary Allowance
[b] Adequate Intake
[a] Vitamin C requirements are 35 mg higher for individuals who smoke.

increased oxidative stress, which affects the brain and nervous system.[10] Thiamin deficiency may present as deficits in neurocognition, peripheral neuropathy, and muscle weakness—or "dry beriberi."[9] Wernicke encephalopathy is a severe form of dry beriberi, which is characterized by a triad of ocular motility abnormalities, ataxia, and confusion, though all three symptoms may not present concurrently.[10] If not treated promptly, Wernicke encephalopathy can progress to Korsakoff syndrome, a complication associated with memory loss and psychosis, and is less likely to be reversible with thiamin repletion.[11]

Nearly 50% of total body thiamin is found in cardiac tissue[2]; therefore, deficiency can also present as "wet beriberi," or high-output cardiac failure.[2,9] In patients who already have a history of heart failure, thiamin deficiency may worsen their clinical status.[12] However, more research is needed to examine the association between thiamin status and clinical outcomes in patients with heart failure.

## Screening and Assessment

Multiple factors may precede the development of thiamin deficiency, including alcohol-use disorders, malnutrition, peritoneal dialysis, hemodialysis, and impaired absorption from the gastrointestinal tract. Inadequate dietary intake, increased metabolic demand, and nutrient losses in cases of hyperemesis gravidarum increase the risk for thiamin deficiency during pregnancy.[10] Acute deficiency symptoms may develop in malnourished individuals in response to refeeding, because of the rapid increases in thiamin utilization for aerobic glycolysis.[18] Disruptions in energy availability resulting from thiamin deficiency may also affect other organ systems, including the respiratory system, the gastrointestinal tract, and accessory organs. Because of the varying severity and (sometimes) overlap of symptoms from different forms of thiamin deficiency, the term *thiamin deficiency disorders* has also been used in the literature.[10]

Erythrocyte transketolase activity and thiamin pyrophosphate levels are sensitive and specific indicators of thiamin status, though testing may be costly, not as readily available to clinicians, and take several days for results to process.[2,9] Because of the barriers clinicians face in obtaining laboratory indexes of thiamin status, prophylactic supplementation is reasonable in patients deemed to be at high risk for deficiency, and empirical treatment should be initiated in patients with clinical symptoms. This is routine practice in patients at risk for or showing signs of refeeding syndrome.[14] If erythrocyte transketolase activity or thiamin pyrophosphate is being assessed, practitioners should obtain blood samples to get an accurate picture of baseline thiamin status before initiating vitamin supplementation. Laboratory results should serve as a diagnostic confirmation to guide further management. Thiamin toxicity is unlikely, even at high supplement doses, and a tolerable upper limit has not been set for thiamin.[12] Delayed diagnosis or misdiagnosis of thiamin deficiency is a concern, as clinical symptoms may mimic those of other medical diagnoses.[10] Thus, empirical thiamin supplementation may be appropriate for individuals exhibiting clinical symptoms and who have known risk factors for deficiency when laboratory assessment is not practical or timely.

# Riboflavin

Riboflavin plays numerous metabolic roles, as its cofactors catalyze enzymatic reactions and transfer electrons throughout aerobic energy pathways.[15] Riboflavin-derived cofactors also promote iron utilization and conversion of vitamin B6 to its active form.[16,17] Hence, anemia resulting from iron or vitamin B6 deficiencies may be more effectively treated by adding riboflavin to the repletion regimen in cases when concurrent deficiencies are likely to exist. This finding has been supported in iron supplementation trials,[15,16] but trials involving vitamin B6 are lacking. Because glutathione reductase (GR) requires a riboflavin cofactor to reduce glutathione, which allows glutathione to function as an antioxidant, riboflavin deficiency may lead to increased oxidative stress, though further research is needed.[15]

## Screening and Assessment

Risk factors for riboflavin deficiency are similar to other water-soluble vitamin deficiencies, but consumption of dairy or meat-free diets pose an additional risk as these are key dietary sources of riboflavin (see Appendix).[15,17]

Laboratory assessment of functional riboflavin deficiency is determined by the erythrocyte GR activation coefficient, which is obtained by calculating the ratio of stimulated enzyme activity—from addition of the cofactor flavin adenine dinucleotide (FAD) to GR in vitro—to the unstimulated enzyme activity.[17] Although this has been used as a biomarker of riboflavin deficiency in population studies, it may not be available in many practice settings. Erythrocyte FAD, which research has shown to be a better measure of riboflavin status compared to plasma riboflavin and does not seem to be influenced by inflammation, may be an alternative approach.[18,19]

# Niacin

Like several other B vitamins, niacin serves as a precursor for coenzymes involved in metabolic pathways, including nicotinamide adenine dinucleotide (NAD) and nicotinamide adenine dinucleotide phosphate (NADP).

## Screening and Assessment

Aside from poor dietary intake and excessive urinary or gastrointestinal excretion, several other factors may be linked to niacin deficiency. Taking immunosuppressive and antituberculosis medications may interfere with niacin metabolism, thus increasing the risk for deficiency.[20] Hartnup disease, a disorder affecting tryptophan metabolism, may contribute to niacin deficiency, as physiological niacin requirements are met through a combination of dietary niacin intake and endogenous synthesis from tryptophan.[21] Pellagra, a disease characterized by the "three Ds"—dermatitis, diarrhea, and dementia—is also associated with niacin deficiency.[20] A 24-hour urine N1-methylnicotinamide level or ratio of whole blood NAD to NADP may be used as a laboratory marker of poor niacin status, but most often deficiency is diagnosed based on clinical presentation.[20]

# Vitamin B6, Vitamin B12, and Folate

Vitamin B6, vitamin B12, and folate are all necessary for the metabolism of homocysteine (refer to Figure 6.1).[22,23] Altered homocysteine metabolism that leads to elevated plasma levels of homocysteine plays a role in the pathogenesis of cancers, neurological disease, bone demineralization, and cardiovascular and cerebrovascular diseases.[24] Although elevated homocysteine levels may be a functional marker of deficiency, additional laboratory assessment is often required to determine whether one or multiple micronutrients are depleted and contributing to hyperhomocysteinemia. Nondietary factors may be associated with elevated homocysteine, including enzymatic defects, thyroid disorders, chronic renal failure, and the use of certain medications.[25]

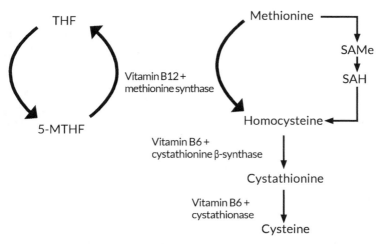

FIGURE 6.1 Utilization of vitamin B6, vitamin B12, and folate in homocysteine metabolism[22,23]

Abbreviations: 5-MTHF, 5-methyltetrahydrofolate; SAH, S-adenosylhomocysteine; SAMe, S-adenosylmethionine; THF, tetrahydrofolate.

# Vitamin B6

The main tissue form of vitamin B6, pyridoxal 5⬚-phosphate (PLP), supports more than 100 metabolic processes, including the synthesis of glycogen, proteins, lipids, hemoglobin, and neurotransmitters.[26] It is also essential for homocysteine catabolism by facilitating the conversion of homocysteine to cysteine.[27,28] Several medications may interfere with vitamin B6 absorption or metabolism including isoniazid, hydralazine, and combination levodopa and carbidopa.[29] In patients receiving levodopa-carbidopa, deficiency risk appears to increase as medication dose increases,[30] as well as when the medication is administered as an intestinal gel infusion.[28] Prophylactic monthly courses of vitamin B6 therapy four to six times per year have been suggested for patients with preexisting peripheral neuropathy or advanced Parkinson disease who are also receiving levodopa-carbidopa intestinal gel.[28]

## Screening and Assessment

Peripheral neuropathy, microcytic anemia, and, less frequently, seizures have been shown to develop in relation to vitamin B6 deficiency.[28,29,31] The possibility of vitamin B6 deficiency should be considered in cases of seizures refractory to antiepileptic therapy, particularly when risk factors for deficiency are present.[31] The onset of neurological symptoms of deficiency tend to be gradual, appearing after several years.[30]

Plasma PLP and 4-pyridoxine acid are most often used clinically to assess biochemical status of vitamin B6 as they reflect liver stores.[26,28] An enzyme-linked immunosorbent assay that directly measures plasma or tissue vitamin B6 concentration is also available.

# Vitamin B12

Vitamin B12 deficiency is the leading cause of macrocytic megaloblastic anemia.[32] Neurologic dysfunction, manifested by ataxia and paresthesia, has also been associated with vitamin B12 deficiency. Natural dietary sources of vitamin B12 are protein-bound and must be released by gastric acid and pepsin in the stomach during digestion. Secretion of intrinsic factor by gastric parietal cells is also required. Vitamin B12 binds to intrinsic factor in the duodenum and is ultimately absorbed via ileal enterocytes.

## Screening and Assessment

Routine vitamin B12 screening is recommended for patients at high risk for deficiency, including those with a history of bariatric surgery (Chapter 14), Crohn's disease with ileal involvement or terminal ileal resection (Chapter 9), or impaired production of intrinsic factor due to gastrectomy or autoimmune process. The American Diabetes Association recommends periodic screening for vitamin B12 deficiency with long-term use of metformin, as deficiency may exacerbate neuropathy.[33] Use of acid-suppressant medications, particularly proton pump inhibitors, could increase risk for deficiency; however, research is conflicting. In theory, small intestinal bacterial overgrowth (SIBO) may be another risk factor for deficiency, as bacteria can interfere with the absorption of vitamin B12.[34] Factors associated with inadequate dietary intake of vitamin B12, such as following a vegan diet, alcoholism, and older age, should also be considered.[33]

It may take several months for changes in red blood cell (RBC) count and characteristics of anemia to develop; thus, the absence of anemia does not exclude the presence of vitamin B12 deficiency.[35] In addition, concurrent iron deficiency may conceal any expected macrocytosis.[36] Therefore, screening for vitamin B12 deficiency, regardless of hematologic profile in high-risk patients, is warranted. A plasma or serum vitamin B12 level is commonly used as a biochemical measure of vitamin B12 status. However, it may not be adequate to identify short-term deficiency, as depletion of circulating vitamin B12 levels occurs gradually. Results may also be confounded by hepatic dysfunction, leading to falsely elevated vitamin B12 concentrations.[37] Because methylmalonate conversion to succinate is dependent on vitamin B12 adequacy, an elevated serum methylmalonic acid (MMA) level is a marker of functional vitamin B12 deficiency and is used to confirm depletion when the serum vitamin B12 level is low to normal (150–400 pg/mL).[33] However, MMA can also be elevated in response to excessive propionate production by gut bacteria in SIBO instead of vitamin B12 deficiency.[34,38] Case reports of SIBO in short bowel syndrome have described patients with normal serum vitamin B12, homocysteine, and hematologic indexes yet elevated MMA who did not respond to vitamin B12 supplementation[34,38]; MMA concentrations only normalized once the course of antibiotics used to treat SIBO was completed. Hyperhomocysteinemia may also be a marker of deficiency but is not specific to vitamin B12 (see sections on vitamin B6 and folate).

# Folate

Folate (or the synthetic form, folic acid) supports cellular processes such as DNA synthesis and serves as a coenzyme for numerous reactions involving transmethylation. To do the latter, folate must be converted to 5-methyltetrahydrofolate (5-MTHF). Folate deficiency can result from malabsorption or from alterations in utilization. For example, experts have recognized that there are increased demands for folate during pregnancy.[39] Folic acid supplementation in the preconception period and during pregnancy optimizes folate status and reduces the risk for neural tube defects. Antifolate medications used for oncology, rheumatoid arthritis, and psoriasis, such as methotrexate, interfere with the conversion of folate to its active form. Concurrent folic acid supplementation may prevent deficiency and hyperhomocysteinemia while decreasing the risk for drug-related side effects and hepatotoxicity.[40] Folate metabolism is dependent on adequacy of vitamin B12; thus, a secondary folate deficiency may also develop in response to vitamin B12 depletion.[36,41] In this situation, serum folate levels may potentially be elevated as 5-MTHF becomes "trapped," or unable to participate further in metabolic processes.[36,41]

## Screening and Assessment

As with vitamin B12 deficiency, macrocytic anemia may or may not be present under conditions of folate deficiency, due to the extent of depletion required to produce changes in erythropoiesis.[42] However, red cell macrocytosis should prompt assessment of folate status in at-risk individuals. Disagreement exists over what laboratory test should be applied to detect folate deficiency. An RBC folate test may reflect folate status over the previous 3 to 4 months and is less susceptible than serum folate testing to recent changes in dietary intake,[43] yet it is more costly, requires sample pretreatment, and takes more time to process compared to serum folate testing.[44] In conjunction with vitamin B12, 5-MTHF facilitates the conversion of homocysteine to methionine. When the serum folate level is low to normal, and obtaining an RBC folate level is not feasible, an elevated homocysteine level strengthens the likelihood that deficiency is present.[36,43]

# Vitamin C

Though relatively uncommon in developed countries, overt signs of vitamin C deficiency have been documented in patients who are critically ill, recovering from bariatric surgery, and receiving dialysis, in whom increased losses occur.[45] Chapters 13, 14, and 10, respectively, discuss these populations.

## Screening and Assessment

Individuals with poor diet quality, such as those with alcoholism or inadequate access to food, are also at risk for deficiency.[46,47] Tobacco use is more widely associated with lower vitamin C status than is nonuse[48,49]; the influence of oxidative stress on vitamin C metabolism is a proposed etiology, though more research is needed.[49] Consequently, the DRI for vitamin C is higher for tobacco users.[48,49] The practitioner should consider the patient's ability to meet increased vitamin C requirements through diet alone when determining the need for supplementation. Most published case reports of micronutrient deficiency in children with autism spectrum disorder involve vitamin C deficiency resulting from extreme food selectivity associated with lack of fruit and vegetable intake; however, it is unclear whether this persists into adulthood.[50] Supplementation is often routinely implemented in patients with wounds (Chapter 11) and burns (Chapter 15) because they have increased nutrient demands and because vitamin C has antioxidant properties. On the other hand, supplementation at extremely high doses (>3 g/d) presents concerns for the potential pro-oxidant effect of vitamin C, though studies are conflicting.[49]

Vitamin C deficiency manifests as scurvy.[6,51] Anemia also commonly co-occurs due to increased hemolysis, decreased absorption of dietary nonheme iron, or the presence of concurrent micronutrient deficiencies. Physical findings generally reflect altered collagen synthesis, as vitamin C serves as a cofactor for enzymatic reactions that support procollagen production. Considering its role in immune health, vitamin C depletion poses concern for increased susceptibility to infection and poor wound healing. Functional markers of deficiency are unknown. Plasma and leukocyte vitamin C levels serve as conventional measurement approaches. Leukocyte vitamin C levels are more representative of tissue stores, whereas plasma levels are influenced readily by recent dietary intake.

# Deficiency Assessment Strategies and Nutrient Interactions

Box 6.2 summarizes assessment strategies for determining water-soluble vitamin status.[1,6] Box 6.3 on page 109 lists drug-nutrient interactions involving the water-soluble vitamins.[2,31,52-59]

# Treatment, Monitoring, and Evaluation

Box 6.4 on page 111 provides an overview of the available formulations and dosing strategies for treating deficiencies in water-soluble vitamins.[52,60-62] Box 6.5 on page 116 provides monitoring and other considerations for each micronutrient deficiency.[52,60-62] Because there is heterogeneity among the many published dosing strategies, these suggestions do not preclude the use of clinical judgment by health care providers. Oral, parenteral, and intramuscular routes are options for many of the water-soluble vitamins. For more rapid repletion in individuals experiencing overt clinical effects, intravenous micronutrient delivery should be considered. Upper limits have been established for niacin, folate, vitamin B6, and vitamin C, and individuals receiving high doses of these products should be monitored for signs and symptoms of toxicity.[63]

**BOX 6.2 Assessment Strategies for Determining Water-Soluble Vitamin Status[1,6]**

### Thiamin

| | |
|---|---|
| Pertinent biochemical tests | Red blood cell (RBC) or whole blood thiamin pyrophosphate (direct) |
| | Erythrocyte transketolase (indirect) |
| Clinical assessment of deficiency | Ocular motility changes |
| | Peripheral neuropathy |
| | Ataxia |
| | Confusion, memory loss, psychosis |
| Special considerations | Cases of "wet beriberi" may present as high-output cardiac failure, lactic acidosis, or edema. |
| | Empirical treatment is appropriate when laboratory assessment is not feasible but risk factors (eg, alcohol use disorder, refeeding syndrome) and signs or symptoms are present. |

### Riboflavin

| | |
|---|---|
| Pertinent biochemical tests | Erythrocyte glutathione reductase activation coefficient |
| | Erythrocyte flavin adenine dinucleotide |
| Clinical assessment of deficiency | Oral cavity: cheilosis, angular stomatitis, magenta tongue |
| | Skin: seborrheic dermatitis |
| Special considerations | Assess C-reactive protein (CRP)[a] to rule out the influence of inflammation if a serum or plasma riboflavin level is obtained. |

### Niacin

| | |
|---|---|
| Pertinent biochemical tests | 24-hour urine N1-methylnicotinamide |
| | Ratio of whole blood or RBC nicotinamide adenine dinucleotide to nicotinamide adenine dinucleotide phosphate |

*Continued on next page*

---

**BOX 6.2** Assessment Strategies for Determining Water-Soluble Vitamin Status[1,6] (cont.)

## Niacin (cont.)

| | |
|---|---|
| Clinical assessment of deficiency | Skin: dermatitis, hyperpigmentation, hyperkeratotic plaques<br>Diarrhea<br>Dementia |

## Pantothenic acid

| | |
|---|---|
| Pertinent biochemical tests | Whole blood, plasma, or 24-hour urine pantothenic acid |
| Clinical assessment of deficiency | Neuromotor impairment<br>Paresthesia<br>Tachycardia<br>Hypotension<br>Upper respiratory infection |
| Special considerations | Pantothenic acid is not routinely assessed in practice due to the rarity of the deficiency. |

## Vitamin B6

| | |
|---|---|
| Pertinent biochemical tests | Plasma or RBC pyridoxal 5'-phosphate (PLP)<br>CRP[a]<br>Complete blood count (CBC, microcytic anemia) |
| Clinical assessment of deficiency | Oral cavity: cheilosis, angular stomatitis, glossitis<br>Skin: seborrheic dermatitis<br>Peripheral neuropathy<br>Seizures |
| Special considerations | Interpret plasma PLP results with caution if CRP >1.0 mg/dL. |

**BOX 6.2  Assessment Strategies for Determining Water-Soluble Vitamin Status[1,6] (cont.)**

### Biotin

| | |
|---|---|
| Pertinent biochemical tests | Plasma or serum biotin |
| Clinical assessment of deficiency | Skin: seborrheic dermatitis<br>Hair: alopecia<br>Nails: brittle<br>Seizures (observed in infants with inborn errors of biotin metabolism) |
| Special considerations | Except in cases of holocarboxylase synthetase deficiency and biotinidase deficiency, biotin is not routinely assessed in practice due to the rarity of the deficiency and the tendency for it to present in conjunction with other B vitamin deficiencies. |

### Folate

| | |
|---|---|
| Pertinent biochemical tests | RBC or serum folate<br>Plasma or serum homocysteine<br>CBC (macrocytic anemia) |
| Clinical assessment of deficiency | Eyes: conjunctival pallor<br>Oral cavity: glossitis<br>Skin: pallor<br>Peripheral neuropathy |
| Special considerations | Plasma or serum folate concentrations should be obtained from fasting patients, but RBC or whole blood specimens can be obtained without regard to food intake. |

*Deficiencies Water-Soluble Vitamins*

*Continued on next page*

## BOX 6.2  Assessment Strategies for Determining Water-Soluble Vitamin Status[1,6] (cont.)

### *Vitamin B12*

| | |
|---|---|
| Pertinent biochemical tests | Serum vitamin B12 |
| | Plasma or serum methylmalonic acid (MMA) |
| | Plasma or serum homocysteine |
| | CBC (macrocytic anemia) |
| Clinical assessment of deficiency | Eyes: conjunctival pallor |
| | Oral cavity: glossitis |
| | Skin: pallor |
| | Peripheral neuropathy |
| Special considerations | Elevated MMA supports deficiency when serum vitamin B12 is 150 to 400 pg/mL. Normal MMA excludes deficiency when homocysteine is elevated. |
| | Serum vitamin B12 may be falsely inflated with liver dysfunction. |

### *Vitamin C*

| | |
|---|---|
| Pertinent biochemical tests | Leukocyte or plasma vitamin C (ascorbate or ascorbic acid) |
| | CRP[a] |
| | CBC (anemia) |
| Clinical assessment of deficiency | Oral cavity: gingivitis, tooth loss |
| | Skin: petechiae, ecchymosis, purpura, pallor |
| | Hair: corkscrew hairs |
| | Musculoskeletal pain, weakness |
| | Poor wound healing |
| Special considerations | Interpret plasma results with caution if CRP >1.0 mg/dL. |

[a] C-reactive protein (CRP) is listed for select nutrients when there is evidence to suggest that plasma or serum levels of the nutrients are influenced by inflammation.

## BOX 6.3 Drug-Nutrient Interactions for Water-Soluble Vitamins[2,31,52-59]

### Thiamin[2,53-55]

| | |
|---|---|
| Drug | Loop diuretics (eg, furosemide, bumetanide, torsemide) |
| Potential effect of drug interaction | Decreased serum thiamin concentration with potential risk of neurological symptoms. This risk is higher in hospitalized patients receiving intensified diuresis. |
| Suggested actions | Routine monitoring for erythrocyte transketolase activity or empirical supplementation is not necessary for patients with optimal nutrient intake and normal nutritional status. |
| | In patients with reduced oral intake, cachexia, or sarcopenia, supplement with a thiamin-containing multivitamin and continue to monitor for signs and symptoms of thiamin deficiency. |

### Niacin[56,57]

| | |
|---|---|
| Drug | 3-hydroxy-3-methylglutaryl coenzyme A (HMG-CoA) reductase inhibitors (eg, statins) |
| Potential effect of drug interaction | Older reports indicate that niacin may increase the risk of myopathy and rhabdomyolysis in individuals taking statins. The incidence generally is very low and unlikely to be clinically significant in most patients with no other risk factors (eg, drug-drug interactions). |
| | Concurrent niacin and ethanol use may increase flushing and pruritus. |
| Suggested actions | Assess the risks and benefits of niacin therapy concurrent with statin therapy. Dose reduction of statin therapy may be necessary in patients taking other drugs that may interact with statins. Monitor for signs and symptoms of rhabdomyolysis and myopathy. |
| | Avoid concurrent use of alcohol and niacin if possible. |

### Vitamin B6[31,58]

| | |
|---|---|
| Drug | Isoniazid |
| | Levodopa-carbidopa |
| | Phenytoin |

*Continued on next page*

## BOX 6.3 Drug-Nutrient Interactions for Water-Soluble Vitamins[2,31,52-59] (cont.)

### Vitamin B6[31,58] (cont.)

| | |
|---|---|
| Potential effect of drug interaction | Isoniazid can deplete vitamin B6, leading to neuropathy. |
| | Levodopa-carbidopa may decrease vitamin B6 concentration and precipitate neurologic symptoms, such as peripheral neuropathy and gait ataxia. This seems to be more common with the intestinal gel formulation of the drug. |
| | Data for phenytoin interaction are very limited and based solely on a few case reports. The clinical significance is very low. |
| Suggested actions | In patients taking isoniazid, supplement with 25 to 50 mg/d vitamin B6. |
| | Monitor patients taking levodopa-carbidopa for signs and symptoms of neuropathy, especially with dosage increases or use of the intestinal gel formulation. |
| | Monitor patients taking phenytoin for signs and symptoms of polyneuropathy. Empirical B6 supplementation is not warranted. |

### Folate[59]

| | |
|---|---|
| Drug | Methotrexate<br>Phenytoin<br>Sulfasalazine |
| Potential effect of drug interaction | These drugs have been reported to decrease serum folate concentration and precipitate macrocytic anemia or other adverse events such as mucositis. |
| | Supplementation with folic acid may also decrease serum phenytoin concentration. |
| Suggested actions | In patients taking methotrexate, give 1 mg/d folic acid orally. |
| | In patients taking phenytoin, monitor hemoglobin concentration and red blood cell indexes. If folic acid supplementation is initiated, check serum phenytoin concentration in 1 week. |
| | In patients taking sulfasalazine, supplement with 1 mg/d of folic acid. |

**BOX 6.4  Available Treatment Forms and Suggested Regimens for Treating Water-Soluble Vitamin Deficiencies[a,52,60-62]**

## *Thiamin*

### Treatment forms

Oral — Tablets in various strengths (10 mg, 25 mg, 50 mg, 100 mg)

Should be taken with food to increase absorption

Injection — Thiamin hydrochloride, 100 mg/mL solution

May be administered as intravenous (IV) push, IV infusion after dilution, or intramuscular (IM) injection

### Treatment regimens[b]

*Coadministration of IV dextrose (in patients with depleted thiamin status)*

100 mg in each of the first few liters of IV fluid

*Acute alcohol withdrawal syndrome*

100 mg, IV, per 25 g dextrose concurrently with IV dextrose

*Beriberi*

10 to 20 mg, IM or IV infusion, three times daily for up to 2 weeks; then by mouth (PO) maintenance with therapeutic multivitamin preparation containing 5 to 10 mg/d for 1 month

*Peripheral neuritis or severe vomiting in pregnancy*

5 to 10 mg/d, IM

*Wernicke-Korsakoff syndrome*

100 to 500 mg/d, IV, for 5 to 7 days or until symptoms resolve in hospitalized individuals

*Neurological symptoms not related to Wernicke-Korsakoff syndrome*

50 to 100 mg/d, PO, in two or three divided doses to maximize absorption

*Prevention of Wernicke encephalopathy in patients with limited intake*

100 to 300 mg, IV or PO, before feeding or infusion of dextrose-containing IV fluids in at-risk individuals; continue for 5 to 7 days

*Deficiencies Water-Soluble Vitamins*

*Continued on next page*

## BOX 6.4  Available Treatment Forms and Suggested Regimens for Treating Water-Soluble Vitamin Deficiencies[a,52,60-62] (cont.)

### *Riboflavin*

#### Treatment forms

Riboflavin in oral and parenteral vitamins; riboflavin 5-phosphate in ophthalmic products

| | |
|---|---|
| Oral | Tablets and capsules in various strengths (25 mg, 50 mg, 100 mg, 400 mg) |
| Injection | Not available as a standalone product in the United States |
| Ophthalmic solution | Ophthalmic solution for progressive keratoconus |

#### Treatment regimens[b]

*Riboflavin deficiency*

5 to 10 mg/d, PO

Alternative regimen: 15 mg every 2 weeks in lactating or pregnant individuals to increase adherence

*Congenital methemoglobinemia*

20 to 120 mg/d, PO, followed by maintenance doses of 10 to 30 mg/d has been reported to be effective in recessive congenital methemoglobinemia secondary to red blood cell (RBC) reduced nicotinamide adenine dinucleotide (NADH) reduced diaphorase or NADH methemoglobin reductase deficiency

### *Niacin*
#### Treatment forms

| | |
|---|---|
| Oral | Tablets and capsules in various strengths (50 mg, 100 mg, 250 mg, 500 mg, 750 mg, 1,000 mg) |
| | Over-the-counter (OTC) supplement and prescription drug |
| | Formulated as immediate-release or extended-release tablets and capsules |
| | Extended-release and immediate-release formulations are not interchangeable. Doses should be retitrated. |
| Injection | Not available as a standalone product in the United States |

---

**BOX 6.4  Available Treatment Forms and Suggested Regimens for Treating Water-Soluble Vitamin Deficiencies[a,52,60-62] (cont.)**

**Treatment regimens[b]**

*Hypertriglyceridemia*

Immediate-release formulation: 250 mg/d, PO, following the evening meal; titrate up weekly as needed to 3 g/d or a target low-density lipoprotein cholesterol (LDL-C). Typical adult daily dose is 2 to 3 g in two to three divided doses.

*Hyperlipidemia*

Immediate-release formulation: 250 mg/d, PO; titrate up every 2 to 4 weeks to 1 to 2 g two to three times daily, not to exceed 6 g/d

Extended-release formulation: 500 mg, PO, once daily at bedtime; titrate up every 4 weeks as needed, not to exceed 2 g/d

*Pellagra*

Immediate-release formulation: 50 to 100 mg, PO, three to four times daily

## Pantothenic acid

**Treatment forms**

| | |
|---|---|
| Oral | OTC supplement tablets in various strengths (100 mg, 200 mg, 500 mg) |
| Injection | Not available as a standalone product in the United States |

**Treatment regimens[b]**

*Pantothenic acid deficiency*

Optimal treatment regimen has not been established. Doses that match or exceed the average daily intake should be considered, depending on individual presentation, risk factors, and clinical responses.

## Vitamin B6

**Treatment forms**

| | |
|---|---|
| Oral | Pyridoxine hydrochloride tablets and capsules as OTC supplements in various strengths (25 mg, 50 mg, 100 mg, 200 mg, 250 mg, 500 mg) |
| Injection | Pyridoxine hydrochloride solution for IV or IM use |

*Deficiencies Water-Soluble Vitamins*

*Continued on next page*

---

**BOX 6.4  Available Treatment Forms and Suggested Regimens for Treating Water-Soluble Vitamin Deficiencies[a,52,60-62] (cont.)**

## Vitamin B6 (cont.)

### Treatment regimens[b]

*Pyridoxine deficiency*

   10 to 20 mg/d, IM or IV, for 3 weeks, followed by daily PO therapy (up to 5 mg/d) for several weeks

*Pyridoxine-dependency seizure*

   Acute seizure: 100 to 600 mg, IV, IM, or PO

   Maintenance therapy: 30 mg/d, PO

*Peripheral polyneuropathy, including concurrent use of isoniazid*

   Treatment: 50 to 300 mg/d, PO

   Prophylaxis: 25 to 50 mg/d, PO

## Biotin

### Treatment forms

Oral            Tablets and capsules as OTC supplements in various strengths (5 mg, 10 mg)

Injection       Not available as a standalone product in the United States

### Treatment regimens[b]

*Biotinidase deficiency*

   The most effective regimen has not been established; clinical data suggest dosing ranges from 10 to 40 mg/d, PO

## Folate

### Treatment forms

Oral            Folic acid tablets or capsules as OTC supplements or prescription drug in various strengths (400 mcg, 800 mcg, 1 mg, 5 mg, 20 mg)

Injection       Folic acid sodium solution for IV, IM, or subcutaneous (SC)

                Doses up to 5 mg can be administered as IV push.

                Larger doses should be diluted in IV fluid and infused over at least 30 minutes.

**BOX 6.4  Available Treatment Forms and Suggested Regimens for Treating Water-Soluble Vitamin Deficiencies[a,52,60-62] (cont.)**

**Treatment regimens[b]**

*Megaloblastic anemias caused by folate deficiency*

   0.4 to 1.0 mg/d, PO or IV

*Adjunctive therapy for alcohol withdrawal syndrome*

   0.4 to 1.0 mg/d, IV or PO, until no longer at risk for alcohol withdrawal

*Homocysteinemia*

   0.5 to 5.0 mg/d, PO

*Prevention of methotrexate-associated adverse effects (eg, stomatitis)*

   1 mg/d, PO; or 5 mg/wk, PO

## Vitamin B12

**Treatment forms**

Most common salt form is cyanocobalamin; also available as methylcobalamin and hydroxocobalamin.

| | |
|---|---|
| Oral | Tablets and lozenges for ingestion or sublingual use |
| Injection | Cyanocobalamin solution (1,000 mcg/mL; 2,000 mcg/mL) for IM or deep SC injection |
| | IV administration **not** recommended |
| Inhalation | Nasal spray (500 mcg/0.1 mL) |

**Treatment regimens[b]**

*Cobalamin deficiency (including anemia)*

   Injection: 500 to 1,000 mcg, IM or SC, once daily for 1 week; then 1,000 mcg, IM or SC, once weekly for 4 to 8 weeks

   Nasal spray: product-specific regimen; one spray in one nostril once weekly, or as directed based on manufacturer information

   Oral: 500 to 2,000 mcg/d, PO; higher doses as needed with decreased intestinal absorption

Note that hydroxocobalamin is also approved by the US Food and Drug Administration as an antidote for cyanide poisoning.

*Continued on next page*

BOX 6.4  Available Treatment Forms and Suggested Regimens for Treating Water-Soluble Vitamin Deficiencies[a,52,60-62] (cont.)

## Vitamin C

**Treatment forms**

Oral      Tablet, capsules, liquids, powders, lozenges, and troches as OTC supplements

Injection    Prescription solution for IM, SC, or IV use; IV route given as a slow infusion

**Treatment regimens[b]**

*Vitamin C deficiency*

Oral: Up to 1 to 2 g/d for 2 days, followed by 500 mg/d for 1 week (off-label dosage)

Injection: 200 mg IV infusion at 33 mg/min once daily for a maximum of 7 days; may retreat until symptoms resolve (FDA-approved regimen for IV product)

[a] For specific gastrointestinal surgery, renal care, critical care, and bariatric surgery guidelines, refer to Chapters 9, 10, 13, and 14, respectively.
[b] Based on published literature; not all are FDA-approved indications.

BOX 6.5  Monitoring and Other Considerations for Water-Soluble Vitamins[a,52,60-62]

## Thiamin

Biochemical: Routine assessment is not recommended.

Concurrent therapy: Magnesium is required as a cofactor for thiamin metabolism.

Serum magnesium status should be assessed and hypomagnesemia corrected alongside thiamin replacement.

## Niacin

High-fat foods may decrease bioavailability.

Flushing and pruritus are common adverse effects of niacin and may be attenuated with a gradual increase in dose or by administering with food.

Extended-release formulation appears to cause less flushing.

Gastrointestinal discomfort, including nausea and vomiting, is common with higher doses.

## BOX 6.5 Monitoring and Other Considerations for Water-Soluble Vitamins[a,52,60-62] (cont.)

### Vitamin B6

Vitamin B6, in combination with doxylamine, has been used to treat pregnancy-associated nausea and vomiting, or morning sickness.

### Vitamin B12

Serum methylmalonic acid concentration or plasma vitamin B12 concentration, or both, should be monitored. Also monitor changes in hemoglobin concentration and clinical symptoms (eg, neurological symptoms such as neuropathy).

Data supporting reliable absorption from the sublingual route are lacking; available evidence is more consistent with the use of orally disintegrated tablets, which dissolve in the mouth and are swallowed for absorption in the small intestine.

### Vitamin C

Intramuscular administration can cause soreness and pain at the injection site. Rapid intravenous administration can cause dizziness or temporary faintness.

High doses (>1 g/d) may lead to elevated plasma ascorbate concentrations, which can interfere with the accuracy of a glucometer, including a continuous glucose monitor; high doses can also result in diarrhea and decreased oral absorption of copper and cobalamin.

Supplemental vitamin C should be used with caution in patients with high risk for or history of kidney stone and hypernatremia. See chapter 10 for information on renal disease and vitamin C.

In patients with known or suspected glucose-6-phosphate dehydrogenase (G6PD) deficiency, hemoglobin concentrations should be monitored when high doses are given because of reports of hemolytic anemia in this population.

[a] Frequency of biochemical monitoring varies based on severity of depletion, presence of overt symptoms, and underlying disease.

Deficiencies Water-Soluble Vitamins

# References

1. Berger MM, Shenkin A, Schweinlin A, et al. ESPEN micronutrient guideline. *Clin Nutr.* 2022;41(6):1357-1424. doi:10.1016/j.clnu.2022.02.015

2. Frank LL. Thiamin in clinical practice. *JPEN J Parenter Enteral Nutr.* 2015;39(5):503-520. doi:10.1177/0148607114565245

3. Monsen ER. Dietary Reference Intakes for the antioxidant nutrients: vitamin C, vitamin E, selenium, and carotenoids. *J Am Diet Assoc.* 2000;100(6):637-640. doi:10.1016/S0002-8223(00)00189-9

4. Polegato BF, Pereira AG, Azevedo PS, et al. Role of thiamin in health and disease. *Nutr Clin Pract.* 2019;34(4):558-564. doi:10.1002/ncp.10234

5. DiBaise M, Tarleton SM. Hair, nails, and skin: differentiating cutaneous manifestations of micronutrient deficiency. *Nutr Clin Pract.* 2019;34(4):490-503. doi:10.1002/ncp.10321

6. Esper DH. Utilization of nutrition-focused physical assessment in identifying micronutrient deficiencies. *Nutr Clin Pract.* 2015;30(2):194-202. doi:10.1177/0884533615573054

7. McMillan DC, Maguire D, Talwar D. Relationship between nutritional status and the systemic inflammatory response: micronutrients. *Proc Nutr Soc.* 2019;78(1):56-67. doi:10.1017/S0029665118002501

8. Duncan A, Talwar D, McMillan DC, Stefanowicz F, O'Reilly DS. Quantitative data on the magnitude of the systemic inflammatory response and its effect on micronutrient status based on plasma measurements. *Am J Clin Nutr.* 2012;95(1):64-71. doi:10.3945/ajcn.111.023812

9. DiNicolantonio JJ, Liu J, O'Keefe JH. Thiamine and cardiovascular disease: a literature review. *Prog Cardiovasc Dis.* 2018;61(1):27-32. doi:10.1016/j.pcad.2018.01.009

10. Smith TJ, Johnson CR, Koshy R, et al. Thiamine deficiency disorders: a clinical perspective. *Ann N Y Acad Sci.* 2021;1498(1):9-28. doi:10.1111/nyas.14536

11. Latt N, Dore G. Thiamine in the treatment of Wernicke encephalopathy in patients with alcohol use disorders. *Intern Med J.* 2014;44(9):911-915. doi:10.1111/imj.12522

12. Wooley JA. Characteristics of thiamin and its relevance to the management of heart failure. *Nutr Clin Pract.* 2008;23(5):487-493. doi:10.1177/0884533608323430

13. Friedli N, Stanga Z, Culkin A, et al. Management and prevention of refeeding syndrome in medical inpatients: an evidence-based and consensus-supported algorithm. *Nutrition.* 2018;47:13-20. doi:10.1016/j.nut.2017.09.007

14. da Silva JSV, Seres DS, Sabino K, et al. ASPEN consensus recommendations for refeeding syndrome. *Nutr Clin Pract.* 2020;35(2):178-195. doi:10.1002/ncp.10474

15. Thakur K, Tomar SK, Singh AK, Mandal S, Arora S. Riboflavin and health: a review of recent human research. *Crit Rev Food Sci Nutr.* 2017;57(17):3650-3660. doi:10.1080/10408398.2016.1145104

16. Fishman SM, Christian P, West KP. The role of vitamins in the prevention and control of anaemia. *Public Health Nutr.* 2000;3(2):125-150. doi:10.1017/s1368980000000173

17. Jungert A, McNulty H, Hoey L, et al. Riboflavin is an important determinant of vitamin B-6 status in healthy adults. *J Nutr.* 2020;150(10):2699-2706. doi:10.1093/jn/nxaa225

18. Hustad S, McKinley MC, McNulty H, et al. Riboflavin, flavin mononucleotide, and flavin adenine dinucleotide in human plasma and erythrocytes at baseline and after low-dose riboflavin supplementation. *Clin Chem.* 2002;48(9):1571-1577.

19. Vasilaki AT, McMillan DC, Kinsella J, Duncan A, O'Reilly DS, Talwar D. Relation between riboflavin, flavin mononucleotide and flavin adenine dinucleotide concentrations in plasma and red cells in patients with critical illness. *Clin Chim Acta.* 2010;411(21-22):1750-1755. doi:10.1016/j.cca.2010.07.024

20. Hołubiec P, Leończyk M, Staszewski F, Łazarczyk A, Jaworek AK, Wojas-Pelc A. Pathophysiology and clinical management of pellagra—a review. *Folia Med Cracov.* 2021;61(3):125-137. doi:10.24425/fmc.2021.138956

21. Fukuwatari T, Shibata K. Nutritional aspect of tryptophan metabolism. *Int J Tryptophan Res.* 2013;6(suppl 1):3-8. doi:10.4137/IJTR.S11588

22. Carlsson CM. Homocysteine lowering with folic acid and vitamin B supplements: effects on cardiovascular disease in older adults. *Drugs Aging.* 2006;23(6):491-502. doi:10.2165/00002512-200623060-00004

23. Robinson K. Homocysteine, B vitamins, and risk of cardiovascular disease. *Heart.* 2000;83(2):127-130. doi:10.1136/heart.83.2.127

24. Koklesova L, Mazurakova A, Samec M, et al. Homocysteine metabolism as the target for predictive medical approach, disease prevention, prognosis, and treatments tailored to the person. *EPMA J.* 2021;12(4):477-505. doi:10.1007/s13167-021-00263-0

25. Kim J, Kim H, Roh H, Kwon Y. Causes of hyperhomocysteinemia and its pathological significance. *Arch Pharm Res.* 2018;41(4):372-383. doi:10.1007/s12272-018-1016-4

26. Spinneker A, Sola R, Lemmen V, Castillo MJ, Pietrzik K, González-Gross M. Vitamin B6 status, deficiency and its consequences—an overview. *Nutr Hosp.* 2007;22(1):7-24.

27. Strain JJ, Dowey L, Ward M, Pentieva K, McNulty H. B-vitamins, homocysteine metabolism and CVD. *Proc Nutr Soc*. 2004;63(4):597-603. doi:10.1079/pns2004390

28. Taher J, Naranian T, Poon YY, et al. Vitamins and infusion of levodopa-carbidopa intestinal gel. *Can J Neurol Sci*. 2022;49(1):19-28. doi:10.1017/cjn.2021.78

29. Gwathmey KG, Grogan J. Nutritional neuropathies. *Muscle Nerve*. 2020;62(1):13-29. doi:10.1002/mus.26783

30. Rojo-Sebastián A, González-Robles C, García de Yébenes J. Vitamin B6 deficiency in patients with Parkinson disease treated with levodopa/carbidopa. *Clin Neuropharmacol*. 2020;43(5):151-157. doi:10.1097/WNF.0000000000000408

31. Gerlach AT, Thomas S, Stawicki SP, Whitmill ML, Steinberg SM, Cook CH. Vitamin B6 deficiency: a potential cause of refractory seizures in adults. *JPEN J Parenter Enteral Nutr*. 2011;35(2):272-275. doi:10.1177/0148607110384118

32. Nagao T, Hirokawa M. Diagnosis and treatment of macrocytic anemias in adults. *J Gen Fam Med*. 2017;18(5):200-204. doi:10.1002/jgf2.31

33. Langan RC, Goodbred AJ. Vitamin B12 deficiency: recognition and management. *Am Fam Physician*. 2017;96(6):384-389.

34. Sentongo TA, Azzam R, Charrow J. Vitamin B12 status, methylmalonic acidemia, and bacterial overgrowth in short bowel syndrome. *J Pediatr Gastroenterol Nutr*. 2009;48(4):495-497. doi:10.1097/MPG.0b013e31817f9e5b

35. Metz J. A high prevalence of biochemical evidence of vitamin B12 or folate deficiency does not translate into a comparable prevalence of anemia. *Food Nutr Bull*. 2008;29(2 suppl):S74-S85. doi:10.1177/15648265080292S111

36. Green R, Datta Mitra A. Megaloblastic anemias: nutritional and other causes. *Med Clin North Am*. 2017;101(2):297-317. doi:10.1016/j.mcna.2016.09.013

37. Baker H, Leevy CB, DeAngelis B, Frank O, Baker ER. Cobalamin (vitamin B12) and holotranscobalamin changes in plasma and liver tissue in alcoholics with liver disease. *J Am Coll Nutr*. 1998;17(3):235-238. doi:10.1080/07315724.1998.10718752

38. Jimenez L, Stamm DA, Depaula B, Duggan CP. Is serum methylmalonic acid a reliable biomarker of vitamin B12 status in children with short bowel syndrome: a case series. *J Pediatr*. 2018;192:259-261. doi:10.1016/j.jpeds.2017.09.024

39. Ferrazzi E, Tiso G, Di Martino D. Folic acid versus 5-methyl tetrahydrofolate supplementation in pregnancy. *Eur J Obstet Gynecol Reprod Biol*. 2020;253:312-319. doi:10.1016/j.ejogrb.2020.06.012

40. Whittle SL, Hughes RA. Folate supplementation and methotrexate treatment in rheumatoid arthritis: a review. *Rheumatology (Oxford)*. 2004;43(3):267-271. doi:10.1093/rheumatology/keh088

41. Smulders YM, Smith DE, Kok RM, et al. Cellular folate vitamer distribution during and after correction of vitamin B12 deficiency: a case for the methylfolate trap. *Br J Haematol*. 2006;132(5):623-629. doi:10.1111/j.1365-2141.2005.05913.x

42. De Bruyn E, Gulbis B, Cotton F. Serum and red blood cell folate testing for folate deficiency: new features? *Eur J Haematol*. 2014;92(4):354-359. doi:10.1111/ejh.12237

43. Sobczyńska-Malefora A, Harrington DJ. Laboratory assessment of folate (vitamin B9) status. *J Clin Pathol*. 2018;71(11):949-956. doi:10.1136/jclinpath-2018-205048

44. Farrell CJ, Kirsch SH, Herrmann M. Red cell or serum folate: what to do in clinical practice? *Clin Chem Lab Med*. 2013;51(3):555-569. doi:10.1515/cclm-2012-0639

45. Panchal S, Schneider C, Malhotra K. Scurvy in a hemodialysis patient. Rare or ignored? *Hemodial Int*. 2018;22(S2):S83-S87. doi:10.1111/hdi.12705

46. Marik PE, Liggett A. Adding an orange to the banana bag: vitamin C deficiency is common in alcohol use disorders. *Crit Care*. 2019;23(1):165. doi:10.1186/s13054-019-2435-4

47. Mosdøl A, Erens B, Brunner EJ. Estimated prevalence and predictors of vitamin C deficiency within UK's low-income population. *J Public Health (Oxf)*. 2008;30(4):456-460. doi:10.1093/pubmed/fdn076

48. Schleicher RL, Carroll MD, Ford ES, Lacher DA. Serum vitamin C and the prevalence of vitamin C deficiency in the United States: 2003-2004 National Health and Nutrition Examination Survey (NHANES). *Am J Clin Nutr*. 2009;90(5):1252-1263. doi:10.3945/ajcn.2008.27016

49. Food and Nutrition Board, Institute of Medicine. *Dietary Reference Intakes for Vitamin C, Vitamin E, Selenium, and Carotenoids*. National Academies Press; 2000.

50. Yule S, Wanik J, Holm EM, et al. Nutritional deficiency disease secondary to ARFID symptoms associated with autism and the broad autism phenotype: a qualitative systematic review of case reports and case series. *J Acad Nutr Diet*. 2021;121(3):467-492. doi:10.1016/j.jand.2020.10.017

51. Kothari P, Tate A, Adewumi A, Kinlin LM, Ritwik P. The risk for scurvy in children with neurodevelopmental disorders. *Spec Care Dentist*. 2020;40(3):251-259. doi:10.1111/scd.12459

52. Micromedex (database). Merative. 2023. Accessed December 15, 2022. www.micromedexsolutions.com

53. Bicer I, Dizdar OS, Dondurmacı E, et al. Furosemide-related thiamine deficiency in hospitalized hypervolemic patients with renal failure and heart failure. *Nefrologia (Engl Ed)*. 2023;43(1):111-119. doi:10.1016/j.nefroe.2022.11.013

54. Gundogan K, Akbudak IH, Bulut K, et al. Thiamin status in adults receiving chronic diuretic therapy prior to admission to a medical intensive care unit: a pilot study. *Nutr Clin Pract*. 2019;34(4):565-571. doi:10.1002/ncp.10241

55. Teigen LM, Twernbold DD, Miller WL. Prevalence of thiamine deficiency in a stable heart failure outpatient cohort on standard loop diuretic therapy. *Clin Nutr*. 2016;35(6):1323-1327. doi:10.1016/j.clnu.2016.02.011

56. Tsui L, Chen L, Ye P, et al. Adverse drug reactions of non-statin antihyperlipidaemic drugs in China from 1989 to 2019: a national database analysis. *BMJ Open*. 2023;13(5):e068915. doi:10.1136/bmjopen-2022-068915

57. Alsheikh-Ali AA, Karas RH. Safety of lovastatin/extended release niacin compared with lovastatin alone, atorvastatin alone, pravastatin alone, and simvastatin alone (from the United States Food and Drug Administration adverse event reporting system). *Am J Cardiol*. 2007;99(3):379-381. doi:10.1016/j.amjcard.2006.08.044

58. Loens S, Chorbadzhieva E, Kleimann A, Dressler D, Schrader C. Effects of levodopa/carbidopa intestinal gel versus oral levodopa/carbidopa on B vitamin levels and neuropathy. *Brain Behav*. 2017;7(5):e00698. doi:10.1002/brb3.698

59. Jansen G, van der Heijden J, Oerlemans R, et al. Sulfasalazine is a potent inhibitor of the reduced folate carrier: implications for combination therapies with methotrexate in rheumatoid arthritis. *Arthritis Rheum*. 2004;50(7):2130-2139. doi:10.1002/art.20375

60. Facts and Comparisons: drug referential resource. Wolters Kluwer. Accessed December 15, 2022. www.wolterskluwer.com/en/solutions/lexicomp/facts-and-comparisons

61. Drugs@FDA: FDA-approved drugs. US Food and Drug Administration. Accessed December 15, 2022. www.accessdata.fda.gov/scripts/cder/daf/index.cfm

62. Drug information. UpToDate. Accessed December 15, 2022. www.uptodate.com/contents/table-of-contents/drug-information

63. Rogovik AL, Vohra S, Goldman RD. Safety considerations and potential interactions of vitamins: should vitamins be considered drugs? *Ann Pharmacother*. 2010;44(2):311-324. doi:10.1345/aph.1M238

# CHAPTER 7

# Iron Deficiency

Kyle Hampson, PharmD, MPH, BCNSP, BCPPS, CNSC, FASPEN and Marcia Nahikian-Nelms, PhD, RDN, FAND

## Introduction

Iron deficiency is a global public health challenge and is the leading cause of anemia worldwide.[1] Iron is a key micronutrient, critical for the production and function of hemoglobin and red blood cells (RBCs). A well-nourished adult has approximately 3 g iron stored in the liver.[2] All people require iron, but children and premenopausal females are the most affected by deficiency. The recommended dietary intake varies by sex and age, as outlined in Table 7.1 on page 124.[3-5] *Iron deficiency* refers to a reduction in iron stores; whereas *iron-deficiency anemia* refers to a major complication of iron deficiency in which microcytic, hypochromic RBCs are present.[1] This chapter explores the complex absorption and recycling of iron in the human body, explains the deficiency states for iron, and provides an overview of treatment strategies.

Iron
Deficiency

## TABLE 7.1 Recommended Iron Intake[3-5]

| Group | Dietary Reference Intake |
| --- | --- |
| Infants, term-6 mo | Adequate Intake, 0.27 mg/d |
| Infants, 7-12 mo | 11 mg/d |
| Children, 1-3 y | 7 mg/d |
| Children, 4-8 y | 10 mg/d |
| Children, 9-13 y | 8 mg/d |
| Males, 14-18 y | 11 mg/d |
| Females, 14-18 y | 15 mg/d |
| Males, 19 y and older | 8 mg/d |
| Premenopausal females, 19-50 y | 18 mg/d |
| Postmenopausal females, 51 y and older | 8 mg/d |
| Pregnant females | 27 mg/d |
| Lactating females, 19-50 y | 9 mg/d |
| Adolescents and all adults, >14 y | Tolerable Upper Intake Level, 45 mg/d |

# Iron Absorption and Metabolism

## Absorption

Excess iron is toxic to the body and, therefore, only 1 to 2 mg are absorbed through the gastrointestinal (GI) tract per day to replenish physiologic turnover. Iron homeostasis is tightly controlled through absorptive pathways and through hepcidin-based homeostatic controls to prevent the formation of hydroxyl radicals that can cause systemic toxicity, such as oxidative damage.[1,6] Numerous factors may enhance or impede iron absorption, meaning that clinicians must evaluate each patient's complete medical and dietary history in order to diagnose iron deficiency and to support the patient's treatment plan.

Iron Deficiency

Hepcidin, a peptide hormone, is produced in the liver and functions by inducing the degradation of ferroportin-1, the transport protein that releases iron from the enterocyte into the plasma. Hepcidin expression increases in response to high levels of circulating or tissue iron, displaying an inverse relationship to iron concentration. Hepcidin is also an acute-phase reactant, showing increased expression in response to inflammation and high levels of inflammatory cytokines (eg, interleukin-6) and the Janus kinase–signal transducer and activator of transcription (JAK-STAT) pathway activation.[1,7] Production of hepcidin is inhibited by iron deficiency, increased erythropoiesis, and tissue hypoxia.[1] Because of the relationship between hepcidin and iron absorption, a growing body of evidence suggests that oral iron absorption may be enhanced using less frequent dosing (eg, alternate day dosing).[8] Although initial studies validate this theory, larger, more robust trials are needed to determine the optimal strategies for maximizing efficacy and minimizing adverse events. Table 7.2 on page 126 summarizes the factors that affect absorption of iron and, consequently, iron status.[6,7,9-12]

# Metabolism and Elimination

After absorption, ferrous iron is bound to transferrin and transported for use to tissues throughout the body. Iron is used in the mitochondria predominantly for the synthesis of heme, which is then transported to the cytosol for integration into proteins, such as hemoglobin.[6,10] Excess ferrous iron that is not bound to transferrin is incorporated into ferritin and stored in the liver.

Iron overload causes harm: excess heme is toxic to the body and may induce cellular apoptosis.[6] Because absorption is limited, iron is not typically removed from the body under normal physiology and is thus continually recycled from aged or damaged RBCs, which contain iron in the heme form. These old and damaged cells are taken up by macrophages, where elemental iron is released through the action of heme oxygenase-1 in the endoplasmic reticulum.[6,7] The action of heme oxygenase-1 serves as the rate-limiting step in the catabolism of heme and is the major regulator of intracellular heme levels.[8] This iron is then

Iron
Deficiency

| TABLE 7.2 Factors Affecting Iron Absorption[6,7,9-12] | | |
| --- | --- | --- |
| Factor | Impact on iron absorption | Comments |
| Type of dietary iron (heme)[6,10] | ↑: absorbed at a rate of 15%-35% | Found in animal food sources |
| Type of dietary iron (nonheme)[6,10] | ↓: absorbed at a rate of 2%-20% | Found in plant food sources |
| Hepcidin[7] | ↓ | Induces degradation of iron transport protein; inverse relationship to iron status |
| Iron status[6] | ↑↓ | Gastrointestinal absorption increases during iron deficiency |
| Vitamin C[11] | ↑ | Reduces ferric to ferrous iron to increase absorption of nonheme iron |
| Zinc[12] | ↓ | May compete for transport molecules |
| Antacids, proton pump inhibitors | ↓ | Medication results in higher pH and reduces absorption |
| Foods high in calcium, phytate, polyphenols[11] | ↓ | May compete for transport molecules |
| Normal gastrointestinal tract and physiology[11] | ↑ | Gastrointestinal surgery, malabsorptive syndromes, inflammatory bowel disease, and liver disease all have the potential to reduce absorption of iron |

bound to transferrin or incorporated into ferritin and stored in the liver. This recycling pathway conserves iron within the body.[1]

The physiological requirement for iron is approximately 25 mg/d. However, 1 to 2 mg iron are lost per day through the turnover of enterocytes in the GI tract and through the urine. In individuals with normal menses, an additional 1 mg/d is lost during menstruation.[2,12,13] In the absence of an excretion pathway, if iron overload is a concern, chelator therapy can be provided.

# Pathophysiology of Deficiencies

Infants older than 6 months, young children (up to 4 years of age), and young females are at the highest risk for iron deficiencies; however, individuals with low dietary iron intake, those experiencing rapid growth with subsequent increased requirements, and those with underlying disease states associated with malabsorption or blood loss are also at risk. Aside from the anemia that is classically described, iron deficiency can have far-reaching impacts on health outcomes. Severe iron deficiency during pregnancy can lead to preterm delivery, low birthweight, and infant and maternal mortality. Iron is also critical for neurologic development in infants, and iron deficiency has been linked to impaired cognitive function in children.[1]

## Dietary Deficiency

Insufficient or poor dietary intake is one potential cause of iron deficiency. A common scenario of dietary iron deficiency is in children who obtain a large portion of their energy intake from cow's milk. Cow's milk contains minimal iron, and children whose diets largely consist of cow's milk will not have sufficient iron intake to meet their needs.[14] Vegetarian diets, vegan diets, or diets low in red meat may induce iron deficiency through insufficient intake. However, this is a less common cause of iron deficiency, as many meat substitutes (eg, tofu) are now fortified with iron. Those individuals who are already malnourished are at a greater risk of iron deficiency.[1]

## Iron Loss

Iron deficiency secondary to underlying disease is common and is typically associated with blood loss or malabsorption. Blood loss may occur after trauma or surgery, from intestinal parasites (eg hookworm colonization), or from inflammatory bowel disease (IBD), and may contribute to iron deficiency.[1] Because iron is incorporated into hemoglobin and myoglobin in RBCs, if blood loss occurs, the iron contained in these blood cells will be lost as well. Peptic ulcer disease may cause bleeding in the GI tract, negatively affecting iron stores. Athletes who experience exercise-induced intravascular hemolysis have increased excretion of iron in the urine. On the other hand, extravascular hemolysis is not associated with iron loss. Perhaps the most common form of iron loss is that seen in menstruating people, who may experience an iron loss of 1 mg/d, commonly exceeding individual dietary intake. Over time, chronic blood loss may be substantial enough to cause iron deficiency.[15]

# Malabsorption

Disorders that cause malabsorption in the GI tract can prevent iron from being adequately absorbed. For example, patients who have undergone surgical resections may develop iron deficiency; various bariatric surgeries, duodenal bypass, or gastrectomy can all reduce iron absorption by altering the exposure of iron to an acidic environment, reducing the release of heme iron from foods, and reducing the activity of ferrireductase. Patients with uncontrolled IBD, especially Crohn's disease, are at higher risk of oral iron malabsorption; this is due to a combination of factors that include decreased oral intake, increased hepcidin expression from chronic inflammation, and decreased absorptive surface and functional iron transport units in the small intestine.[16,17] Patients with intestinal failure and celiac disease may develop iron deficiency secondary to malabsorption.[1]

# Increased Iron Demand

The body has increased iron demands during periods of rapid growth and development, such as infancy, adolescence, and pregnancy. The combination of a complex absorption process and inability for dietary intake to accommodate increased need places individuals in these periods of life at higher risk for deficiency. Iron needs during pregnancy are heightened during the third trimester, when most iron is transferred from mother to child.[1,15] In the third trimester, the plasma volume expands by approximately 50%; however, RBC production only increases by 25%, resulting in a dilutional reduction in hemoglobin.[18] Individuals of childbearing age also have increased demand during menstruation, above and beyond what may be lost during menses.

# Drug-Induced Causes

Some medications can alter the physiologic absorption of iron. Medications that increase the gastric pH, such as proton pump inhibitors or histamine-2 receptor blockers, will reduce iron availability and uptake. Glucocorticoids, salicylates, and nonsteroidal anti-inflammatory drugs may cause gastritis and GI blood loss, which can lead to an increased risk for iron deficiency.[1] In addition, erythropoiesis-stimulating agents (eg, erythropoietin) increase iron utilization and can induce deficiency if iron is not provided in sufficient amounts.

# Genetic Causes

Any genetic alteration that affects the complex absorption process of iron has the capacity to cause substantial deficiency. The most common genetic mutation that leads to iron deficiency is in the gene called transmembrane protease, serine 6 (*TMPRSS6*), which codes for the protease TMPRSS6 (commonly referred to as matripase-2), a hepatocyte plasma membrane protease that degrades hemojuvelin (HJV). HJV is a coreceptor for bone morphogenetic protein 6 (BMP6), the central pathway for regulating hepcidin expression.[19] When a mutation in *TMPRSS6* is present, the BMP6-HJV pathway is unable to regulate hepcidin expression. Hepcidin levels are consequently high, reducing ferroportin expression, which ultimately reduces the influx of iron into the body.[7] Mutations in *TMPRSS6* have been associated with refractory iron-deficiency anemia, a clinical condition that leads to profound anemia. Other defects in the iron absorption process that lead to reduced intestinal iron absorption, including mutations in genes coding for divalent metal ion transporter 1, ferroportin, hephaestin (an intestinal iron oxidase), and transferrin receptor 2, have been reported.[19]

# Physical and Laboratory Assessment Strategies

Some cases of iron deficiency and iron-deficiency anemia are asymptomatic, with patients showing few or no clinical signs. Abnormalities in hematologic parameters or iron study laboratory findings precede clinical signs or symptoms of iron deficiency and are often the most important indications to initiate treatment before the deficiency becomes symptomatic.[1] Deficiency syndromes are commonly characterized as follows[1,3,10,15]:

- iron deficiency without anemia (subclinical)
- iron deficiency with mild anemia that presents with some changes in laboratory values and some clinical signs
- iron deficiency with severe anemia that presents with overt changes in laboratory values and observable signs and symptoms

Ferritin is a positive acute phase reactant, making it challenging to interpret during the presence of active inflammation. Hepcidin also increases in response to inflammation, inhibiting iron absorption from the intestinal tract and promoting the sequestration of iron within macrophages, leading to a functional iron deficiency.[20] Thus, some practice guidelines have included recommendations regarding the interpretation of iron studies within the setting of an elevated C-reactive protein. For example, the European Crohn's and Colitis Organization recommends using a serum ferritin of 100 ng/mL or less to identify iron deficiency in patients with IBD. In cases where ferritin exceeds 100 ng/mL but transferrin saturation is below 20%, a functional iron deficiency may be present.[21]

The physical and clinical symptoms of iron status are summarized in Box 7.1.[1,3,16,18]

## Hemoglobin and Hematocrit

The most common and important hematologic sign of iron deficiency is downtrending hemoglobin and hematocrit values. Hemoglobin is a polypeptide complex with a ferrous ion in the center that forms the heme group. It is the main protein in RBCs and is what enables them to carry oxygen. When iron supply and storage in the body are insufficient, hemoglobin cannot be adequately synthesized. Consequently, this decreases the number of RBCs being produced by the bone marrow and put into circulation, which in turn causes a decrease in hemoglobin concentration in the blood. Hemoglobin concentration, therefore, is a surrogate marker of the number of functional RBCs in circulation,

---

**BOX 7.1  Physical and Clinical Symptoms of Low Iron Status[1,3,16,18]**

### *Physical symptoms*

Skin[a] (pallor and rough, dry patches)

Oral cavity[a] (angular chelitis [inflammation and breakdown at corners of the mouth], glossitis [red swollen tongue], decreased papillation [decreased size and number of taste buds])

Esophagus (esophageal webs)

Abdomen (chronic gastritis)

Scalp (hair loss)

Nails (koilonychia [spooning of the nails])

### *Clinical symptoms*

Dysphagia[b] (difficulty swallowing)

Dysgeusia[b] (impaired or loss of taste)

Loss of appetite[b]

Pica[b] (consumption or craving of nonfood substances [eg, clay, dirt, ice, paper])

Weakness

Fatigue[c]

Poor body temperature regulation

Dyspnea on exertion[c]

Difficulty with concentration[c]

[a] Rule out deficiencies in B vitamins such as riboflavin and niacin.
[b] Rule out other diagnoses and medical interventions that can result in similar symptoms.
[c] Dyspnea, fatigue, and difficulty concentrating are linked to reduced oxygenation of tissues.

Iron
Deficiency

---

and a decreased concentration implies a reduced capacity of the body to carry oxygen. Hematocrit is a measure of the percentage of blood volume (per 100 mL) made up of RBCs. If the hematocrit concentration is decreased, the total number of functional RBCs usually decreases as well. Therefore, a decrease in a patient's hematocrit value may also suggest a decrease in total RBC count and a reduction in oxygen-carrying capacity in relation to blood volume.[15,22]

These parameters are sensitive to vascular fluid status—values increase during dehydration (due to hemoconcentration) and decrease during volume overload (due to hemodilution). Hematocrit is particularly sensitive to changes in plasma volume and total body water. A small change in plasma volume can have a major effect on the hematocrit value. Hemoglobin concentration is the gold standard for diagnosis of anemia.[1,22]

# Red Blood Cell Indexes

RBC indexes, such as the mean corpuscular volume (MCV), mean corpuscular hemoglobin (MCH), and mean corpuscular hemoglobin concentration (MCHC), are also altered with iron deficiency. These indexes describe the characteristics of RBCs.

- The MCV indicates RBC size and can be directly measured by an automated hematology analyzer.[22] Iron-deficiency anemia manifests as a *microcytic anemia*, meaning that RBCs are smaller than when iron is present in sufficient amounts, and is characterized by a low MCV.[15,18]

- The MCH indicates RBC color and is calculated by dividing the hemoglobin level by the RBC count.[22] Iron-deficiency anemia manifests with a reduced MCH, indicating hypochromic RBCs (pale red rather than the robust red seen when iron stores are adequate).

- Although the MCHC is not useful clinically, iron-deficiency anemia is the only type of nutritional anemia in which the MCHC is routinely low. The MCHC is calculated by dividing the hemoglobin value by the hematocrit value.[22]

# Ferritin

Iron is incorporated into the cellular and serum protein ferritin for storage. Serum ferritin level is a reliable indicator of the total iron pool in the body and the most used clinical screening test for the adequacy of iron stores. A low serum ferritin concentration suggests iron deficiency.[1] However, this laboratory value should be interpreted in the context of the individual, as ferritin is an acute-phase reactant and is elevated during times of inflammation.[22] Ferritin level and transferrin saturation (TSAT) are directly measured from the serum and tend to shift in the same direction as iron status in the body. Total iron-binding capacity (TIBC), being an ex vivo test that requires mixing serum in iron solution and washing, is more difficult for clinicians to conceptualize. The clinician can determine iron status with ferritin and TSAT, without TIBC as a validation. In selected disease states (eg, chronic kidney disease), interventions involve supplementing iron until a specific TSAT is reached.[18,22]

# Serum Iron

Serum iron concentration lacks sensitivity for assessing iron stores in the body and is not the primary or exclusive laboratory test for determining iron deficiency or iron-deficiency anemia.[15,22] When iron is deficient, stores become depleted, and serum values of ferritin are reduced. The body mobilizes iron from these stores and attempts to scavenge free iron from the bloodstream by increasing levels of transferrin, the iron-protein complex responsible for transporting iron. Transferrin binds to circulating iron and is imported into cells after binding to special transferrin receptors on their surfaces for iron utilization at the cellular level. The percentage of iron-binding sites on transferrin that are occupied by iron is clinically expressed as TSAT; a low TSAT is another surrogate marker suggesting iron deficiency.[1,19,23] When transferrin increases, the TIBC, or number of binding sites on transferrin, also increases. The serum iron concentration is usually well controlled by the body and remains relatively stable. Oral iron intake transiently increases serum iron concentration, but the iron is quickly redistributed and excess iron is converted to ferritin to prevent toxicity.

## Soluble Transferrin Receptor

Although not routinely used in the assessment of iron deficiency or iron-deficiency anemia in the United States, the soluble transferrin receptor (sTfR) can help delineate between iron-deficiency anemia and anemia of chronic inflammation. This fragment of a membrane receptor is present at elevated levels in iron-deficiency anemia but is unaffected in anemia of chronic inflammation.[15,18] sTfR concentration is employed more widely outside the United States and is included in the World Health Organization recommendations for assessing iron status.[24] Some academic medical centers are starting to use it, but clinicians' experience with this marker is still limited in the United States.[25]

## Hepcidin

Although not routinely used to assess iron deficiency or iron-deficiency anemia in the United States, hepcidin concentration has been endorsed by the European Society for Clinical Nutrition and Metabolism, with a grade A recommendation to include it in the assessment for iron-deficiency anemia in conjunction with STfR.[26] Because hepcidin affects iron absorption and distribution, it is logical to continue to investigate it as a biomarker of iron status in patients experiencing inflammation. Table 7.3 on page 136 summarizes the key laboratory tests for iron status.[1,15,18,22,23,27-29]

# Treatment, Monitoring, and Evaluation

In addition to increased dietary intake of iron, iron repletion is a key component in managing iron deficiency or iron-deficiency anemia. Historically, oral supplements have been used before advancing to intravenous replacement products. Although new data for certain patient populations (eg, those with active IBD) suggest that intravenous products may be used as first-line replacement therapy, these findings may not extend to other patient populations.[30] Intravenous repletion carries the risk of hyperchromatosis because iron does not leave the body once administered. More important, most established intravenous iron regimens were developed in the context of patients with chronic kidney disease (CKD) who were receiving hemodialysis, and hematopoietic responses in that population differ from those in patients with IBD and other illnesses unrelated to CKD.

# Treatment: Oral Iron

Numerous oral forms of nonheme iron have been developed. Three—ferrous fumarate, ferrous sulfate, and ferrous gluconate—are widely used in the United States. These provide readily absorbable iron, as ferrous iron does not need to be reduced by ferrireductase for absorption in the duodenum. In addition, these products are less expensive than newer products such as polysaccharide-iron complex.[30,31] Clinical responses to them are also more predictable, and dose modification strategies are better understood.

Polysaccharide-iron complex is a trivalent iron supplement that is highly water soluble and associated with fewer adverse effects.[31] Despite the favorable adverse-effect profile of this preparation, a single-center, randomized, double-blind, superiority trial comparing polysaccharide-iron complex with ferrous sulfate for the treatment of nutritional anemia (with dosages providing equal amounts of elemental iron) showed that infants and young children had a substantially lower hemoglobin response with polysaccharide-iron complex. Interestingly, however, this study showed a substantial improvement in successful administration with the complex, possibly due to its improved taste and better adverse-effect profile.[32]

In 2019, ferric maltol, a nonsalt oral iron preparation, was approved by the US Food and Drug Administration (FDA) for use in adults.[25,30] This newer formulation is a complex of ferric iron and the carbohydrate trimaltol. Trimaltol increases the bioavailability of the iron, allowing for administration of lower doses of elemental iron that still provide therapeutic effects.[30,33]

Oral heme iron products are also available but head-to-head comparative trials between heme and nonheme supplements are lacking.

**TABLE 7.3 Laboratory Tests for Iron Status**[1,15,18,22,23,27-29]

| Test | Reference range[a] | Iron deficiency without anemia[b] | Iron deficiency with mild anemia[b] | Iron deficiency with severe anemia | Comments[c] |
|---|---|---|---|---|---|
| Hemoglobin (Hb) | M: 14.0-17.5 g/dL<br>F: 12.3-15.3 g/dL | M: 14.0-17.5 g/dL<br>F: 12.3-15.3 g/dL | 9 to 12 g/dL | 6-7 g/dL | A measure of the oxygen-carrying capacity of blood<br>Sensitive to fluid status<br>Gold standard for the diagnosis of anemia but does not indicate the cause |
| Hematocrit (Hct) | M: 42%-50%<br>F: 36%-45% | M: 42%-50%<br>F: 36%-45% | NA | NA | Percentage of the volume of blood that is composed of red blood cells<br>Generally three times the Hb concentration in a stable person without fluid disorders<br>Sensitive to fluid status<br>May indicate anemia but does not indicate the cause and is less reliable than Hb |
| Red blood cell (RBC) count | M: 4.5-5.9 x 10⁶ cells/mcL<br>F: 4.1-5.1 x 10⁶ cells/mcL | Normal | Normal or low | Low | Number of RBCs in a given amount of blood<br>May be abnormal for reasons other than iron deficiency<br>Sensitive to fluid status |
| Mean corpuscular volume (MCV) | 80-100 fL | Normal | Normal or low | Low | Measure of the size or cell volume of RBCs<br>In addition to iron, may be low in other forms of microcytic anemia |

| | | Normal | Normal or low | Low | |
|---|---|---|---|---|---|
| Mean corpuscular hemoglobin (MCH) | 26-34 pg/cell | | | Low | Measure of the concentration of hemoglobin in RBCs, as indicated by RBC color |
| Ferritin | 12-300 ng/mL | <30 ng/mL[d] | <12-15[d] ng/mL | <12 ng/mL | Storage form of iron; not sensitive for iron deficiency<br>Positive acute-phase reactant (increases with inflammation) |
| Transferrin | 300-360 mcg/dL | 300-390 mcg/dL | 350-400 mcg/dL | >410 mcg/dL | Iron transport protein<br>Not specific for iron-deficiency anemia<br>Negative acute-phase reactant (decreases with inflammation) |
| Transferrin saturation (TSAT) | 20%-50% | 20% | <15% | <10% | (Serum iron/TIBC) x 100<br>Percentage of iron-binding sites occupied with iron<br>Responsive to inflammation |
| Mean corpuscular hemoglobin concentration (MCHC) | 33-36 g/dL | Normal | Normal or low | Low | Only consistently low in iron-deficiency anemia, not in other types |
| Total iron-binding capacity (TIBC) | 300-360 mcg/dL | 300-390 mcg/dL | 350-400 mcg/dL | >410 mcg/dL | Capacity for transferrin to bind iron<br>Not specific for iron-deficiency anemia; also elevated in anemia of inflammation |

*Continued on next page*

**TABLE 7.3 Laboratory Tests for Iron Status**[1,15,18,22,23,27,29] (cont.)

| Test | Reference range[a] | Iron deficiency without anemia[b] | Iron deficiency with mild anemia[b] | Iron deficiency with severe anemia | Comments[c] |
|------|------|------|------|------|------|
| Serum iron | 60-160 mcg/dL | Normal or low | Low | Low | Not used to identify iron deficiency or iron-deficiency anemia; Not specific for iron-deficiency anemia; may be normal or elevated in anemia of inflammation |
| Soluble transferrin receptor (sTfR) | M: 1.8-4.6 mg/L F: 1.9-4.4 mg/L | High | High | High | Not commonly used in the United States; more widely used outside the country, primarily as a screening test for iron deficiency or iron-deficiency anemia |
| Hepcidin[e] | M: 18.2-81.5 ng/mL F: 17.2-91.2 ng/mL | Unknown | Low | Low | Not FDA-approved for evaluation of iron deficiency in the United States; reference ranges established from the Namibia population |

Abbreviations: FDA, US Food and Drug Administration; F, females; M, males; NA, not applicable.

[a] May vary based on institutional laboratory.

[b] For gastrointestinal surgery, renal care, critical care and bariatric surgery guidelines, see Chapters 9, 10, 13, and 14, respectively.

[c] Frequency of biochemical monitoring varies based on severity of depletion, presence of overt symptoms, and underlying disease.

[d] Practitioners of adult hematology often use a cutoff of 30 ng/mL, which is supported by bone marrow correlations and international guidelines.

[e] Available research suggests a potential role for hepcidin to diagnosis iron-deficiency anemia; however, more research is needed to understand the fluctuations of hepcidin with various stages of anemia.

Oral heme iron products are usually expensive and may not be acceptable for patients who are vegan.

Impaired oral absorption may occur with a number of medications when taken concurrently with oral iron supplements. The clinician should carefully review the patient's history and medication list before initiating oral iron therapy and should collaborate with other clinicians (eg, a pharmacist) to optimize treatment outcomes. See Box 7.2 on page 140 for a summary of oral iron treatments.[30-35]

# Treatment: Intravenous Iron Repletion

Intravenous iron preparations bypass enteric iron absorption and the complex regulatory process mediated by hepcidin; therefore, they can provide rapid repletion of iron stores. However, because intravenous iron administration results in 100% bioavailability and there is no intrinsic mechanism by the body to effectively remove iron once administered, practitioners must take caution to prevent acute and chronic iron overdose. Although intravenous iron products have different characteristics that affect their clinical use, the structure of these products is the same. They are all colloidal suspensions of spherical particles that contain a polynuclear iron-oxyhydroxide gel core and a polymer shell, which is often made of carbohydrate derivatives.[30,31] Once in the bloodstream, the iron-carbohydrate complexes undergo phagocytosis by macrophages, are released into an intracellular iron pool, and are incorporated into transferrin or ferritin.[36] Despite having a common structure, intravenous iron preparations vary in their chemical properties, the size of their polymer shell, the size of their core, and the strength of the bond between their polymer shell and iron-containing core.[30,36,37]

The challenge for most intravenous iron products is that the FDA-approved indications and regimens were developed for patients with CKD, and the dosages are determined using hemoglobin concentration. Although some studies have used iron deficit as the basis for dosing, the results have been inconsistent. More important, using many of these products in patients without CKD is technically an "off-label" use. Table 7.4 on page 142 provides a comparison of intravenous iron products.[38-44]

## BOX 7.2  Common Oral Iron Preparations[30-35]

### *Ferrous fumarate*

| | |
|---|---|
| **Dosing** | 106 mg iron[a] one to three times per day |
| | New data may support lower or alternate-day dosing |
| **Features** | Readily absorbable |
| | Provides ferrous iron |
| | Provides 33% elemental iron based on the strength listed on the product label |
| | Increased chance of gastrointestinal side effects |

### *Ferrous sulfate*

| | |
|---|---|
| **Dosing** | 65 mg iron[a] one to three times per day |
| | New data may support lower or alternate-day dosing |
| **Features** | Provides ferrous iron |
| | Provides 20% elemental iron based on the strength listed on the product label |
| | Increased chance of gastrointestinal side effects |
| | Used in patients on dialysis |

### *Ferrous gluconate*

| | |
|---|---|
| **Dosing** | 35 mg iron[a] one to three times per day |
| | New data may support lower or alternate-day dosing |
| **Features** | Provides ferrous iron |
| | Provides 11.6% elemental iron based on the strength listed on the product label |
| | Increased chance of gastrointestinal side effects |

### *Polysaccharide-iron complex*

| | |
|---|---|
| **Dosing** | 50 to 200 mg[a] daily |
| **Features** | Provides 100% elemental iron based on the strength listed on the product label |

**BOX 7.2  Common Oral Iron Preparations[30-35] (cont.)**

**Ferric maltol**

| | |
|---|---|
| **Dosing** | 30 mg[a] twice daily |
| **Features** | Nonsalt iron-trimaltol (carbohydrate) complex |
| | Absorbed within enterocyte |
| | Fewer gastrointestinal side effects because it provides ferric iron |
| | Provides 30 mg elemental iron and 201.5 mg maltol based on the strength listed on the product label |

[a] The amount of elemental iron provided is based on the strength of the formulation. For example, if a product labeled iron sulfate, 240 mg, is listed as 20% elemental iron, 48 mg elemental iron is provided per tablet.

## Adverse Effects

Intravenous iron products are notorious for their adverse-effect profile. The quantity and severity of these adverse reactions is inversely proportional to the size of the iron polymer and strength of the iron-polymer complex.[36] Among the available intravenous products, the rate of iron release into the systemic circulation varies with the type of carbohydrate coating used and the technology used in incorporating the iron within the complex. Formulations with a less stable bond will release some iron into the bloodstream before the complex undergoes phagocytosis by macrophages.[30,36,37] If more iron is released than can be bound by circulating transferrin, this free iron can produce oxidative stress, hypotension, and other adverse effects.[30,36,37] Experts postulate that free iron is the cause of multiple reactions including arthralgias, myalgias, back pain, flushing, headache, chest pressure, nausea, diarrhea, and low-grade fever.[34]

Adverse effects can be acute (occurring immediately after infusion), delayed (occurring hours up to 1 day after infusion), or long-term (occurring days after the infusion). Acute reactions are most likely to be caused by the effects of labile free iron and are generally mild and transient. The most common delayed reactions are arthralgias and myalgias. Data supporting long-term reactions are weak but may support an increase in

Iron
Deficiency

**TABLE 7.4 Comparison of Intravenous Iron Products**[38-44]

| Product | Polymer shell (size in daltons) | Black box warning / Test dose required? | Dosing (adult unless noted) | Comments |
|---|---|---|---|---|
| Low-molecular-weight iron dextran | Dextran polysaccharides (150,000-165,000) | Yes/Yes | Based on iron deficit[a] Can use total dose repletion | Black box warning for anaphylaxis |
| Iron sucrose | Sucrose (34,000-60,000) | No/No | Based on iron deficit[a] Maximum dose (adults): 200 mg per infusion Maximum dose (pediatrics): 100 mg per infusion Prescribed in eight doses of 125 mg for adults and 0.5 mg per kilogram of body weight for children | Commonly used in patients with gastrointestinal disease |
| Sodium ferric gluconate | Gluconate (289,000-444,000) | No/No | 125 mg for eight doses | Commonly used for patients receiving dialysis |
| Ferumoxytol | Polyglucose sorbitol carboxymethylether (750,000) | Yes/No | 510 mg for one dose, followed by 510 mg 3-8 d later | Black box warning for hypersensitivity (symptomatic hypotension) May interfere with magnetic resonance imaging |

| | | | | |
|---|---|---|---|---|
| Ferric carboxymaltose | Carboxymaltose (150,000) | No/No | 15 mg per kilogram of body weight (maximum 750 mg per dose), repeat 7 d later if necessary | Strong iron-carbohydrate complex that allows for larger dose infusions<br><br>May cause transient hypophosphatemia because of induction of fibroblast growth factor 23, which regulates phosphate |
| Ferric derisomaltose | Derisomaltose (155,000) | No/No | 1,000 mg per dose | Marketed in Europe as iron isomaltoside<br><br>New iron matrix structure allows for slower release |

[a] Iron deficit is estimated using many different equations. Preferred equations may vary between products and institutions.

mortality if cumulative doses exceed 1 g iron intravenously in 6 months.[37] The iron-oxyhydroxide complex may trigger the release of complement. This will activate other immune-related cells (eg, mast cells) to release vasoactive mediators (eg, histamine).[17] This is considered a complement activation–related pseudoallergy, which is generally mild and self-limiting but may lead to rash, pruritis, headache, flushing, or nausea and vomiting.[17,37] Most of these reactions subside with a reduction in the infusion rate or after stopping the infusion. If patients experience these symptoms, future infusions are not contraindicated, but patients may benefit from a slower infusion rate or a more dilute infusion.[17] Premedication with diphenhydramine, hydrocortisone, or epinephrine, alone or in combination, has historically been used but has fallen out of favor, as these medications may cause vasoactive reactions that can be falsely attributed to the intravenous iron infusion.[25] Rare cases of anaphylaxis have been reported, with symptoms including urticaria, angioedema, bronchospasm, hypotension, and bradycardia. If this occurs, resuscitation measures should be taken and the patient should not receive infusions of the causative formulation in the future.[37]

# Monitoring and Evaluation

Once iron therapy has been initiated, the clinician should assess the patient to determine effectiveness of the therapy and periodically reevaluate the need for continued treatment. The patient should also be monitored for iron overload syndrome (ie, hemochromatosis), which is often associated with a genetic condition. However, secondary iron overload may occur when the hepcidin regulation pathway is bypassed, as with intravenous iron products, or if the patient requires RBC transfusions.[38,39] Patients who receive RBC transfusions should be given intravenous iron preparations with the understanding that the iron contained in the donor blood cells will be recycled in the same fashion as in endogenous RBCs, and will be available for hematopoiesis in approximately 60 to 90 days. If iron and RBC transfusions are given concurrently, the delayed availability of iron from transfused RBCs should be considered when calculating iron dosage. Patients with active systemic infections should not receive iron supplementation.[6,45]

Once iron repletion begins, laboratory parameters start to normalize at different rates. The serum reticulocyte count starts to increase within days. A detectable increase in hemoglobin concentration is usually seen within 2 to 3 weeks, indicating a positive response.[10] In general, hemoglobin levels increase more rapidly at the start of therapy (1 to 2 g/dL during the first 2 weeks) and then level out at 0.7 to 1 g/dL per week until concentrations normalize.[10] Depending on the severity of the deficiency, iron stores may take more than 6 months to fully replete.[7] Serum ferritin is the preferred value for monitoring iron stores.[1,18,22,34] Although no consensus exists regarding standardized intervals for monitoring response to therapy, clinicians should check laboratory parameters routinely. Once treatment begins, a complete blood count and iron studies should be conducted every 1 to 3 months, depending on the stability of the patient. In addition, the patient's food records and adherence to supplementation should be assessed. In severe anemia, many clinicians assess the reticulocyte count earlier (after 1 month) to evaluate the current dosing regimen. Although no evidence exists to support this practice, it may provide insight into the direction of RBC production, which serves as a surrogate marker for future development of anemia.

# References

1. Camaschella C. Iron-deficiency anemia. *N Engl J Med*. 2015;372(19): 1832-1843. doi:10.1056/NEJMra1401038

2. Rizvi S, Schoen RE. Supplementation with oral vs. intravenous iron for anemia with IBD or gastrointestinal bleeding: is oral iron getting a bad rap? *Am J Gastroenterol*. 2011;106(11):1872-1879. doi:10.1038/ajg.2011.232

3. Heuberger RA. Diseases of the hematological system. In: Nelms M, Sucher K, eds. *Nutrition Therapy and Pathophysiology*, 4th ed. Cengage; 2022:568-602.

4. Institute of Medicine (US) Panel on Micronutrients. Iron. In: *Dietary Reference Intakes for Vitamin A, Vitamin K, Arsenic, Boron, Chromium, Copper, Iodine, Iron, Manganese, Molybdenum, Nickel, Silicon, Vanadium, and Zinc*. National Academies Press; 2001:chap 9. www.ncbi.nlm.nih.gov/books /NBK222309

5. McKeever L. Vitamins and trace elements. In: Mueller CM, ed. *The ASPEN Adult Core Curriculum*. 3rd ed. American Society for Parenteral and Enteral Nutrition; 2017:139-182.

6.  Chifman J, Laubenbacher R, Torti SV. A systems biology approach to iron metabolism. *Adv Exp Med Biol.* 2014;844:201-225. doi:10.1007/978-1 -4939-2095-2_10

7.  Fuqua BK, Vulpe CD, Anderson GJ. Intestinal iron absorption. *J Trace Elem Med Biol.* 2012;26(2-3):115-119. doi:10.1016/j.jtemb.2012.03.015

8.  Yanatori I, Richardson DR, Toyokuni S, Kishi F. How iron is handled in the course of heme catabolism: integration of heme oxygenase with intracellular iron transport mechanisms mediated by poly (rC)-binding protein-2. *Arch Biochem Biophys.* 2019;672:108071. doi:10.1016/j.abb.2019.108071

9.  Stoffel NU, Zeder C, Brittenham GM, Moretti D, Zimmermann MB. Iron absorption from supplements is greater with alternate day than with consecutive day dosing in iron-deficient anemic women. *Haematologica.* 2020;105(5):1232-1239. doi:10.3324/haematol.2019.220830

10. Chan LN, Mike LA. The science and practice of micronutrient supplementations in nutritional anemia: an evidence-based review. *JPEN J Parenter Enteral Nutr.* 2014;38(6):656-672. doi:10.1177 /0148607114533726

11. Troost FJ, Brummer RJ, Dainty JR, Hoogewerff JA, Bull VJ, Saris WH. Iron supplements inhibit zinc but not copper absorption in vivo in ileostomy subjects. *Am J Clin Nutr.* 2003;78(5):1018-1023. doi:10.1093/ajcn /78.5.1018

12. Hooda J, Shah A, Zhang L. Heme, an essential nutrient from dietary proteins, critically impacts diverse physiological and pathological processes. *Nutrients.* 2014;6(3):1080-1102. doi:10.3390/nu6031080

13. Napolitano M, Dolce A, Celenza G, et al. Iron-dependent erythropoiesis in women with excessive menstrual blood losses and women with normal menses. *Ann Hematol.* 2014;93(4):557-563. doi:10.1007/s00277-013-1901-3

14. Ziegler EE. Consumption of cow's milk as a cause of iron deficiency in infants and toddlers. *Nutr Rev.* 2011;69(suppl 1):S37-S42. doi:10.1111/j.1753 -4887.2011.00431.x

15. DeLoughery TG. Microcytic anemia. *N Engl J Med.* 2014;371(14): 1324-1331. doi:10.1056/NEJMra1215361

16. Mattiello V, Schmugge M, Hengartner H, von der Weid N, Renella R; SPOG Pediatric Hematology Working Group. Diagnosis and management of iron deficiency in children with or without anemia: consensus recommendations of the SPOG Pediatric Hematology Working Group. *Eur J Pediatr.* 2020;179(4):527-545. doi:10.1007/s00431 -020-03597-5

17. Goyal A, Zheng Y, Albenberg LG, et al. Anemia in children with inflammatory bowel disease: a position paper by the IBD Committee of the North American Society of Pediatric Gastroenterology, Hepatology and Nutrition. *J Pediatr Gastroenterol Nutr.* 2020;71(4):563-582. doi:10.1097 /MPG.0000000000002885

Iron
Deficiency

18. Kujovich JL. Evaluation of anemia. *Obstet Gynecol Clin North Am.* 2016;43(2):247-264. doi:10.1016/j.ogc.2016.01.009

19. Anderson GJ, Frazer DM, McLaren GD. Iron absorption and metabolism. *Curr Opin Gastroenterol.* 2009;25(2):129-135. doi:10.1097/MOG.0b013e32831ef1f7

20. Dignass A, Farrag K, Stein J. Limitations of serum ferritin in diagnosing iron deficiency in inflammatory conditions. *Int J Chronic Dis.* 2018;2018:9394060. doi:10.1155/2018/9394060

21. Dignass AU, Gasche C, Bettenworth D, et al. European consensus on the diagnosis and management of iron deficiency and anaemia in inflammatory bowel diseases. *J Crohns Colitis.* 2015;9(3):211-222. doi:10.1093/ecco-jcc/jju009

22. Hutson PR. Hematology: red and white blood cell tests. In: Lee M, ed. *Basic Skills in Interpreting Laboratory Data.* 3rd ed. American Society of Health-System Pharmacists; 2004:441-467.

23. Buttarello M, Pajola R, Novello E, Mezzapelle G, Plebani M. Evaluation of the hypochromic erythrocyte and reticulocyte hemoglobin content provided by the Sysmex XE-5000 analyzer in diagnosis of iron deficiency erythropoiesis. *Clin Chem Lab Med.* 2016;54(12):1939-1945. doi:10.1515/cclm-2016-0041

24. *WHO Guideline on Use of Ferritin Concentrations to Assess Iron Status in Individuals and Populations.* World Health Organization; 2020. www.who.int/publications/i/item/9789240000124

25. Chang J, Bird R, Clague A, Carter A. Clinical utility of serum soluble transferrin receptor levels and comparison with bone marrow iron stores as an index for iron-deficient erythropoiesis in a heterogeneous group of patients. *Pathology.* 2007;39(3):349-353. doi:10.1080/00313020701329732

26. Berger MM, Shenkin A, Schweinlin A, et al. ESPEN micronutrient guideline. *Clin Nutr.* 2022;41(6):1357-1424. doi:10.1016/j.clnu.2022.02.015

27. Pavord S, Daru J, Prasannan N, et al. UK guidelines on the management of iron deficiency in pregnancy. *Br J Haematol.* 2020;188(6):819-830. doi:10.1111/bjh.16221

28. Short MW, Domagalski JE. Iron deficiency anemia: evaluation and management. *Am Fam Physician.* 2013;87(2):98-104.

29. van den Broek NR, Letsky EA, White SA, Shenkin A. Iron status in pregnant women: which measurements are valid? *Br J Haematol.* 1998;103(3):817-824. doi:10.1046/j.1365-2141.1998.01035.x

30. Girelli D, Ugolini S, Busti F, Marchi G, Castagna A. Modern iron replacement therapy: clinical and pathophysiological insights. *Int J Hematol.* 2018;107(1):16-30. doi:10.1007/s12185-017-2373-3

31. Liu T, Liu T, Liu H, et al. Preparation and characterization of a novel polysaccharide-iron (III) complex in *Auricularia auricula* potentially used as an iron supplement. *Biomed Res Int*. 2019:6416941. doi:10.1155/2019/6416941

32. Powers JM, Buchanan GR, Adix L, Zhang S, Gao A, McCavit TL. Effect of low-dose ferrous sulfate vs iron polysaccharide complex on hemoglobin concentration in young children with nutritional iron-deficiency anemia: a randomized clinical trial. *JAMA*. 2017;317(22):2297-2304. doi:10.1001/jama.2017.6846

33. Khoury A, Pagan KA, Farland MZ. Ferric maltol: a new oral iron formulation for the treatment of iron deficiency in adults. *Ann Pharmacother*. 2021;55(2):222-229. doi:10.1177/1060028020941014

34. Kumar A, Sharma E, Marley A, Samaan MA, Brookes MJ. Iron deficiency anaemia: pathophysiology, assessment, practical management. *BMJ Open Gastroenterol*. 2022;9(1):e000759. doi:10.1136/bmjgast-2021-000759

35. Monoferric (ferric derisomaltose). Package insert. Pharmacosmos; January 2020.

36. Mantadakis E. Advances in pediatric intravenous iron therapy. *Pediatr Blood Cancer*. 2016;63(1):11-16. doi:10.1002/pbc.25752

37. Bircher AJ, Auerbach M. Hypersensitivity from intravenous iron products. *Immunol Allergy Clin North Am*. 2014;34(3):707-723, x-xi. doi:10.1016/j.iac.2014.04.013

38. Kumpf VJ. Update on parenteral iron therapy. *Nutr Clin Pract*. 2003;18(4):318-326. doi:10.1177/0115426503018004318

39. Hampson K, Nguyen T. A review of intravenous iron replacement medications for nurse practitioners. *J Nurs Pract*. 2020;16(3):224-227.

40. Accrufer (ferric maltol). Package insert. Shield Pharmaceuticals; July 2019.

41. Iron polysaccharide complex. Lexicomp. Wolters Kluwer. Accessed January 14, 2024. https://online.lexi.com/lco/action/search?q=6800&nq=true&t=globalid&origin=api

42. Iron sucrose. Package insert. American Regent; 2015.

43. Ferrlecit. Package insert. Sanofi Aventis; 2015.

44. Ferumoxytol. Package insert. Patheon Manufacturing; 2015.

45. Baker RD, Greer FR; Committee on Nutrition American Academy of Pediatrics. Diagnosis and prevention of iron deficiency and iron-deficiency anemia in infants and young children (0-3 years of age). *Pediatrics*. 2010;126(5):1040-1050. doi:10.1542/peds.2010-2576

Iron
Deficiency

CHAPTER 8

# Deficiencies in Trace Minerals

Holly Estes-Doetsch, MS, RDN, LD and
Lingtak-Neander Chan, PharmD, BCNSP, FCCP, FASPEN

## Introduction

Trace minerals, including chromium, copper, fluoride, iodine, iron, manganese, selenium, and zinc, are required in small amounts (less than 100 mg/d) and are essential for physiologic function. As many trace mineral deficiencies are relatively rare, this chapter focuses on those that occur most frequently in patients who are not receiving nutrition support—namely, copper, selenium, and zinc. Iron deficiency is covered in detail in Chapter 7.

Copper, selenium, and zinc all function as part of metalloenzymes to facilitate metabolic processes and support antioxidant defense systems. The roles of each are described further in the sections that follow. Absorption occurs in the stomach (copper), duodenum (copper, selenium, zinc), and proximal jejunum (zinc).[1] The Dietary Reference Intakes for trace minerals are presented in Box 8.1.[2]

**BOX 8.1** Dietary Reference Intakes for Trace Minerals for Nonpregnant Adults[2]

## Chromium (Adequate Intake [AI])

**Age 19 to 50 years**
Males: 35 mcg
Females: 25 mcg

**Age over 50 years**
Males: 30 mcg
Females: 20 mcg

## Copper (Recommended Dietary Allowance [RDA])
Males: 900 mcg
Females: 900 mcg

## Fluoride (AI)
Males: 4 mg
Females: 3 mg

## Iodine (RDA)
Males: 150 mcg
Females: 150 mcg

## Manganese (AI)
Males: 2.3 mg
Females: 1.8 mg

## Selenium (RDA)
Males: 55 mcg
Females: 55 mcg

## Zinc (RDA)
Males: 11 mg
Females: 8 mg

# Pathophysiology of Deficiencies

Aside from prolonged inadequate dietary intake, other causes of copper, selenium, or zinc deficiencies include substantial losses secondary to renal replacement therapy,[3] malabsorptive conditions, bariatric surgery (Chapter 14), other gastrointestinal surgery (Chapter 9), and wounds (Chapter 11).[4,5] Menkes disease and primary acrodermatitis enteropathica are genetic conditions that impair intestinal copper[4] and zinc[6] transport, respectively.

# Physical and Biochemical Assessments

A range of clinical signs and symptoms affecting the eyes, hair, skin, nails, gastrointestinal tract, immune function, and nervous system have been associated with trace mineral deficiency. Obtaining a serum or plasma concentration is the most common biochemical assessment strategy for trace mineral status in clinical practice settings. However, clinicians should be familiar with the limitations of this strategy in order to interpret test results appropriately; low plasma concentrations may not accurately reflect the functional status of these trace elements. Inflammatory processes, through altering hepatic production of select carrier proteins, influence serum levels of most trace elements (refer to Chapter 4); thus, C-reactive protein levels should routinely be monitored in conjunction with blood trace mineral concentrations.[7] Additional points regarding inflammation and trace minerals include:

- Approximately 90% of circulating copper is bound to ceruloplasmin, which is upregulated in the setting of systemic inflammation. This promotes elevations in serum copper and may mask a functional deficiency.[4]

- Serum zinc decreases rapidly with inflammation, likely because of an increased intracellular uptake of zinc, zinc's reliance on albumin for circulatory transport, and reduced hepatic albumin production within the setting of metabolic stress.

- Decreased hepatic synthesis of selenoprotein P, the primary selenium transport protein, has also been noted during inflammatory states.

# Copper Deficiency

Copper-dependent metalloenzymes ("cuproenzymes") serve as cofactors for growth and connective tissue development, energy metabolism, neurotransmitter synthesis, myelination of the nervous system, and melanin production.[4,8,9] As a component of superoxide dismutase enzymes 1 and 2, copper plays a critical role in combating oxidative stress.[10] Copper is also integrated into the ferroxidase enzymes hephaestin and ceruloplasmin, which regulate iron absorption and mobilization, respectively.[4,8] As a result, copper deficiency may interfere with hemoglobin synthesis, leading to anemia. Research has shown that copper deficiency–induced anemia resolves with copper repletion, as has leukopenia, another hematologic alteration associated with copper depletion.[8] Myeloneuropathy has been described in case reports of copper deficiency, but functional deficits may continue to persist after copper replacement therapy.[10] Other reported neurological symptoms of deficiency include optic neuropathy, irritation, psychosis, and ataxia. Less commonly, researchers have noted depigmentation of the hair or skin.[4]

## Screening and Assessment

Copper deficiencies have been reported with long-term jejunal feedings, as most copper absorption is limited to the stomach and duodenum. Interestingly, administration of 10 to 40 g cocoa powder (which contains 0.04 mg copper per gram) has been shown to correct copper levels in some patients fed via jejunostomy.[11,12] Other reports have not observed increased jejunal copper provision to be effective, and patients required gastric or parenteral copper therapy to resolve the deficiency.[13]

Excessive zinc intake, such as through chronic high-dose zinc therapy (>50 mg/d elemental zinc)[14] or the use of zinc-containing denture adhesives or creams,[10] poses risks for copper deficiency by increasing the synthesis of metallothionein in intestinal cells. Metallothionein has a high affinity for copper, and when expressed in high levels in the enterocytes, it decreases the intestinal absorption of copper by trapping it in the cytoplasm of the enterocyte.[8,10] Thus, copper and zinc status should be evaluated concurrently in these cases.

Except under conditions of Wilson disease and aceruloplasminemia, serum or plasma copper and its transport protein, ceruloplasmin, are considered suitable indicators of copper status in practice.[15,16] Impaired activity of superoxide dismutase is a potential functional marker of copper deficiency, but alterations in this enzyme may not manifest until later stages of deficiency.[4]

# Selenium Deficiency

In the 1930s, widespread and often fatal cardiac abnormalities were first reported in Keshan County, an area of China with low soil selenium content, though they have since been reported in several other rural and remote areas of China in association with poor selenium intake.[17] Selenium exerts its functional effects as selenocysteine, which is integrated into proteins. Selenoproteins comprise several enzyme systems that combat reactive oxygen species and support immune health, including glutathione peroxidases, thioredoxin reductases, and methionine sulfoxide reductases.[18,19] Experts theorize that selenoprotein P, a major transporter of selenium in plasma, possesses antioxidant properties. Glutathione peroxidases, in particular, protect cell function across multiple organ systems.[20] Severe selenium deficiency may promote increased oxidative stress in myocardial cells, leading to heart failure.[21] Several case reports have described patients with cardiomyopathy in the presence of selenium depletion, also known as Keshan disease, which improved following selenium replacement therapy.[21-26] Many of these patients had a history of gastrointestinal disease or surgery.

## Screening and Assessment

Additional symptoms noted in association with selenium deficiency include muscle weakness or pain secondary to skeletal myopathy and lightening of the hair, skin, and nail beds.[27,28] These overt physical manifestations of selenium deficiency are rare and have been primarily described in case reports of patients receiving selenium-free enteral or parenteral nutrition support.[28-30] Other selenoproteins, the iodo-thyronine deiodinases, support the conversion of thyroxine ($T_4$) into triiodothyronine ($T_3$)[18,20]; thus, selenium deficiency may also impair thyroid hormone activity.[31,32] However, limited evidence has not shown either plasma $T_4$ or the ratio of $T_3$ to $T_4$ to be an effective biomarker of selenium status.[33]

The Dietary Reference Intakes for selenium are based on optimal levels of glutathione peroxidase as a functional indicator of selenium status,[34] but in practice, serum, plasma, or whole blood selenium levels are often obtained to monitor patients at high risk of deficiency.[7] Alopecia, brittle nails, diarrhea, garlic breath odor, and impaired memory and mental focus have been reported as symptoms of selenium toxicity[19,35]; thus, monitoring to assess the appropriateness of selenium replacement therapy is essential.

# Zinc Deficiency

The consequences of zinc deficiency are vast, which may be attributed to its multifaceted actions in maintaining human health. As a constituent of approximately 300 metalloenzymes, a structural component of proteins and transcription factors, and a nutrient with several regulatory roles, zinc is vital in catalyzing the metabolic reactions needed for energy pathways, tissue accretion and maintenance, gut mucosa support, and immune function.[5]

## Screening and Assessment

Adverse effects of deficiency include seborrheic dermatitis, delayed wound healing, hair loss, anorexia, decreased reproductive function, and increased risk for infection. Though the mechanism is unclear, zinc deficiency impairs sensory function, leading to altered or reduced taste or smell. Studies have noted a high prevalence of zinc deficiency in hospitalized patients with anorexia nervosa (24%–64.3%).[31,36] In light of the adverse effects of zinc deficiency on taste perception and appetite, this finding may have potential implications for refeeding and weight restoration in these individuals, but more research is needed. Zinc also promotes the secretion of growth factors, and deficiency is associated with poor linear growth in children, independent of energy and protein intake.[5]

Although gastrointestinal zinc losses may be substantial in individuals with high-output fistulas, ostomies, reduced functional length of the gastrointestinal tract, or diarrheal illnesses, diarrhea may also develop in response to zinc deficiency and perpetuate zinc losses. A Cochrane review found that zinc supplementation of 10 to 20 mg/d may reduce the duration of acute and persistent diarrhea in young children (<5 years) in developing countries,[37] though the effects in adults are unknown.

Serum or plasma zinc are common laboratory markers of zinc status in practice, but due to homeostatic mechanisms, these concentrations may not accurately reflect the functional status of zinc in the body.[5] Hair zinc concentration has been investigated as a marker of total body zinc status, but is not routinely used as contamination of the sample is a concern.[38] A low level of alkaline phosphatase, a zinc-dependent enzyme, in conjunction with risk factors (eg, increased zinc losses) may trigger suspicion for zinc deficiency. Alkaline phosphatase is associated with zinc status and studies have shown that it increases in response to zinc supplementation in pediatric studies.[39-41] However, these findings have not been consistently replicated in adults.[42]

Supplemental zinc may be more effectively absorbed when taken on an empty stomach and apart from iron supplementation. Phytic acids chelate with zinc in the intestinal lumen and inhibit its absorption, whereas iron and zinc compete for intestinal uptake.[5] Though zinc toxicity is somewhat rare due to intestinal regulation of zinc homeostasis, practitioners should take care to avoid long-term use of supplemental zinc because of its adverse effect on copper absorption. In individuals requiring long-term zinc therapy, concurrent copper supplementation with routine laboratory monitoring of both micronutrients may be warranted.

# Summary of Assessment Strategies

Assessment strategies for copper, selenium, and zinc are summarized in Box 8.2.[28-30,38,43]

## BOX 8.2 Assessment Strategies for Trace Mineral Status[28-30,38,43]

### *Copper*

**Pertinent biochemical tests**

Copper (serum or plasma)

Ceruloplasmin

C-reactive protein

Complete blood count (anemia, leukopenia, thrombocytopenia)

**Clinical assessment of deficiency**

Hair: depigmentation

Skin: depigmentation

Altered gait, peripheral neuropathy, vision loss

**Special considerations**

Copper is a positive acute-phase reactant.

Include a serum zinc test if supplemental zinc is used for more than 3 months. Determine if zinc therapy should be discontinued.

If the patient is symptomatic, check vitamin B12 and folate statuses to rule out other deficiencies. Include iron studies if anemia is present.

### *Selenium*

**Pertinent biochemical tests**

Glutathione peroxidase (erythrocyte or plasma), if available

Selenium (serum, plasma, or whole blood)

C-reactive protein

**Clinical assessment of deficiency**

Hair: depigmentation

Skin: depigmentation

Nails: whitening of nail bed

Skeletal muscle or cardiac myopathy, gait ataxia

**Special considerations**

Selenium is a negative acute-phase reactant.

Consider thiamin deficiency as an alternative diagnosis in patients at high risk who present with cardiac symptoms.

*Continued on next page*

**BOX 8.2   Assessment Strategies for Trace Mineral Status[28-30,38,43] (cont.)**

### Zinc

**Pertinent biochemical tests**

Zinc (serum or plasma)

C-reactive protein

Albumin

**Clinical assessment of deficiency**

Hair: alopecia

Skin: acrodermatitis enteropathica, impaired wound healing

Hypogeusia, dysgeusia, hyposmia, anorexia, diarrhea, growth failure (in infants and young children), hypogonadism

**Special considerations**

Zinc is a negative acute-phase reactant.

Zinc levels are falsely low with hypoalbuminemia.

If level is elevated with supplemental zinc use, discontinue zinc therapy and check serum copper.

# Treatment, Monitoring, and Evaluation

Boxes 8.3 on page 158  and 8.4 on page 159 provide an overview of available treatment formulations, dosing strategies, and monitoring considerations for copper, selenium, and zinc therapy.[44-46] Because there is heterogeneity among published dosing strategies, these suggestions do not preclude the use of clinical judgment by health care providers. Oral and parenteral routes are options for trace mineral delivery. For more rapid repletion in individuals experiencing overt symptoms, intravenous micronutrient provision should be considered. Tolerable upper limits have been established for trace minerals, and individuals receiving high doses of these products should be monitored for signs and symptoms of toxicity.

**BOX 8.3   Available Treatment Forms and Suggested Regimens for Treating
Trace Mineral Deficiencies[a,44-46]**

## Copper
### Treatment forms

Oral          Tablets, capsules in various strengths as over-the-counter (OTC)
              dietary supplements

Injection     Cupric chloride or cupric sulfate

### Treatment regimens

*For prevention of copper deficiency*

   0.3 to 0.5 mg/d

*For treatment of hypocupremia*

   Elemental copper, 2 to 8 mg/d, by mouth (PO), in two to three divided doses for
   2 to 3 weeks

   1 to 4 mg mixed in 0.9% sodium chloride, intravenous (IV), daily for 6 to 7 days;
   concentration 0.02 mg/mL or less; infuse over at least 2 hours

## Selenium
### Treatment forms

Oral          Tablets, capsules, and oral liquids in organic and inorganic
              salt forms and various strengths (50 mcg, 100 mcg, 125 mcg,
              200 mcg, oral drops) as OTC dietary supplements

Injection     Selenious acid injection (United States Pharmacopeia) to be
              administered as IV infusion after dilution

### Treatment regimens

For prevention of selenium deficiency: 60 to 100 mcg/d, IV or PO; higher for
at-risk patient populations, such as those with burn injuries

## Zinc
### Treatment forms

Oral          Tablets, capsules in various strengths as OTC dietary supplements

Injection     Multiple salt forms available in the United States

*Continued on next page*

---

**BOX 8.3  Available Treatment Forms and Suggested Regimens for Treating Trace Mineral Deficiencies[a,44-46] (cont.)**

### Treatment regimens

*For treatment of zinc deficiency*

Elemental zinc, 0.5 to 1 mg/kg body weight per day, PO, up to 60 mg two to three times daily

IV zinc in 0.9% sodium chloride; final concentration 0.2 mg/mL or less; infuse over 1 hour via central line

Zinc sulfate is the preferred IV product, based on a large volume of published data. Initial dose should be 250 to 500 mcg/kg/d, divided in two to three doses.

If zinc sulfate is unavailable, zinc chloride can be used with lower concentration (not to exceed 25 mg in 250 mL, or 0.1 mg/mL final concentration).

[a] For specific gastrointestinal surgery, wound, critical care, and bariatric surgery guidelines, see Chapters 9, 11, 13, and 14, respectively.

---

**BOX 8.4  Monitoring and Other Considerations for Trace Mineral Deficiencies[a,44-46]**

## *Copper*

### Monitoring

Monitor serum copper and ceruloplasmin concentrations.

Elevated serum copper and ceruloplasmin alongside normal C-reactive protein (CRP) may indicate toxicity. Biliary disease or obstruction increases toxicity risk.

### Other considerations

With long-term zinc supplement use (>3 months) for prophylaxis, consider supplementing zinc and copper in a ratio of 10:1 (eg, 10 mg zinc for every 1 mg copper).

Regimen should be based on elemental copper. If the total weight of the salt is listed instead, elemental copper can be calculated based on the salt form:

- Copper gluconate, 14%
- Copper chloride, 37%

> **BOX 8.4  Monitoring and Other Considerations for Trace Mineral
> Deficiencies[a,44-46] (cont.)**

## *Selenium*

### Monitoring

Blood selenium is required to determine status. Preferred laboratory test is
plasma glutathione peroxidase 3. Simultaneous determination of CRP and albumin is required for interpretation.

### Other considerations

Continuous infusion provides higher selenium retention by the tissues over a
short infusion time (2–4 hours).

## *Zinc*

### Monitoring

Plasma zinc concentration drops in response to inflammation. Monitor CRP to
guide the interpretation of plasma zinc concentration.

### Other considerations

Regimen should be based on elemental zinc. If the total weight of the salt is listed
instead, elemental zinc can be calculated based on the salt form:

- Zinc gluconate, 14.3%
- Zinc sulfate, 23%
- Zinc acetate, 30%
- Zinc picolinate, 35%
- Zinc chloride, 48%
- Zinc oxide, 81%

[a] Frequency of biochemical monitoring varies based on severity of depletion, presence of
overt symptoms, and underlying disease.

# References

1. Kiela PR, Ghishan FK. Physiology of intestinal absorption and secretion. *Best Pract Res Clin Gastroenterol.* 2016;30(2):145-159. doi:10.1016/j.bpg.2016.02.007

2. Food and Nutrition Board, National Academies. Dietary Reference Intakes (DRIs): Recommended Dietary Allowances and Adequate Intakes, elements [table]. In: National Academies of Sciences, Engineering, and Medicine; Health and Medicine Division; Food and Nutrition Board; Committee to Review the Dietary Reference Intakes for Sodium and Potassium; Oria M, Harrison M, Stallings VA, eds. *Dietary Reference Intakes for Sodium and Potassium.* National Academies Press; 2019. Accessed March 25, 2023. www.ncbi.nlm.nih.gov/books/NBK545442/table/appJ_tab3

3. Berger MM, Broman M, Forni L, Ostermann M, De Waele E, Wischmeyer PE. Nutrients and micronutrients at risk during renal replacement therapy: a scoping review. *Curr Opin Crit Care.* 2021;27(4):367-377. doi:10.1097/MCC.0000000000000851

4. Altarelli M, Ben-Hamouda N, Schneider A, Berger MM. Copper deficiency: causes, manifestations, and treatment. *Nutr Clin Pract.* 2019;34(4):504-513. doi:10.1002/ncp.10328

5. Livingstone C. Zinc: physiology, deficiency, and parenteral nutrition. *Nutr Clin Pract.* 2015;30(3):371-382. doi:10.1177/0884533615570376

6. Krebs NF. Update on zinc deficiency and excess in clinical pediatric practice. *Ann Nutr Metab.* 2013;62(suppl 1):19-29. doi:10.1159/000348261

7. Berger MM, Talwar D, Shenkin A. Pitfalls in the interpretation of blood tests used to assess and monitor micronutrient nutrition status. *Nutr Clin Pract.* 2023;38(1):56-69. doi:10.1002/ncp.10924

8. Myint ZW, Oo TH, Thein KZ, Tun AM, Saeed H. Copper deficiency anemia: review article. *Ann Hematol.* 2018;97(9):1527-1534. doi:10.1007/s00277-018-3407-5

9. Burkhead JL, Collins JF. Nutrition information brief—copper. *Adv Nutr.* 2022;13(2):681-683. doi:10.1093/advances/nmab157

10. Jamal R, Dihmis OW, Carroll LS, Pengas G. Hypocupraemia-induced anaemia, sensory ataxia and cognitive impairment secondary to zinc-containing dental adhesive. *BMJ Case Rep.* 2021;14(7):e239375. doi:10.1136/bcr-2020-239375

11. Barraclough H, Cooke K. Are patients fed directly into the jejunum at risk of copper deficiency? *Arch Dis Child.* 2019;104(8):817-819. doi:10.1136/archdischild-2019-316969

12. Nishiwaki S, Iwashita M, Goto N, et al. Predominant copper deficiency during prolonged enteral nutrition through a jejunostomy tube compared to that through a gastrostomy tube. *Clin Nutr.* 2011;30(5): 585-589. doi:10.1016/j.clnu.2011.04.008

13. Osland EJ, Polichronis K, Madkour R, Watt A, Blake C. Micronutrient deficiency risk in long-term enterally fed patients: a systematic review. *Clin Nutr ESPEN.* 2022;52:395-420. doi:10.1016/j.clnesp.2022.09.022

14. Moon N, Aryan M, Westerveld D, Nathoo S, Glover S, Kamel AY. Clinical manifestations of copper deficiency: a case report and review of the literature. *Nutr Clin Pract.* 2021;36(5):1080-1085. doi:10.1002/ncp.10582

15. Kumar N, Butz JA, Burritt MF. Clinical significance of the laboratory determination of low serum copper in adults. *Clin Chem Lab Med.* 2007;45(10):1402-1410. doi:10.1515/CCLM.2007.292

16. Bost M, Houdart S, Oberli M, Kalonji E, Huneau JF, Margaritis I. Dietary copper and human health: current evidence and unresolved issues. *J Trace Elem Med Biol.* 2016;35:107-115. doi:10.1016/j.jtemb.2016.02.006

17. Shi Y, Yang W, Tang X, Yan Q, Cai X, Wu F. Keshan disease: a potentially fatal endemic cardiomyopathy in remote mountains of China. *Front Pediatr.* 2021;9:576916. doi:10.3389/fped.2021.576916

18. Labunskyy VM, Hatfield DL, Gladyshev VN. Selenoproteins: molecular pathways and physiological roles. *Physiol Rev.* 2014;94(3):739-777. doi:10.1152/physrev.00039.2013

19. Fairweather-Tait SJ, Bao Y, Broadley MR, et al. Selenium in human health and disease. *Antioxid Redox Signal.* 2011;14(7):1337-1383. doi:10.1089/ars.2010.3275

20. Brown KM, Arthur JR. Selenium, selenoproteins and human health: a review. *Public Health Nutr.* 2001;4(2B):593-599. doi:10.1079/phn2001143

21. Boldery R, Fielding G, Rafter T, Pascoe AL, Scalia GM. Nutritional deficiency of selenium secondary to weight loss (bariatric) surgery associated with life-threatening cardiomyopathy. *Heart Lung Circ.* 2007;16(2):123-126. doi:10.1016/j.hlc.2006.07.013

22. Munguti CM, Al Rifai M, Shaheen W. A rare cause of cardiomyopathy: a case of selenium deficiency causing severe cardiomyopathy that improved on supplementation. *Cureus.* 2017;9(8):e1627. doi:10.7759/cureus.1627

23. Massoure PL, Camus O, Fourcade L, Simon F. Bilateral leg oedema after bariatric surgery: a selenium-deficient cardiomyopathy. *Obes Res Clin Pract.* 2017;11(5):622-626. doi:10.1016/j.orcp.2017.05.004

24. Sirikonda NS, Patten WD, Phillips JR, Mullett CJ. Ketogenic diet: rapid onset of selenium deficiency-induced cardiac decompensation. *Pediatr Cardiol.* 2012;33(5):834-838. doi:10.1007/s00246-012-0219-6

25. Saliba W, El Fakih R, Shaheen W. Heart failure secondary to selenium deficiency, reversible after supplementation. *Int J Cardiol.* 2010;141(2):e26-e27. doi:10.1016/j.ijcard.2008.11.095

26. Burke MP, Opeskin K. Fulminant heart failure due to selenium deficiency cardiomyopathy (Keshan disease). *Med Sci Law.* 2002;42(1): 10-13. doi:10.1177/002580240204200103

27. Chariot P, Bignani O. Skeletal muscle disorders associated with selenium deficiency in humans. *Muscle Nerve.* 2003;27(6):662-668. doi:10.1002 /mus.10304

28. Yagi M, Tani T, Hashimoto T, et al. Four cases of selenium deficiency in postoperative long-term enteral nutrition. *Nutrition.* 1996;12(1):40-43. doi:10.1016/0899-9007(95)00062-3

29. Abrams CK, Siram SM, Galsim C, Johnson-Hamilton H, Munford FL, Mezghebe H. Selenium deficiency in long-term total parenteral nutrition. *Nutr Clin Pract.* 1992;7(4):175-178. doi:10.1177 /0115426592007004175

30. Etani Y, Nishimoto Y, Kawamoto K, et al. Selenium deficiency in children and adolescents nourished by parenteral nutrition and/ or selenium-deficient enteral formula. *J Trace Elem Med Biol.* 2014;28(4):409-413. doi:10.1016/j.jtemb.2014.09.001

31. Kodali V. Selenium deficiency in mineral-rich mid-Western Australia. *Rural Remote Health.* 2018;18(2):4350. doi:10.22605/RRH4350

32. Pizzulli A, Ranjbar A. Selenium deficiency and hypothyroidism: a new etiology in the differential diagnosis of hypothyroidism in children. *Biol Trace Elem Res.* 2000;77(3):199-208. doi:10.1385/BTER:77:3:199

33. Ashton K, Hooper L, Harvey LJ, Hurst R, Casgrain A, Fairweather-Tait SJ. Methods of assessment of selenium status in humans: a systematic review. *Am J Clin Nutr.* 2009;89(6):2025S-2039S. doi:10.3945/ajcn.2009 .27230F

34. Thomson CD. Assessment of requirements for selenium and adequacy of selenium status: a review. *Eur J Clin Nutr.* 2004;58(3):391-402. doi:10 .1038/sj.ejcn.1601800

35. Aldosary BM, Sutter ME, Schwartz M, Morgan BW. Case series of selenium toxicity from a nutritional supplement. *Clin Toxicol (Phila).* 2012;50(1):57-64. doi:10.3109/15563650.2011.641560

36. Hanachi M, Dicembre M, Rives-Lange C, et al. Micronutrients deficiencies in 374 severely malnourished anorexia nervosa inpatients. *Nutrients.* 2019;11(4):792. doi:10.3390/nu11040792

37. Lazzerini M, Wanzira H. Oral zinc for treating diarrhoea in children. *Cochrane Database Syst Rev.* 2016;12(12):CD005436. doi:10.1002/14651858 .CD005436.pub5

38. Berger MM, Shenkin A, Schweinlin A, et al. ESPEN micronutrient guideline. *Clin Nutr*. 2022;41(6):1357-1424. doi:10.1016/j.clnu.2022.02.015

39. Imamoğlu S, Bereket A, Turan S, Taga Y, Haklar G. Effect of zinc supplementation on growth hormone secretion, IGF-I, IGFBP-3, somatomedin generation, alkaline phosphatase, osteocalcin and growth in prepubertal children with idiopathic short stature. *J Pediatr Endocrinol Metab*. 2005;18(1):69-74. doi:10.1515/jpem.2005.18.1.69

40. Rocha ÉDM, de Brito NJN, Dantas MMG, Silva AA, Almeida MG, Brandão-Neto J. Effect of zinc supplementation on GH, IGF1, IGFBP3, OCN, and ALP in non-zinc-deficient children. *J Am Coll Nutr*. 2015;34(4):290-299. doi:10.1080/07315724.2014.929511

41. Bui VQ, Marcinkevage J, Ramakrishnan U, et al. Associations among dietary zinc intakes and biomarkers of zinc status before and after a zinc supplementation program in Guatemalan schoolchildren. *Food Nutr Bull*. 2013;34(2):143-150. doi:10.1177/156482651303400203

42. Lowe NM, Fekete K, Decsi T. Methods of assessment of zinc status in humans: a systematic review. *Am J Clin Nutr*. 2009;89(6):2040S-2051S. doi:10.3945/ajcn.2009.27230G

43. Esper DH. Utilization of nutrition-focused physical assessment in identifying micronutrient deficiencies. *Nutr Clin Pract*. 2015;30(2):194-202. doi:10.1177/0884533615573054

44. Facts and Comparisons: drug referential resource. Wolters Kluwer. Accessed December 15, 2022. www.wolterskluwer.com/en/solutions/lexicomp/facts-and-comparisons

45. Drugs@FDA: FDA-approved drugs. US Food and Drug Administration. Accessed December 15, 2022. www.accessdata.fda.gov/scripts/cder/daf/index.cfm

46. Micromedex (database). Merative. 2023. Accessed December 15, 2022. www.micromedexsolutions.com

# CHAPTER 9

# Gastrointestinal Surgery

Kristen M. Roberts, PhD, RDN, LD, CNSC, FASPEN, FAND,
and David C. Evans, MD, FACS, FCCM, FASPEN

## Introduction

Gastrointestinal (GI) surgeries involving the lumen or the accessory organs (eg, the pancreas) increase a patient's risk of developing suboptimal micronutrient status because these surgeries disrupt the normal physiology of digestion and absorption. Many patients undergoing surgery, particularly those with short bowel syndrome and intestinal failure, require home parenteral nutrition (PN), enteral nutrition (EN), or intravenous fluids. Resources for micronutrient and electrolyte dosing and repletion in patients on nutrition support are reported elsewhere.[1-3] In addition, information on micronutrient assessment and repletion after bariatric surgery is covered in Chapter 14.

There are many limitations to understanding micronutrient management in patients recovering from GI surgery. The literature lacks defined guidelines for the routine assessment and treatment of micronutrient status, leaving clinicians to rely on their clinical experience and an understanding of the postsurgical anatomy to establish repletion regimens that account for the specialized function of a GI tract that has been resected, bypassed, or otherwise altered. Published literature focuses on center-specific strategies or case presentations that may not be appropriate for all surgical patients. The lack of clinical trials assessing repletion strategies after GI surgical procedures means few evidence-based guidelines are available for the clinician to consult when assessing micronutrient needs. This chapter highlights the status of micronutrient treatment strategies for patients undergoing surgery who do not require nutrition support (PN or EN).

# Surgical Procedures

Several GI surgeries affect micronutrient absorption, including the esophagectomy, small and large bowel resections, and the pancreato-duodenectomy (Whipple procedure). Before reviewing the literature on micronutrient management in a subset of surgical cases, a review of each surgical procedure and a discussion of the impact on intestinal nutrient absorption are necessary. Figure 9.1 on page 168 reviews the location of micronutrient absorption throughout an intact GI tract.

## Esophagectomy With Reconstructive Conduit

An esophagectomy is a commonly used surgical treatment for esophageal cancer, achalasia, congenital abnormalities, and caustic injuries. The procedure consists of a partial or full resection of the esophagus and the formation of a conduit created preferably from the stomach but alternatively consisting of jejunum or colon. Selection of the conduit is dependent on the preoperative diagnosis and the availability of healthy tissue to serve as the conduit. The minimally invasive esophagectomy with a gastric pull-up as the replacement conduit is the most common and preferred esophagectomy, as this procedure requires a single anastomosis (refer to Figure 9.2 on page 168). A jejunal conduit is more surgically challenging, requiring several bowel and vascular anastomoses, but the natural peristalsis present in that tissue is suitable for reconstructing the esophageal conduit. Similarly to the jejunal conduit, the colonic

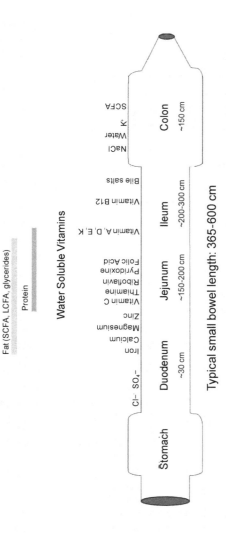

FIGURE 9.1  Absorption of macronutrients and micronutrients in the intact gut

Abbreviations: LCFA, long-chain fatty acid; SCFA, short-chain fatty acid.

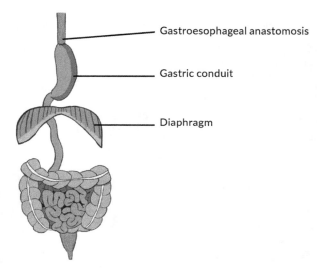

FIGURE 9.2 Esophagectomy with gastric conduit

Printed with permission from artist Gretchen Murray.

interposition requires multiple bowel anastomoses but no vascular anastomosis. Although the colonic interposition can contribute to fluid and electrolyte malabsorption (mostly due to the now shortened remnant colon left at the terminus of the GI tract), the acid resistance in patients with reflux provides a substantial advantage.[4] The performing surgeon is responsible for determining which of these procedures will produce the best outcomes for the patient based on the patient's anatomy and the surgeon's expertise. Adults with jejunal or colonic conduits typically lack a remnant stomach. Patients who underwent reconstruction as children may have an intact stomach.

An esophagectomy can alter micronutrient intake and absorption because of a change in the acidic environment related to proton pump inhibitors (needed to control acid reflux), dumping syndrome, malabsorption related to changes in intestinal transit (all esophagectomies include division of the vagus nerves), and loss of absorptive capacity. The vagus nerve is the longest cranial nerve that stimulates the involuntary movements of the GI tract and promotes pancreatic enzyme release into the duodenum through the common bile duct. When the vagus nerve is disrupted or denervated, as seen in an esophagectomy, exocrine pancreatic insufficiency may result from the lack of pancreatic stimulation.[5] Exocrine pancreatic insufficiency leads to inadequate fat digestion and absorption, ultimately resulting in an increased risk for fat-soluble vitamin deficiencies, postoperative weight loss, or malnutrition. In addition, many patients undergoing esophagectomy experience some nutritional impacts from malignancy, dysphagia, or the side effects of neoadjuvant chemoradiation even before undergoing surgery. Esophagectomy is also complicated by high leak rates (6%–12% reported), as well as by a high risk of anastomotic stricture (26% in one trial).[6,7] Patients with a leak are unable to resume oral intake until the leak is resolved and may require nutrition support (PN or EN). Strictures may limit oral intake and cause dysphagia. Because of the high risk of complications, some surgeons routinely place jejunostomy tubes, but this practice has remained variable and controversial. In select patients with preoperative malnutrition, a jejunostomy tube may be placed before surgery to optimize the patient's nutrition or to support the patient through chemoradiation treatment. Observational research has identified at least one micronutrient deficiency present up to 2 years after an esophagectomy.[8-10] Nutritional anemias are responsible for the majority of micronutrient deficiencies reported. One study reported data on a cross-sectional cohort and a prospective cohort and estimated that more than 18% of patients developed a vitamin B12 deficiency after esophagectomy.[10] However, other studies have reported deficiencies in vitamin A, vitamin E, iron, and B vitamins as prevalent in the postoperative period.[8-10]

# Intestinal Resections and Ostomies

Intestinal resections are commonly performed to treat obstruction, perforation, trauma, inflammatory disease (eg, Crohn's disease), congenital abnormalities, or malignancy. The GI reconfigurations possible from bowel resections are unlimited due to the variations in preoperative and intraoperative diagnoses. These surgeries can result in numerous anastomoses or an ostomy formation (temporary or permanent). The location, bowel length in continuity, and remaining health of the GI tract are essential factors in determining the risk for micronutrient deficiency. Refer to Figure 9.3 for illustrations of a jejunal resection, an ileal resection, and a small bowel resection with end jejunostomy.

Small bowel resections hold a greater micronutrient deficiency risk than do colonic resections because of the absorption location of most micronutrients (refer to Figure 9.1). The larger the resection, the greater the risk.[11] This is evident in patients with short bowel syndrome, in whom reliance on PN to maintain micronutrient status is common once more than 50% of the intestine is resected. Zinc, fat-soluble vitamins, magnesium, and iron abnormalities are most commonly reported in patients with surgical resections who are reliant on nutrition support.[12-14] In the setting of a total colectomy or partial colectomy, micronutrient digestion and absorption are largely intact, and micronutrient supplementation is less common. However, there are increased risks of vitamin K deficiency because the presence of colonic bacteria for in vivo

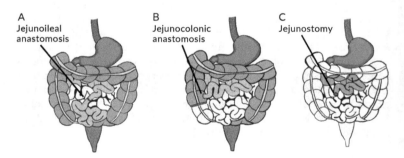

## FIGURE 9.3  Potential intestinal resections

A. Jejunal resection with jejunoileal anastomosis; short segment jejunal and ileal resections often do not cause lasting effects as the body adapts and recovers. B. Ileal resection with jejunocolonic anastomosis. Ileal resection with less than 100 cm of ileum retained results in impaired bile salt and fat malabsorption and is considered type 2 short bowel syndrome (see section on intestinal rehabilitation). C. Massive small bowel resection with an end jejunostomy—type 1 short bowel syndrome.
Printed with permission from artist Gretchen Murray.

production is eliminated or minimized. In patients with high-output stomas (>800 mL/d), maldigestion and malabsorption can increase the risk of developing micronutrient deficiency.[15]

# Pancreaticoduodenectomy (Whipple Procedure)

A pancreaticoduodenectomy, also called a Whipple procedure, is a technically complex surgery involving resection of the pancreatic head, distal stomach, gallbladder, distal common bile duct, and the duodenum (refer to Figure 9.4 on page 172). The procedure requires a pancreaticojejunostomy, choledochojejunostomy, and a gastrojejunostomy. Postoperative complications are reduced when the distal stomach (pylorus) can be preserved.[16] Considerable variations in complications exist, depending on the preoperative and intraoperative diagnoses, and complications can lead to high rates of morbidity (up to 50%) and mortality (approximately 1%).[17] Pancreatic fistula is the leading complication associated with high morbidity and mortality rates[18]; however, delayed gastric emptying, chylous ascites, infectious complications, and hemorrhage have all been reported.[16]

The nutrition-related side effects of pancreaticoduodenectomy, such as dumping syndrome, malabsorption, exocrine pancreatic insufficiency, and malnutrition, further compromise micronutrient status. An analysis of data from a randomized controlled trial compared preoperative and postoperative micronutrient levels in trial participants and identified deficiencies in thiamin, vitamin B6, and iron in 50% of participants.[19] Another study monitored 47 patients who had normal serum zinc status prior to undergoing pancreaticoduodenectomy; at 6 months post procedure, zinc deficiency had developed in 68% of patients, 42% of whom had positive findings on a nutrition focused physical exam.[20] Although there is a lack of randomized, controlled clinical trials investigating pancreatic enzyme replacement therapy (PERT) for the prevention of micronutrient deficiencies, it is clinically reasonable to use these medications when exocrine pancreatic insufficiency is suspected, although PERT does not preclude the risk for micronutrient deficiency. See Box 9.1 on page 173 for PERT dosing strategies.[21]

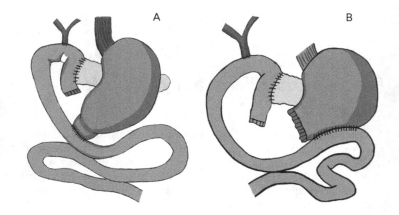

FIGURE 9.4  Anatomical reconfigurations after a
pancreaticoduodenectomy

A. Pylorus-sparing pancreaticoduodenectomy. B. Pancreaticoduodenectomy with pylorus resection.
Printed with permission from artist Gretchen Murray.

# General Micronutrient Concerns Associated With Gastrointestinal Surgeries

Intestinal surgeries can lead to suboptimal micronutrient status in clinical scenarios associated with a reduction in intestinal surface area, pH alterations, poor mixing of intestinal secretions with luminal contents, and the presence of an overgrowth of bacteria (ie, small intestinal bacterial overgrowth, or SIBO). Massive ileal resections cause the most substantial consequences because of the loss of surface area. Ileal resections affect vitamin B12 absorption and disrupt the enterohepatic circulation of bile acids. Following a large ileal resection (>100 cm), a depletion of the bile acid pool is evident after 6 months. At that point, bile

| | |
|---|---|
| **BOX 9.1 Dosing Strategies for Pancreatic Enzyme Replacement Therapy[21]** | |
| **Medication, pancrelipase** | Creon<br>• Creon 6 (6,000 lipase unit [LU])<br>• Creon 12 (12,000 LU)<br>• Creon 24 (24,000 LU)<br>Zenpep (5,000 LU)<br>Pancreaze (4,200 LU) |
| **Formulation** | Tablet |
| **Starting dose** | Tablet dosing: 1 tablet with meals or snacks<br>Weight-based dosing: 500 to 2,500 LU per kilogram of dry body weight |
| **Maximum dose** | 10,000 units or less per kilogram of dry body weight per meal<br>Less than 4,000 units per gram of fat ingested |

salt supplementation can promote fat digestion and absorption, reducing the risk of developing fat-soluble vitamin deficiencies. In a small ileal resection (<100 cm), bile salt reabsorption continues, and there is a lesser effect on fat-soluble vitamin status.[22,23]

In addition to the loss of surface area, pH alterations in the gastric pouch can impede the release of intrinsic factor and prevent the conversion of ferric iron to ferrous, further decreasing the bioavailability of iron and vitamin B12 and increasing the need for treatments to prevent deficiency. Poor mixing of intestinal secretions with luminal contents occurs when the duodenum is bypassed, as in a pancreaticoduodenectomy, or when loss of the terminal ileum disrupts the ileal brake and decreases intestinal transit time.[22,23] PERT may be necessary when fat-soluble vitamin deficiencies are present or when there are overt signs of steatorrhea. Lastly, the loss of the ileocecal valve is strongly associated with an increased risk of colonic microbe migration into the small intestine leading to a diagnosis of SIBO.[24] Although the mechanism for deficiency is poorly understood, the presence of SIBO increases the risk for malnutrition and the development of micronutrient deficiencies (eg, vitamin B12 deficiency).[25]

Box 9.2 summarizes a sample of research studies focused on micronutrient assessment of patients who have undergone GI surgery.[8-10,12-14,19,20,26]

---

**BOX 9.2   Representative Samples of Micronutrient Deficiencies in Gastrointestinal Surgical Cohorts Not Receiving Nutrition Support**[8-10,12-14,19,20,26]

### Esophagectomy

**Janssen et al (2020)[8]**

| | |
|---|---|
| **Study design, time frame, population details** | Design: observational<br>Length of follow-up: 6 to 24 months<br>Sample size: N = 83 |
| **Micronutrient assessment** | Preoperative assessment: none<br>Postoperative assessment: serum iron, ferritin, thiamin, vitamin B6, vitamin B12, vitamin D, folate, and methylmalonic acid<br>Note: Over-the-counter (OTC) supplementation was not tracked. Registered dietitian nutritionist (RDN) was involved in monitoring status. Inflammatory markers were not included in the assessment, which may alter true rates of deficiency. |
| **Outcome** | At 6.1 months:<br>• Patients with one micronutrient deficiency (1 MD): 78%<br>• Patients with more than one micronutrient deficiency (> 1 MD): 37%<br>At 16.5 months:<br>• 1 MD: 41%<br>• > 1 MD: 17%<br>At 24.8 months:<br>• 1 MD: 61%<br>• > 1 MD: 39%<br>Deficiencies in iron, B vitamins, and vitamin D were the most common. Folate deficiency anemia was commonly reported. |

**BOX 9.2  Representative Samples of Micronutrient Deficiencies in Gastrointestinal Surgical Cohorts Not Receiving Nutrition Support[8-10,12-14,19,20,26] (cont.)**

### Heneghan et al (2015)[9]

| | |
|---|---|
| **Study design, time frame, population details** | Design: prospective<br>Follow-up: 1, 6, 18, and 24 months<br>Included patients with gastrectomy<br>Sample size: N = 45 |
| **Micronutrient assessment** | Preoperative and postoperative assessment: vitamin A, vitamin E, vitamin D, folate, ferritin, iron<br><br>Note: Inflammatory markers were not included in the assessment, which may alter the rates of true deficiency. |
| **Outcome** | At 18 to 24 months:<br><br>• Vitamin A deficiency in 81.5%<br>• Vitamin E deficiency in 61.5%<br>Iron and vitamin D status were suboptimal at baseline and follow-up but did not change over the study period. |

### Van Hagen et al (2017)[10]

| | |
|---|---|
| **Study design, time frame, population details** | Design: cross-sectional and prospective<br>Length of follow-up: 1 to 3 years<br>Sample size: N = 99 preoperatively, cross-sectional; and N = 88 prospectively |
| **Micronutrient assessment** | Serum transcobalamin and methylmalonic acid |
| **Outcome** | Cross-sectional: Vitamin B12 deficiency in 11%<br>Prospective: Vitamin B12 deficiency in 5.6% at baseline and in 10.2% postoperatively<br>The authors estimated that 18.2% would develop a vitamin B12 deficiency. |

*Continued on next page*

> **BOX 9.2** Representative Samples of Micronutrient Deficiencies in
> Gastrointestinal Surgical Cohorts Not Receiving Nutrition
> Support[8-10,12-14,19,20,26] (cont.)

## Small and large bowel resections

### Feng et al (2020)[12]

| | |
|---|---|
| **Study design, time frame, population details** | Design: retrospective |
| | Follow-up: unknown |
| | Sample size: N = 31 pediatric patients transitioning to enteral autonomy |
| **Micronutrient assessment** | Assessment after enteral autonomy: serum zinc, copper, vitamin D, vitamin B12, folate |
| | Note: Inflammatory markers were not included in the assessment, which may alter the rates of true deficiency. |
| **Outcome** | After achieving enteral autonomy: |

- Zinc deficiency in 51.6%
- Copper deficiency in 38.7%
- Vitamin D deficiency in 32.3%
- Iron deficiency in 6.5%
- Vitamin B12 deficiency in 6.5%

### Soares-Mota et al (2015)[13]

| | |
|---|---|
| **Study design, time frame, population details** | Design: cross-sectional |
| | Follow-up: none |
| | Sample size: N = 71; cross-sectional n = 38 with Crohn's disease and n = 33 controls |
| | Excluded patients with < 180 cm of remaining intestine |
| **Micronutrient assessment** | Assessment: C-reactive protein (CRP); serum vitamin A and hepatic vitamin A stores |
| | Note: Dietary vitamin A was quantified using a food frequency questionnaire. |

**BOX 9.2  Representative Samples of Micronutrient Deficiencies in Gastrointestinal Surgical Cohorts Not Receiving Nutrition Support[8-10,12-14,19,20,26] (cont.)**

### Soares-Mota et al (2015)[13] (cont.)

| | |
|---|---|
| **Outcome** | Biochemical findings: |
| | • Vitamin D deficiency in 29% of Crohn's group, regardless of surgical history |
| | • Vitamin A: Decreased retinol stores in liver in 37% of Crohn's group; low serum vitamin A levels with normal retinol stores in 5% of Crohn's group; low serum vitamin A associated with lower BMI and lower body fat weight; CRP not associated with low serum vitamin A levels |
| | Dietary assessment: |
| | • Low vitamin A status in 29% of Crohn's group |
| | • No association between dietary vitamin A and serum or storage retinol levels |

### Naber et al (1998)[14]

| | |
|---|---|
| **Study design, time frame, population details** | Design: cross-sectional |
| | Follow-up: none |
| | Sample size: N = 31 with Crohn's disease, including n = 16 with a history of small bowel resection |
| **Micronutrient assessment** | Biochemical assessment: serum zinc, serum alkaline phosphatase activity, and zinc concentration in erythrocytes, mononuclear cells, and polymorphonuclear cells |
| | Note: Inflammatory markers were not included in the assessment, which may alter the rates of true deficiency. |
| **Outcome** | Serum zinc concentration declined as the length of small bowel resection increased. |

*Continued on next page*

BOX 9.2  Representative Samples of Micronutrient Deficiencies in
Gastrointestinal Surgical Cohorts Not Receiving Nutrition
Support[8-10,12-14,19,20,26] (cont.)

## *Pancreaticoduodenectomy*

### Tabriz et al (2021)[19]

| | |
|---|---|
| **Study design, time frame, population details** | Design: prospective randomized controlled trial<br>Follow-up: 1 week, 3 months, 6 months, 12 months<br>Sample size: N = 47 with pancreatic cancer |
| **Micronutrient assessment** | Preoperative and postoperative assessment: iron, ferritin, transferrin, vitamin A, thiamin, vitamin B6, vitamin B12, folate, trace elements<br>Note: RDN was consulted to assist with management. Inflammatory markers were not included in the assessment, which may alter the rates of true deficiency. |
| **Outcome** | Preoperatively and postoperatively: Poor vitamin D status<br>Postoperatively: Thiamin, vitamin B6, and iron deficiencies in 50% |

### Braga et al (2012)[26]

| | |
|---|---|
| **Study design, time frame, population details** | Design: prospective randomized clinical trial<br>Follow-up: 1 day, 3 days, and 7 days after an oral nutritional supplement<br>Sample size: N = 36 without severe malnutrition |
| **Micronutrient assessment** | Preoperative and postoperative assessment: vitamin C, E, zinc, selenium<br>Note: Inflammatory markers were not included in the assessment, which may alter the rates of true deficiency. |

> **BOX 9.2  Representative Samples of Micronutrient Deficiencies in Gastrointestinal Surgical Cohorts Not Receiving Nutrition Support**[8-10,12-14,19,20,26] **(cont.)**

**Braga et al (2012)[26] (cont.)**

| | |
|---|---|
| **Outcome** | Preoperatively: |

- Normal selenium and zinc status
- Low vitamin C status
- Higher-than-normal vitamin E status

Postoperatively:

- Within 1 to 3 days of surgery, all micronutrients dropped from baseline levels.
- Patients receiving an oral nutritional supplement had higher vitamin C, zinc, and selenium levels compared to those receiving a placebo.

**Yu et al (2011)[20]**

| | |
|---|---|
| **Study design, time frame, population details** | Design: retrospective cross-sectional, case-control study<br>Follow-up: none<br>Sample size: n = 47 with normal preoperative zinc status compared to an n = 21 non–pylorus-sparing Whipple procedure and n = 27 pylorus-sparing Whipple procedure |
| **Micronutrient assessment** | Preoperative and postoperative (6 months) assessment: zinc<br>Note: Inflammatory markers were not included in the assessment, which may alter the rates of true deficiency. |
| **Outcome** | No detection of zinc deficiency preoperatively<br>Biochemical assessment: |

- Postoperative zinc deficiency in 68%
- Iron deficiency in 14.4%

Nutrition focused physical exam:

- Postoperative zinc deficiency (in 42%) associated with skin rash
- Photophobia
- Glossitis

# Intestinal Rehabilitation

Intestinal rehabilitation is a process for enhancing the absorptive capacity of the gut, improving nutritional status, and reducing the need for PN through diet, medications, and reconstructive surgery.[27] After a surgical resection or reconfiguration of the GI tract, the intestine goes through phases of intestinal adaptation. Intestinal adaptation has been best described in the literature on short bowel syndrome as occurring in three distinct phases following an intestinal resection[23,28,29]:

- Phase 1 is characterized by intestinal hypersecretion leading to poor micronutrient absorption and steatorrhea, and the patient often requires nutrition support to maintain nutritional status. Generally, this phase lasts for up to 6 months postoperatively.

- Phase 2 occurs within the first 2 years of an intestinal resection and is the optimal time for intestinal rehabilitation, as there is a substantial reduction in steatorrhea and a reduced dependency on micronutrient treatments, especially the need for additional fat-soluble vitamins.

- Phase 3 occurs in a small subset of patients. This phase is characterized by prolonged intestinal failure, and the patient requires nutrition support to sustain nutritional status. It may be appropriate to evaluate these patients for intestinal transplantation if other medical, nutritional, and surgical procedures to restore optimal nutrition are unavailable. Given the possibility of serious complications associated with long-term nutrition support and the small number of intestinal transplant programs in the United States, early referral is imperative to improve surgical outcomes in this subset of patients.[30]

# Perioperative Micronutrient Concerns

## Anemia

Suboptimal vitamin and mineral status in the perioperative period can lead to nutritional concerns. Iron deficiency anemia is common in the United States and is identified in up to 40% of patients preoperatively and up to 90% of patients postoperatively.[31] Deficits in iron, vitamin B12, folate, copper, and vitamin C are the most common micronutrient deficiencies that contribute to anemia. Preoperative anemia is associated with an increased need for blood transfusions, longer length of hospital stay, and increased mortality.[32] The clinician should be aware of this risk for patients undergoing elective procedures and assess micronutrient status as part of the preoperative evaluation. In individuals requiring emergent surgery, assessment can be completed postoperatively, but the clinician must consider the inflammatory response and its impact on the biochemical assessment (Chapter 4). If treatment for iron deficiency anemia in the immediate postoperative period is necessary, intravenous iron replacement is preferred over oral replacement because of the poor tolerance and absorption of oral preparations.[31,32] Chapter 7 provides more information on iron deficiency.

## Vitamin D Deficiency

Deficiencies in fat-soluble vitamins can be seen in patients with decreased intestinal surface area, the presence of steatorrhea, and inadequate oral intake (Chapter 5). A 2015 systematic review highlighted that 84% of included studies (26 of 31) suggested worse surgical outcomes in the presence of low vitamin D levels.[33] Only two of these studies took place in a GI cohort, however, and further evaluation is needed to establish whether additional assessment and treatment tactics are necessary. Patients at risk should be given a preoperative assessment. In an earlier study, researchers reviewed vitamin D status in a postoperative GI cohort of pediatric patients with inflammatory bowel disease (IBD) and found that vitamin D deficiency increased as the length of intestinal resection increased. Three treatment strategies for repletion of vitamin D status were selected, and participants were randomly assigned to receive one of three treatments: (1) 2,000 IU vitamin D2 by mouth daily for 6 weeks; (2) 2,000 IU vitamin D3 by mouth daily for 6 weeks; or (3) 50,000 IU vitamin D2 by mouth weekly for 6 weeks. The group receiving weekly dosing had a statistically significant greater increase in their serum 25-hydroxyvitamin D levels ($P<.0001$), and this was the preferred strategy.[11] Unfortunately, this finding was not duplicated in an adult IBD cohort.

# Micronutrient Assessment

After reviewing the details of the relevant GI surgical procedure and considering the risk factors for suboptimal micronutrient status associated with that procedure, the clinician should perform a thorough, procedure-specific micronutrient assessment of the patient. Chapters 5 through 8 cover the basic micronutrient assessment of physical and biochemical findings. This chapter focuses on the components of assessment unique to patients undergoing GI surgery who are not receiving nutrition support. The important components of assessment include reviewing operative and pathology reports, assessing the patient's intestinal transit time, and identifying complications through dietary and stool assessments.

## Operative and Pathology Reports

It is imperative for practitioners to review the operative and pathology reports after a GI surgery to understand a patient's risk for micronutrient deficiency. Operative reports should describe the health and length of the remaining tissue and the presence of disease, adhesions, and strictures. Although the remaining intestinal length is essential to understanding micronutrient deficiency risk, it is often undocumented. If that is the case, a conversation with the surgical team can provide insights into the health and length of the remaining intestine. In the absence of that, the clinician should review the pathology reports to ascertain the length of resected bowel. This measure can, in turn, be used to estimate remaining bowel length. However, because the GI tract can range anywhere from 300 to 600 cm, knowing the length of resected bowel might not be sufficient to determine micronutrient deficiency risk.

# Intestinal Transit Studies

Intestinal transit studies contribute to understanding micronutrient deficiency risk by providing information on the exposure of luminal contents to the epithelial cells lining the GI tract. Unfortunately, the commonly used transit studies—hydrogen breath testing, GI scintigraphy, radiopaque markers, and wireless motility capsules—all have limitations in surgical patients that may decrease the specificity of the results.[34] The hydrogen breath test is easy to administer and relatively inexpensive,[35] but the results are influenced by SIBO, which is a risk factor in many GI surgeries.[24] GI scintigraphy and radiopaque marker tests typically involve ingestion of a labeled meal followed by frequent imaging to determine transit time. Although liquids and solids empty at various times, a mixed-meal small bowel transit time has been reported to range from 72 to 392 minutes.[36] As intestinal transit time decreases, intestinal length or health (or both) is thought to decline as well. However, clinicians should use their judgment, as this is not always true: patients with dumping syndrome may empty their intestines within 30 minutes and have sufficient intestinal length.

# Plasma Citrulline Level

Citrulline is an amino acid secreted by the enterocytes lining the GI tract. It appears to be a sensitive marker of intestinal absorption and length in various postsurgical conditions, such as short bowel syndrome.[37] It is possible that patients with a low citrulline level (eg, <20 mcmol/L) may be at an increased risk for micronutrient deficiency, but this has not been established.[27]

# Dietary and Stool Assessment

In patients who have undergone GI surgery, assessing the diet through a 24-hour recall or daily food record is not sufficient to determine exposure to micronutrients. Concomitant assessment of dietary intake and stool characteristics—including consistency, color, presence of undigested foods, and transit time—is imperative to understanding true micronutrient exposure. Consider a patient with an ileostomy and lactose intolerance. The patient's reported dairy intake may be sufficient to meet the Recommended Dietary Allowance for calcium. However, suppose the dietary assessment reveals that after ingesting 1 cup of lactose-containing milk, the patient empties a milky substance into the ileostomy bag within 15 minutes. The patient is likely not absorbing adequate calcium from this beverage. The clinician may need to consider alternative dietary sources of calcium or initiate a calcium supplement.

Stool characteristics can enhance the understanding of the absorptive and digestive capacity of the GI tract and are critical to assessing and evaluating micronutrient status in surgical patients. Stool consistency can be described using the Bristol stool scale, which categorizes consistency from hard lumps (type 1) to watery (type 7).[38,39] Reviewing changes in stool consistency throughout the day and in correlation with dietary intake increases the understanding of transit time and foods that may be contributing to malabsorption.[39] Assessments such as yellow and orange-pigmented stools that are greasy or oily are clear signs of steatorrhea, increasing the risk of fat-soluble vitamin deficiencies.[40] Dietary fat adjustments or initiation of PERT are appropriate considerations in those with steatorrhea.[21] The appearance of undigested foods in the stool indicates maldigestion but can also assist the clinician in determining intestinal transit time. As with the milk example, timing between ingestion and excretion in the stool is a surrogate marker for intestinal transit. Abnormalities in stool characteristics, consistency, and transit increase a patient's risk of developing a micronutrient deficiency and warrant further consideration for prevention. Box 9.3 lists stool characteristics and suspected etiologies for consideration in the assessment process.[41]

| BOX 9.3 Stool Characteristics Utilized in the Assessment of Gastrointestinal Function | |
|---|---|
| *Stool color/appearance* | *Indication* |
| Green | Bile/pancreatic secretions |
| Yellow | Bile/pancreatic secretions/malabsorption of dietary fat |
| White or gray | Biliary obstruction |
| Brown | Normal |
| Watery | Osmotic or secretory process |
| Oily, greasy | Malabsorption, maldigestion, or rapid transit |
| Frothy | Small intestinal bacterial overgrowth or steatorrhea |
| Detectable food particles | Maldigestion |
| Foul smelling | Steatorrhea |
| Blood | Melena, occult, hematochezia, inflammatory process, possible malignancy |
| Elevated electrolyte composition | Secretory diarrhea |
| Leukocytes | Inflammatory process |
| Mucus | Secretory or infectious etiology |

Reprinted with permission from Roberts KM. Diseases of the lower gastrointestinal tract. In: Nelms M, Sucher KP, eds. *Nutrition Therapy and Pathophysiology.* 4th ed. Cengage Learning; 2020:393. See source 41.

Gastrointestinal Surgery

# Micronutrient Dosing Strategies

Without definitive guidelines for the prevention and treatment of micronutrient abnormalities in surgical patients, clinicians are challenged with reviewing the published literature and staying current in their knowledge of postsurgical anatomy. This chapter has provided information on selected surgical procedures and the available research relating to these procedures. This information, together with Chapters 5 through 8, can guide micronutrient dosing strategies. Box 9.4 summarizes the findings of the current research on micronutrient assessment and treatment strategies for GI surgical patients not receiving nutrition support.[20,28,42,43] It is not a substitute for clinical judgment, and more research is needed to develop definitive dosing strategies.

---

**BOX 9.4  Suggestions for Monitoring and Treating Micronutrient Deficiency in Gastrointestinal Surgical Patients Not Receiving Nutrition Support[20,28,42,43]**

### Esophagectomy

| | |
|---|---|
| Micronutrients of concern | Iron, B vitamins, folate, vitamin D |
| Published considerations for micronutrient treatment strategies | No suggested prevention or treatment strategies are indicated in the literature. Review Chapters 5 through 8 for considerations for repletion if needed. |

### Small bowel resection

| | |
|---|---|
| Micronutrients of concern | In patients with steatorrhea or bile salt malabsorption or who are taking a bile acid sequestrant: vitamins A, D, E, and K |
| | In patients with end jejunostomy: zinc, copper |
| | In patients with ileal resection: vitamin B12, iron, folate, calcium, copper, zinc, vitamin B6 |

**BOX 9.4  Suggestions for Monitoring and Treating Micronutrient Deficiency in Gastrointestinal Surgical Patients Not Receiving Nutrition Support[20,28,42,43] (cont.)**

| | |
|---|---|
| **Considerations for micronutrient treatment strategies** | Pharmacotherapy:<br>• Consider pancreatic enzyme replacement therapy (PERT) to enhance absorption.<br>• Consider antidiarrheal or antisecretory medications to enhance absorption in patients with short bowel syndrome.<br><br>For suboptimal micronutrient status:<br>• Fat-soluble vitamins<br>  ○ Vitamin A<br>    ■ If no corneal changes, 10,000 to 25,000 IU/d (3,000–7,500 mcg RAE/d), by mouth (PO), for 1 to 2 weeks.<br>    ■ With corneal changes, 50,000 to 100,000 IU (15,000–30,000 mcg RAE), intramuscular (IM), followed by 50,000 IU (15,000 mcg RAE), IM, daily for 2 weeks.<br>  ○ Vitamin D<br>    ■ 1,250 mcg (50,000 IU), PO, every other day until level normalizes.<br>    ■ If no response, consider higher doses up to 3,750 mcg (150,000 IU), PO, three to five times weekly.<br>    ■ If required, provide calcitriol, PO.[a]<br>  ○ Vitamin E: 80 to 100 IU, PO, divided into three doses, when deficiency is detected (see Chapter 5)<br>  ○ Vitamin K: 5 mg/d, PO, until prothrombin time normalizes<br>• Water-soluble vitamins: vitamin B12: 1,000 mcg/d, IM or subcutaneous (SC), for 5 days, followed by 1,000 mcg/mo, IM; or consider 1,000 or 2,000 mcg/d, PO; or consider 1,000 mcg/wk, IM. Consider IM injections when ileal resections are >100 cm. |

*Continued on next page*

**BOX 9.4  Suggestions for Monitoring and Treating Micronutrient Deficiency in Gastrointestinal Surgical Patients Not Receiving Nutrition Support[20,28,42,43] (cont.)**

| Considerations for micronutrient treatment strategies (continued) | |
|---|---|

Considerations for micronutrient treatment strategies (continued)

- Minerals
  - Zinc[b]: Zinc sulfate equivalent to 22.5 to 45 mg elemental zinc, PO (as effervescent tablets or capsules), three times daily. For each 8 to 15 mg elemental zinc, add 1 mg copper.
  - Calcium: 1,500 mg elemental calcium daily with multivitamin
  - Thiamin: For treatment of Wernicke encephalopathy, 500 mg, IV, three times daily for 2 to 3 days; or 250 mg/d or more, IV, for 5 days; or 30 mg, PO, twice daily
  - Copper: Copper sulfate equivalent to 2.4 mg elemental copper in 100 mL 0.9% sodium chloride, IV, administered over 1 hour daily for 5 days
  - Iron: Parenteral iron until hemoglobin and hematocrit normalize

For prevention in high-risk populations:
- Fat-soluble vitamins
  - Vitamin A: 10,000 to 50,000 IU/d (3,000–15,000 mcg RAE/d), PO, if normal liver function
  - Vitamin D (ergocalciferol or cholecalciferol): 10 to 20 mcg/d (400–800 IU/d), PO; or 2,500 mcg (100,000 IU), PO, every 3 to 6 months
- Water-soluble vitamins
  - Vitamin B12: IM: 1,000 mcg every 2 to 3 months, or 3,000 mcg every 6 months. PO: 1,000 mcg/wk or 250 to 350 mcg/d.
  - Thiamin: If active vomiting, 100 mg/d, PO, for 7 to 14 days
- Minerals
  - Zinc[b]
    - If draining fistula or high-output diarrhea or stoma: elemental zinc, 12 mg/d, PO.
    - Otherwise, elemental zinc, 3 to 4 mg/d, PO.

BOX 9.4  Suggestions for Monitoring and Treating Micronutrient Deficiency in Gastrointestinal Surgical Patients Not Receiving Nutrition Support[20,28,42,43] (cont.)

  - Calcium: Calcium citrate, 1,200 to 2,000 mg/d, PO, in divided doses
  - Copper: Copper gluconate, oxide, or sulfate equivalent to 2 mg elemental copper daily, PO; 1 mg copper for each 8 to 15 mg zinc supplemented
  - Iron: Maximum of 100 to 150 mg, PO, daily or every other day

### Large bowel resection

| | |
|---|---|
| Micronutrients of concern | Vitamin K, biotin |
| Published considerations for micronutrient treatment strategies | For suboptimal micronutrient status, Vitamin K: 10 mg/wk, PO |

### Biliopancreatic diversion

| | |
|---|---|
| Micronutrients of concern | Zinc, vitamin A, vitamin D, vitamin C, selenium, thiamin, vitamin B6 |
| Published considerations for micronutrient treatment strategies | Pharmacotherapy<br>• Consider PERT to enhance absorption.<br>• Consider antidiarrheal medications to enhance absorption in patients with rapid transit.<br>• Consider oral nutritional supplements immediately after surgery.<br>For suboptimal micronutrient status: zinc sulfate equivalent to 12 mg elemental zinc when diarrhea is present[b] |

[a] Consider use of calcitriol with chronic renal dialysis, hyperparathyroidism in chronic kidney disease without dialysis, hypoparathyroidism, and pseudohypoparathyroidism.
[b] 50 mg elemental zinc is equivalent to approximately 220 mg zinc sulfate.

# References

1. Malone A, Carney LN, Carrera AL, Mays A, eds. *ASPEN Enteral Nutrition Handbook*. 2nd ed. American Society for Parenteral and Enteral Nutrition; 2019.

2. Ayers P, Bobo ES, Hunt RT, Mays AA, Worthington PH, eds. *ASPEN Parenteral Nutrition Handbook*. 3rd ed. American Society for Parenteral and Enteral Nutrition; 2020.

3. Bruno J, Canada T, Canada N, Tucker AM, Ybarra JV, eds. *ASPEN Fluids, Electrolytes, and Acid-Base Disorders Handbook*. 2nd ed. American Society for Parenteral and Enteral Nutrition; 2020.

4. Fajardo R, Abbas AE, Petrov RV, Bakhos CT. Salvage esophagectomy. *Surg Clin North Am*. 2021;101(3):467-482. doi:10.1016/j.suc.2021.03.008

5. Huddy JR, Macharg FM, Lawn AM, Preston SR. Exocrine pancreatic insufficiency following esophagectomy. *Dis Esophagus*. 2013;26(6): 594-597. doi:10.1111/dote.12004

6. Ryan CE, Paniccia A, Meguid RA, McCarter MD. Transthoracic anastomotic leak after esophagectomy: current trends. *Ann Surg Oncol*. 2017;24(1):281-290. doi:10.1245/s10434-016-5417-7

7. Nguyen NT, Hinojosa MW, Smith BR, Chang KJ, Gray J, Hoyt D. Minimally invasive esophagectomy: lessons learned from 104 operations. *Ann Surg*. 2008;248(6):1081-1091. doi:10.1097/SLA.0b013e31818b72b5

8. Janssen HJB, Fransen LFC, Ponten JEH, Nieuwenhuijzen GAP, Luyer MDP. Micronutrient deficiencies following minimally invasive esophagectomy for cancer. *Nutrients*. 2020;12(3):778. doi:10.3390/nu12030778

9. Heneghan HM, Zaborowski A, Fanning M, et al. Prospective study of malabsorption and malnutrition after esophageal and gastric cancer surgery. *Ann Surg*. 2015;262(5):803-808. doi:10.1097/SLA.0000000000001445

10. van Hagen P, de Jonge R, van Berge Henegouwen MI, et al. Vitamin B12 deficiency after esophagectomy with gastric tube reconstruction for esophageal cancer. *Dis Esophagus*. 2017;30(12):1-8. doi:10.1093/dote/dox102

11. Leichtmann GA, Bengoa JM, Bolt MJ, Sitrin MD. Intestinal absorption of cholecalciferol and 25-hydroxycholecalciferol in patients with both Crohn's disease and intestinal resection. *Am J Clin Nutr*. 1991;54(3): 548-552. doi:10.1093/ajcn/54.3.548

12. Feng H, Zhang T, Yan W, et al. Micronutrient deficiencies in pediatric short bowel syndrome: a 10-year review from an intestinal rehabilitation center in China. *Pediatr Surg Int.* 2020;36(12):1481-1487. doi:10.1007/s00383-020-04764-3

13. Soares-Mota M, Silva TA, Gomes LM, et al. High prevalence of vitamin A deficiency in Crohn's disease patients according to serum retinol levels and the relative dose-response test. *World J Gastroenterol.* 2015;21(5):1614-1620. doi:10.3748/wjg.v21.i5.1614

14. Naber TH, van den Hamer CJ, Baadenhuysen H, Jansen JB. The value of methods to determine zinc deficiency in patients with Crohn's disease. *Scand J Gastroenterol.* 1998;33(5):514-523. doi:10.1080/00365529850172098

15. Cresci GA. Gastrointestinal tract surgery. In: Matarese L, Raymone JL, Mullin GE, eds. *The Health Professional's Guide to Gastrointestinal Nutrition.* Academy of Nutrition and Dietetics; 2015:168-181.

16. Simon R. Complications after pancreaticoduodenectomy. *Surg Clin North Am.* 2021;101(5):865-874. doi:10.1016/j.suc.2021.06.011

17. Cameron JL, Riall TS, Coleman J, Belcher KA. One thousand consecutive pancreaticoduodenectomies. *Ann Surg.* 2006;244(1):10-15. doi:10.1097/01.sla.0000217673.04165.ea

18. Kawaida H, Kono H, Hosomura N, et al. Surgical techniques and postoperative management to prevent postoperative pancreatic fistula after pancreatic surgery. *World J Gastroenterol.* 2019;25(28):3722-3737. doi:10.3748/wjg.v25.i28.3722

19. Tabriz N, Uslar VN, Obonyo D, Weyhe D. Micronutritional status after pylorus preserving duodenopancreatectomy: analysis of data from a randomized controlled trial. *Sci Rep.* 2021;11(1):18475. doi:10.1038/s41598-021-97438-6

20. Yu HH, Yang TM, Shan YS, Lin PW. Zinc deficiency in patients undergoing pancreatoduodenectomy for periampullary tumors is associated with pancreatic exocrine insufficiency. *World J Surg.* 2011;35(9):2110-2117. doi:10.1007/s00268-011-1170-z

21. Prescott J. Pancreatic enzyme replacement therapy: a view from behind the counter. *Pharmacy Times.* 2016;82(10).

22. Matarese LE, Harvin G. Nutritional care for patients with intestinal failure. *Gastroenterol Clin North Am.* 2021;50(1):201-216. doi:10.1016/j.gtc.2020.10.004

23. Jeppesen PB, Fuglsang KA. Nutritional therapy in adult short bowel syndrome patients with chronic intestinal failure. *Gastroenterol Clin North Am.* 2018;47(1):61-75. doi:10.1016/j.gtc.2017.10.004

24. Cresci GA, Bawden E. Gut microbiome: what we do and don't know. *Nutr Clin Pract.* 2015;30(6):734-746. doi:10.1177/0884533615609899

25.  Quigley EMM, Murray JA, Pimentel M. AGA clinical practice update on small intestinal bacterial overgrowth: expert review. *Gastroenterology*. 2020;159(4):1526-1532. doi:10.1053/j.gastro.2020.06.090

26.  Braga M, Bissolati M, Rocchetti S, Beneduce A, Pecorelli N, Di Carlo V. Oral preoperative antioxidants in pancreatic surgery: a double-blind, randomized, clinical trial. *Nutrition*. 2012;28(2):160-164. doi:10.1016/j.nut.2011.05.014

27.  Rhoda KM, Parekh NR, Lennon E, et al. The multidisciplinary approach to the care of patients with intestinal failure at a tertiary care facility. *Nutr Clin Pract*. 2010;25(2):183-191. doi:10.1177/0884533610361526

28.  Aksan A, Farrag K, Blumenstein I, Schröder O, Dignass AU, Stein J. Chronic intestinal failure and short bowel syndrome in Crohn's disease. *World J Gastroenterol*. 2021;27(24):3440-3465. doi:10.3748/wjg.v27.i24.3440

29.  Ber Y, García-Lopez S, Gargallo-Puyuelo CJ, Gomollón F. Small and large intestine (II): inflammatory bowel disease, short bowel syndrome, and malignant tumors of the digestive tract. *Nutrients*. 2021;13(7):2325. doi:10.3390/nu13072325

30.  Pironi L, Sasdelli AS. New insights into the indications for intestinal transplantation. *Curr Opin Organ Transplant*. 2021;26(2):186-191. doi:10.1097/MOT.0000000000000846

31.  Gómez-Ramírez S, Bisbe E, Shander A, Spahn DR, Muñoz M. Management of perioperative iron deficiency anemia. *Acta Haematol*. 2019;142(1):21-29. doi:10.1159/000496965

32.  Muñoz M, Acheson AG, Bisbe E, et al. An international consensus statement on the management of postoperative anaemia after major surgical procedures. *Anaesthesia*. 2018;73(11):1418-1431. doi:10.1111/anae.14358

33.  Iglar PJ, Hogan KJ. Vitamin D status and surgical outcomes: a systematic review. *Patient Saf Surg*. 2015;9:14. doi:10.1186/s13037-015-0060-y

34.  Lin HC, Prather C, Fisher RS, et al. Measurement of gastrointestinal transit. *Dig Dis Sci*. 2005;50(6):989-1004. doi:10.1007/s10620-005-2694-6

35.  von der Ohe MR, Camilleri M. Measurement of small bowel and colonic transit: indications and methods. *Mayo Clin Proc*. 1992;67(12):1169-1179. doi:10.1016/s0025-6196(12)61147-1

36.  Maurer AH, Krevsky B. Whole-gut transit scintigraphy in the evaluation of small-bowel and colon transit disorders. *Semin Nucl Med*. 1995;25(4):326-338. doi:10.1016/s0001-2998(95)80006-9

37.  Fragkos KC, Forbes A. Citrulline as a marker of intestinal function and absorption in clinical settings: a systematic review and meta-analysis. *United European Gastroenterol J*. 2018;6(2):181-191. doi:10.1177/2050640617737632

38. Lewis SJ, Heaton KW. Stool form scale as a useful guide to intestinal transit time. *Scand J Gastroenterol*. 1997;32(9):920-924. doi:10.3109 /00365529709011203

39. Saad RJ, Rao SS, Koch KL, et al. Do stool form and frequency correlate with whole-gut and colonic transit? Results from a multicenter study in constipated individuals and healthy controls. *Am J Gastroenterol*. 2010;105(2):403-411. doi:10.1038/ajg.2009.612

40. Min M, Patel B, Han S, et al. Exocrine pancreatic insufficiency and malnutrition in chronic pancreatitis: identification, treatment, and consequences. *Pancreas*. 2018;47(8):1015-1018. doi:10.1097/MPA .0000000000001137

41. Roberts KM. Diseases of the lower gastrointestinal tract. In: Nelms M, Sucher KP, eds. *Nutrition Therapy and Pathophysiology*. 4th ed. Cengage Learning; 2020.

42. Sundaram A, Koutkia P, Apovian CM. Nutritional management of short bowel syndrome in adults. *J Clin Gastroenterol*. 2002;34(3):207-220. doi:10 .1097/00004836-200203000-00003

43. Lung BE, Mowery ML, Komatsu DE. Calcitriol. In: *StatPearls* (online). StatPearls Publishing; 2022. NCBI Bookshelf. Accessed January 19, 2023. www.ncbi.nlm.nih.gov/books/NBK526025

# CHAPTER 10

# Chronic Kidney Disease

Melissa Mroz-Planells, DCN, RDN, and
Lance Kruger, PharmD, RPh

## Introduction

The primary causes of chronic kidney disease (CKD) are hypertension and diabetes. Consequently, patients with CKD have a higher risk for cardiovascular disease, due to these comorbidities. Hyperhomocysteinemia, reported as occurring in 85% to 100% of patients with CKD, also contributes to cardiovascular disease risk.[1-4] As kidney function declines, as measured by the glomerular filtration rate (GFR), plasma homocysteine levels increase and may reach high levels by the time a patient has end-stage renal disease.[4] Vitamin and mineral deficiencies are also common in CKD.[5]

In addition to comorbidities, other reported causes of micronutrient deficiencies in CKD include loss of kidney function, drug-nutrient interactions, renal replacement therapy (RRT), medical nutrition therapies resulting in restrictive dietary patterns, altered digestion and absorption, and illness.[6] Much of the literature on micronutrient deficiencies in CKD focuses on the role of RRT. A 2022 study reported that more than

90% of patients receiving continuous renal replacement therapy (CRRT) had at least one micronutrient deficiency diagnosed through serum values.[7] See Chapter 13 for more on CRRT in critical care. Approximately 70% of people treated with maintenance hemodialysis are routinely prescribed vitamin and mineral supplements; however, consistent evidence that would provide exact guidance for supplementation and help determine specific requirements is lacking.[5,6,8] Micronutrient requirements for patients in other stages of CKD, patients receiving peritoneal dialysis, and patients who have undergone a transplant have not been fully explored. These individuals may be deficient in thiamin, folate, calcium, iron, copper, and vitamins A, B6, C, D, or K.[6,8,9] Despite observational studies indicating a high prevalence of deficiencies in patients with CKD, micronutrient intervention studies are lacking, which prohibits the development of micronutrient-specific guidelines for managing deficiencies in these patients. The National Kidney Foundation's Kidney Disease Outcomes Quality Initiative (KDOQI)[9] and Kidney Disease: Improving Global Outcomes (KDIGO)[10] are long-standing publishers of clinical practice guidelines that provide evidence-based recommendations for the management of kidney disease.

This chapter reviews the roles played by selected micronutrients in CKD. Though the focus is on prevention of micronutrient deficiencies, concerns regarding elevated serum levels are discussed when relevant. Each section includes a review and summary of the literature and available guidelines, as well as a discussion of treatment strategies for consideration. Assessment and treatment strategies for all micronutrients are then summarized in a table at the end of the chapter. This information should be used alongside clinical judgment.

Box 10.1 on page 195 lists the distinguishing characteristics for each stage of CKD.[10]

# Micronutrient Assessment

Registered dietitian nutritionists (RDNs), in collaboration with physicians or other medical providers, are responsible for assessing patients with CKD for micronutrient deficiencies and prescribing repletion or supplementation as needed, based on disease stage, available evidence,

| BOX 10.1 Stages of Chronic Kidney Disease[10] | | |
|---|---|---|
| **Stage** | **Description** | **Glomerular filtration rate (GFR) (mL/min/1.73 m²)** |
| | At increased risk | ≥60 (with risk factors for chronic kidney disease) |
| 1 | Kidney damage with normal or increased GFR | ≥90 |
| 2 | Mild reduction in GFR | 60-89 |
| 3a | Moderate reduction in GFR | 45-59 |
| 3b | Moderate reduction in GFR | 30-44 |
| 4 | Severe reduction in GFR | 15-29 |
| 5 | Kidney failure | <15 (or dialysis) |

and clinical judgment.[1,2] Through patient interview, which can incorporate tools such as food records or diet recalls, the RDN can determine whether the patient is taking over-the-counter vitamin or mineral supplements, eating fortified foods, and consuming adequate amounts of micronutrients. The patient is examined for clinical signs and symptoms of deficiencies and also undergoes a biochemical assessment (when appropriate) and a nutrition focused physical exam.[6] Because patients with CKD are at high risk for micronutrient abnormalities, special multivitamin supplements have been formulated for this population to facilitate a preventive approach. Table 10.1 compares the micronutrient content of such renal-specific multivitamin supplements to that of a standard multivitamin/mineral supplement.[11-13]

**TABLE 10.1  Adult Renal Multivitamin Supplements vs Standard Multivitamin/Mineral Supplement[11-13]**

| Micronutrient | Renal gel formulation[11] | Renal tablet formulation[12] | Standard multivitamin/mineral supplement[13] |
|---|---|---|---|
| Vitamin C | 100 mg | 60 mg | 60 mg |
| Thiamin | 1.5 mg | 1.5 mg | 1.5 mg |
| Riboflavin | 1.7 mg | 1.7 mg | 1.7 mg |
| Niacin | 20 mg | 20 mg | 20 mg |
| Vitamin B6 | 10 mg | 10 mg | 2 mg |
| Folate | 1 mg | 1 mg | 667 mcg of dietary folate equivalents |
| Vitamin B12 | 6 mcg | 6 mcg | 6 mcg |
| Biotin | 150 mcg | 300 mcg | 30 mcg |
| Pantothenic acid | 5 mg | 10 mg | 10 mg |
| Vitamin A | 0 | 0 | 1,050 mcg |
| Vitamin D3 | 0 | 0 | 25 mcg (1,000 IU) |
| Vitamin E | 0 | 0 | 13.5 mg |
| Vitamin K | 0 | 0 | 25 mcg |
| Calcium | 0 | 0 | 200 mg |
| Iron | 0 | 0 | 18 mg |
| Phosphorous | 0 | 0 | 20 mg |
| Iodine | 0 | 0 | 150 mcg |
| Magnesium | 0 | 0 | 50 mg |
| Zinc | 0 | 0 | 11 mg |
| Selenium | 0 | 0 | 55 mcg |
| Copper | 0 | 0 | 0.5 mg |
| Manganese | 0 | 0 | 2.3 mg |
| Chromium | 0 | 0 | 35 mcg |

*Continued on next page*

| Micronutrient | Renal gel formulation[11] | Renal tablet formulation[12] | Standard multivitamin/mineral supplement[13] |
|---|---|---|---|
| Molybdenum | 0 | 0 | 45 mcg |
| Chloride | 0 | 0 | 72 mg |
| Potassium | 0 | 0 | 80 mg |

# Water-Soluble Vitamins

## B Vitamins

Homocysteine is a nonessential, sulfur-containing amino acid that is regulated by vitamin B6, vitamin B12, and folate as methyl donors.[1,2] Folate is a methyl provider, and vitamin B12 acts as a regulator of DNA methylation and the epigenetic network.[2] Hyperhomocysteinemia impairs endothelial function, stimulates the inflammatory process, oxidizes low-density lipids, and increases the proliferation of smooth muscle cells.[1-3] In the presence of uremia, hyperhomocysteinemia targets methyltransferases, which leads to changes in the genes that control methylation.[2-4] Epigenetic dysregulation in CKD includes alterations in nutritional status, increased oxidative stress, enhanced inflammation, changes to the gut microbiome, and production of uremic toxins.[1-4]

Researchers reported thiamin deficiency in CKD as a result of losses from RRT (primarily hemodialysis), losses associated with diuretics, and malnutrition.[14] Reduced renal clearance for the vitamin metabolites in CKD stages 1 through 4 (prior to dialysis) may result in higher than normal metabolite plasma or cellular levels.[4,15] Furthermore, erythrocyte transketolase and whole blood thiamin pyrophosphate values are sensitive and specific to assessing thiamin status but may be impaired in CKD because of the impact of uremic metabolites. Assessment of these values may be confirmed by the presence of clinical symptoms.[5]

## Treatment Strategies

Maximizing nutrient intake is a crucial component of the treatment plan for micronutrient deficiencies in patients with CKD. The RDN can assist with identifying nutrient-dense foods and planning nutrient-dense meals via the medical nutrition therapy prescription. There is evidence to support folic acid supplementation in patients with hyperhomocysteinemia. However, because routine pharmacologic dosing of folate, with or without a vitamin B complex, has not been definitively shown to reduce adverse cardiovascular outcomes,[5,9] experts do not recommend supplementing folate based solely on hyperhomocysteinemia. In addition, a high intake of folate may mask pernicious anemia.[9]

Supplementation with thiamin, folate, vitamin B12, or a vitamin B complex is recommended when clinical signs and symptoms indicate deficiency or insufficiency of folate or vitamin B12 (see Chapter 6), or it can be used proactively for individuals with CKD stages 1 through 5 and following kidney transplant.[8]

# Vitamin C

Vitamin C deficiency is common in patients with advanced CKD because of nutrient losses from dialysis therapy, dietary restrictions on foods high in potassium but also rich in vitamin C, and increased vitamin C requirements associated with inflammation.[15,16] Plasma vitamin C concentration drives the degree of tubular reabsorption, and in advanced stages of CKD, tubular resorption can be compromised, leading to persistent hypovitaminosis. Supplementation of vitamin C in patients receiving dialysis is of interest because of the potential for vitamin C to support the ongoing treatment of anemia, oxidative stress, and inflammation, despite the limited availability of dosing strategies in the published literature. Research has made it evident that RRT leads to a reduction in plasma vitamin C concentration, but there is insufficient data to guide optimal dosing because the available data does not take into account the risk for vitamin C overdose in those with end-stage renal disease.[15]

## Treatment Strategies

Increased intake of foods rich in vitamin C—such as citrus fruits, bell peppers, strawberries, tomatoes, cruciferous vegetables, and white potatoes—helps maintain vitamin C status and should be encouraged. Individuals in all stages of CKD may safely supplement 60 to 100 mg vitamin C per day. KDOQI guidelines suggest that for adults with CKD stages 1 through 5D, a reasonable vitamin C prescription would be at least 90 mg/d for males and 75 mg/d for females.[3,17] There are concerns of toxicity with supplemental doses higher than 500 mg/d, as this may increase the risk for calcium oxalate stones.[18,19]

# Fat-Soluble Vitamins

Dietary intake of fat-soluble vitamins may be insufficient in individuals with certain subclasses of CKD, thus increasing the risk for deficiencies. However, unlike supplementation of water-soluble nutrients, supplementation of fat-soluble vitamins carries with it the added risk of toxicity. Although the focus of this chapter is on prevention and treatment of deficiencies in patients with CKD, clinicians working with this population should be aware of the concern for toxicity.

## Vitamin A

Retinol is the commonly studied form of vitamin A and the predominate vitamin A compound essential for human health; therefore, it is the form discussed here (refer to Chapter 5 for more on vitamin A). Elevated serum retinol concentration has been reported in advanced stages of CKD and during dialysis. Despite this finding, the higher serum levels of retinol do not appear to be consistent with actual vitamin A stores. In CKD, retinol metabolism is altered in two ways[5]:

- Degradation of the retinol carrier protein (apo-retinol-binding protein, or RBP-4) is reduced, which in turn contributes to the higher serum levels of retinol.
- Retinol binding protein (RBP), which transports vitamin A in the

serum, cannot be cleared during dialysis due to the large size of the molecule, leading to higher serum levels of vitamin A.

For this reason, the concern for retinol toxicity is typically low, as the higher serum levels are likely the result of changes in the metabolism of retinol.[4] Although medical nutrition therapy for CKD often reduces the dietary intake of vitamin A, there are no recommendations for supplementation.[4,9]

# Vitamin E

The prevalence of vitamin E deficiency in individuals with CKD is not well known. Vitamin E can interact with anticoagulant and antiplatelet medications that are commonly prescribed to patients with CKD.[6] Note that the potential for toxicity may increase the risk of hemorrhagic stroke and impair platelet aggregation.[9,20-22]

Research into supplementation of vitamin E in patients with CKD has produced conflicting results.[20,21] Furthermore, studies show that in patients receiving maintenance hemodialysis, the effect of vitamin E supplementation at doses ranging from 400 to 800 IU/d is not statistically significant with regard to lowering levels of C-reactive protein and interleukin-6 (indicators of inflammation).[9] This may be related to the fact that vitamin E is not filtered through dialysis. The available evidence does not support a need for vitamin E supplementation in patients with CKD.

## Treatment Strategies

Data are lacking to suggest a need for vitamin E intake exceeding the Dietary Reference Intake in patients with CKD. (Chapter 5 provides a review of the standard assessment, treatment, and monitoring of vitamin E deficiency.) In those requiring supplementation, oral doses of vitamin E in excess of 1,000 to 1,500 IU/d should not be prescribed without close monitoring of serum levels, due to the risk of toxicity and the antithrombotic effects.[20,21] Practitioners should pay attention to over-the-counter supplementation and the risk of drug-nutrient interactions to prevent toxicity.[1]

# Vitamin K

Research suggests that a large percentage of individuals with CKD have suboptimal vitamin K status that is likely linked to both increased needs and lower dietary intake. Vitamin K is an essential component of a carboxylase enzyme used in the synthesis of the coagulation factors II, VII, IX, and X. In addition, the vitamin K–dependent carboxylase enzymes are a constituent step in the synthesis of osteocalcin and the inhibition of vascular calcifications. The pathophysiology of CKD and the complications of the standard medications used to treat CKD result in a higher demand for these processes and may increase the overall requirement for vitamin K.[23-25] For example, phosphate binders, a common element of therapy in CKD, may adversely affect vitamin K status. A 2017 study demonstrated that there is a potential binding of vitamin K with the use of calcium-based phosphate binders.[26] In addition, lower dietary intake of dark leafy vegetables and dairy products by patients receiving RRT could reduce the overall vitamin K status.[23]

Because heart disease is associated with CKD, several studies have assessed the use of vitamin K therapy in reducing risk of heart disease.[27-29] The findings suggest that vitamin K supplementation may reduce calcifications, and more specific recommendations may be developed with future research. At this time, specific guidelines for supplementation are not available. Vitamin K supplementation should not be provided for patients receiving anticoagulant medicines. Chapter 5 provides additional guidance.

# Vitamin D

CKD is associated with increased risk of vitamin D insufficiency (serum levels of 16–30 ng/mL) and deficiency (serum levels of ≤15 ng/mL).[30,31] Vitamin D is activated in the kidneys, and lower levels of vitamin D in patients with CKD are largely driven by a decline in vitamin D metabolism and synthesis as kidney function declines.[30] Calcitriol is the form of vitamin D present after hydroxylation in the liver and kidneys, and it is considered to be the fully functional form of vitamin D.[31]

Secondary hyperparathyroidism is a common complication of CKD. Put simply, it is the disruption of the normal feedback loop that results in parathyroid hormone (PTH) release. Lower serum calcium and higher serum phosphorus levels stimulate an increase in PTH release as the body attempts to correct the abnormal serum levels. Higher PTH levels subsequently reduce the absorption and release of vitamin D. If not controlled, the stimulation of PTH release results in hyperplasia of the parathyroid, and, thus, secondary hyperparathyroidism continues.[32,33] A retrospective study found that hyperparathyroidism was associated with a 1.3-times-higher risk of fractures and death, a 2.2-times-higher risk of major adverse cardiovascular events, and a five-times-higher risk of CKD progression.[34]

Serum 25-hydroxyvitamin D concentration is the most-assessed biochemical level of vitamin D and is preferred over serum 1,25-dihydroxyvitamin D. Ergocalciferol (vitamin D2) and cholecalciferol (vitamin D3) are appropriate for supplementation or repletion, even in patients with a reduced ability to complete the final hydroxylation, as occurs in CKD.[3]

## Treatment Strategies

The use of vitamin D receptor activators, including calcitriol, is a potential strategy for the repletion of vitamin D, as well as for the treatment of hyperparathyroidism. KDOQI guidelines confirm that both vitamin D2 and vitamin D3 are sufficient for treatment of vitamin D deficiency and result in improvements in PTH levels.[9] However, the guidelines lack a specific recommendation for dosing strategies for vitamin D repletion when the goal is to reduce PTH levels.

In addition to dietary supplements containing vitamin D2 or vitamin D3, there are also prescription vitamin D formulations indicated for use in patients with CKD. Calcitriol in its naturally active form can be prescribed for patients with stage 5 CKD; however, it is limited by a risk for hypercalcemia, hypercalciuria, and hyperphosphatemia. Paricalcitol and doxercalciferol are synthetic vitamin D analogues. Like calcitriol, paricalcitol is biologically active, whereas doxercalciferol requires activation in the liver before it can act as an agonist on vitamin D receptors.[34]

# Minerals

The kidneys are responsible for maintaining homeostasis of several key minerals. Calcium, iron, sodium, potassium, phosphorus, and copper are of particular concern in CKD. A healthy functioning kidney adapts to changing dietary intake by excreting or reabsorbing minerals to maintain homeostasis; this balance is lost as kidney function declines. Chapters 7 and 8 provide more detailed information on mineral deficiencies.

## Calcium

Calcium homeostasis in CKD is complex. Reduced kidney function affects the conversion of vitamin D to its active form, and a lower serum vitamin D level may result in hypocalcemia. This begins a feedback loop with the stimulation of PTH to correct the low serum calcium level. As secondary hyperparathyroidism develops, the ongoing risk of hypocalcemia continues to be a concern.[35]

Studies in individuals with moderate CKD indicate that the kidney remains capable of maintaining a neutral calcium balance when the Recommended Dietary Allowance (RDA) for calcium is consumed. However, consumption of excess calcium results in a positive calcium balance. In addition, there may be an increased risk for calcium oxalate stones.[36] Therefore, adults with CKD should maintain a dietary calcium intake of 1,000 to 1,200 mg/d.[37,38]

The serum calcium level should be assessed with consideration of the serum albumin concentration using the following formula:

$$\text{corrected calcium} = 0.8 \times (4 - \text{patient's albumin level}) + \text{serum calcium level}$$

The assessment of calcium status should also include a review and assessment of vitamin D status.

## Treatment Strategies

The RDA for calcium ranges from 1,000 to 1,200 mg/d for adults, dependent on age and sex.[38] Daily calcium needs should be met via a combination of dietary calcium and, if needed, supplemental calcium. Hypocalcemia is typically addressed by increasing the calcium content of the diet if the assessment indicates inadequate oral intake. As CKD progresses, calcium supplementation may be needed in an over-the-counter form such as calcium carbonate, which also serves as a phosphate binder. For example, consumption of a chewable calcium carbonate tablet such as TUMS (500 mg elemental calcium per tablet) at each meal assists with maintaining serum calcium levels while reducing serum phosphorus levels.

Hypercalcemia can first be managed with the elimination of oral calcium supplements or calcium-enriched foods. Other factors to consider include ensuring appropriate hydration status and addressing elevated PTH levels. In patients receiving RRT, the dialysis prescription can also be adjusted to decrease the amount of calcium in the dialysate.[36]

To treat the bone mineral disorder associated with CKD, the medications cinacalcet and etelcalcetide can be administered to manage serum calcium levels and treat hyperparathyroidism.[39,40]

# Phosphorus

The kidneys are responsible for excreting excess phosphorus to maintain homeostasis. Because of compensatory mechanisms, elevations in serum phosphorus concentration do not manifest until the latest stages of CKD. Increased levels of PTH and fibroblast growth factor 23 signal the kidneys to increase phosphorus excretion. These compensatory mechanisms begin to fail and can no longer maintain phosphate excretion in the latest stages of kidney disease, when patients are typically starting dialysis.[41,42]

In some cases, hyperphosphatemia may manifest in earlier stages of CKD and, along with the resulting elevations in PTH and fibroblast growth factor 23, is associated with accelerated progression of CKD. Ultimately, elevations in phosphorus levels are apparent in many patients despite ongoing dialysis, and these elevations are associated with increased risk of mortality.[41,42] Research has shown that elevated serum phosphorus concentration is associated with increased progression of vascular calcification and higher morbidity and mortality due to cardiovascular complications.[43,44]

## Treatment Strategies

Treatment of hyperphosphatemia using phosphorus binders is typically required for patients with stage 5 CKD who are receiving maintenance dialysis. Phosphorus binders must be taken with meals because they work by forming nonabsorbable complexes with phosphate present in the diet. This activity prevents the absorption of phosphorus and lowers serum levels in patients receiving dialysis.[45] Box 10.2 lists the pros and cons of common phosphate binders.[46]

Phosphorus levels are also managed through diet and the regulation of dialysate composition. Depending on serum phosphorus values, patients may be asked to reduce their dietary intake of phosphorus. Caution should be taken with foods high in phosphorus additives, as they are more readily absorbed (bioavailability estimated at 90%–100%) than foods high in natural phosphorus (bioavailability estimated at 30%–60%).[45] Foods high in natural phosphorus include dairy foods, such as milk and cheese, as well as animal proteins. Foods high in phosphorus additives include processed foods, such as sodas and deli meats.[47] KDIGO guidelines recommend that patients receiving dialysis maintain serum phosphorus levels within the normal laboratory ranges (3.0–4.5 mg/dL).[46]

| BOX 10.2 Common Phosphate Binders[46] | |
|---|---|
| **Calcium acetate (PhosLo)** | |
| **Pros** | Generic availability |
| | Increases calcium level to correct hypocalcemia and lower parathyroid hormone level |
| **Cons** | Risk of hypercalcemia and vascular calcification |
| | Constipation |

## BOX 10.2 Common Phosphate Binders[46] (cont.)

### *Sevelamer carbonate (Renvela)*

**Pros**    Generic availability

Lowers low-density lipoprotein cholesterol level

**Cons**    Low potency

Constipation

Binds and decreases absorption of fat-soluble vitamins

### *Lanthanum carbonate (Fosrenol)*

**Pros**    Generic availability

High potency

**Cons**    Must be fully chewed to avoid gastrointestinal risks

Potential systemic absorption and toxicity

### *Sucroferric oxyhydroxide (Velphoro)*

**Pros**    No contraindications

High potency

Very limited systemic iron absorption

**Cons**    No generic availability

Dark stool due to iron content

### *Ferric citrate (Auryxia)*

**Pros**    Indicated in nondialysis chronic kidney disease to treat iron deficiency anemia

**Cons**    No generic availability

Risk of iron overload due to systemic absorption

Dark stool due to iron content

It is also important to recognize that hypophosphatemia may occur in patients after a kidney transplant.

# Potassium

For individuals with normal or preserved kidney function (GFR >60), up to 90% of dietary potassium is excreted. Abnormalities in serum potassium levels occur in 5% to 20% of individuals with CKD when compensatory mechanisms can no longer accommodate the rising serum potassium level.[48] In addition to the decreasing kidney function that affects excretion of potassium, factors such as renin-angiotensin-aldosterone system inhibition, metabolic acidosis, and side effects of medications used after kidney transplantation may also result in hyperkalemia.[49] Angiotensin-converting enzyme (ACE) inhibitors and angiotensin II receptor blockers (ARBs) are commonly used to treat hypertension in patients with CKD, as they provide cardiovascular and kidney protection in addition to their primary mechanism of blood pressure control. A substantial body of literature has examined the benefit of discontinuing the use of ACE inhibitors and ARBs as the first line of treatment for hyperkalemia, but this research has not resulted in consistent recommendations.[50]

Hypokalemia can also be present in people with CKD. Major causes include the use of potassium-wasting diuretic medications, gastrointestinal losses, side effects of other medications, and abnormalities in aldosterone levels.[51,52]

Serum potassium levels should be closely monitored in patients with CKD because hyperkalemia and hypokalemia can result in serious and life-threatening events. The occurrence of cardiovascular events, as well as mortality, increases with both hypokalemia and hyperkalemia.[48,49] In patients with end-stage renal disease who are undergoing hemodialysis, hyperkalemia is a major concern because thrice-weekly hemodialysis is relied on to remove potassium and lower serum potassium levels to the normal range. Despite this, serum potassium levels will again start to increase immediately following dialysis, leading to fluctuations in levels, with a peak just before dialysis and a trough immediately after dialysis. These fluctuations may also be associated with increased mortality and cardiovascular events.[52,53]

## Treatment Strategies

A full investigation into the root cause of hyperkalemia enables the clinician to determine the optimal treatment strategy. A thorough diet recall from the patient can determine high dietary sources of potassium. Dietary potassium is consumed through fruits, vegetables, and dairy products, as well as some food additives.[54]

In addition to dietary restrictions for the control of hyperkalemia, medical management can include the use of diuretics and potassium binders. Potassium-wasting diuretics can be used to decrease serum potassium levels in patients with sufficient kidney function to respond to the diuretic. Potassium binders can be administered in patients with end-stage renal disease or when other options are not effective. These medications are nonabsorbable compounds that exchange a cation for potassium in the gut; potassium is then excreted in the feces. The pros and cons of common potassium binders are listed in Box 10.3 on page 210.[51-53]

# Sodium

As kidney function declines, so does the body's ability to regulate extracellular fluid volume. The imbalance of sodium and chloride results in both edema and the potential for increased blood pressure. In addition, sodium retention may increase the risk of metabolic acidosis.

## Treatment Strategies

In CKD stages 1 through 4, dietary sodium intake should not exceed 2,300 to 2,400 mg/d. As CKD progresses to stage 5, the recommended intake is dependent on urine output but is typically around 2,000 mg/d.[55] Additional interventions may be prescribed within the dialysis prescription, as well as the removal of fluid during RRT.

## BOX 10.3  Common Potassium Binders[51-53]

### *Sodium polystyrene sulfonate (Kayexalate)*

Used primarily for the treatment of acute hyperkalemia

**Pros**   Nonselective: also binds calcium and magnesium[a]

Can be administered rectally if needed

Inexpensive

**Cons**   Gastrointestinal (GI) discomfort with incidence of fatal GI bleeding reported

Nonselective: also binds calcium and magnesium[a]

Variable effect and delayed onset of symptom correction

### *Patiromer (Veltassa)*

Used primarily for the treatment of chronic hyperkalemia

**Pros**   No sodium content

Once-daily dosing

**Cons**   GI discomfort

Nonselective: also binds sodium and magnesium

### *Sodium zirconium cyclosilicate (Lokelma)*

Used primarily for the treatment of chronic hyperkalemia

**Pros**   High selectivity for potassium

Quick onset (within 1 h)

Once-daily or every-other-day dosing

**Cons**   GI discomfort

Edema

[a] Depending on the scenario, calcium and magnesium binding could be a positive or negative effect of potassium binders.

# Iron

Iron deficiency is a reduction in iron stores, whereas iron deficiency anemia is a serious complication of iron deficiency in which microcytic, hypochromic red blood cells are present.[56,57] Anemia is common in patients with CKD. Although it is primarily caused by decreased production of erythropoietin in the kidney, anemia in CKD is also attributed to disruptions in iron metabolism. Patients with CKD can experience blood loss (from repeated blood draws and other factors) and impaired iron absorption, which leads to absolute iron deficiency as iron stores are depleted. In addition, the presence of chronic inflammation in CKD increases hepcidin, which not only impairs iron absorption but also decreases the release of iron from iron stores, leading to functional iron deficiency.[57]

Iron deficiency anemia can be diagnosed by monitoring ferritin levels and transferrin saturation values in patients with CKD. The following are diagnostic criteria for iron deficiency anemia and indicate that iron supplementation may be warranted[58]:

- a ferritin level less than 100 ng/mL in patients not receiving dialysis
- a ferritin level less than 200 ng/mL in patients receiving dialysis
- a transferrin saturation value less than 20%

However, these laboratory test results should be interpreted in the context of the individual patient because ferritin is an acute-phase reactant and is elevated during times of inflammation.[58]

## Treatment Strategies

Oral iron supplementation is commonly used for patients not receiving dialysis. Intravenous iron supplementation is recommended for those receiving dialysis, owing to their higher levels of hepcidin and increased inflammation, both of which impair absorption of oral iron. Oral formulations include over-the-counter supplements such as ferrous sulfate, ferrous gluconate, ferrous fumarate, and iron polysaccharide, in addition to prescription ferric citrate. Although the ferrous formulations are less expensive and more readily available, the overall dose that can be administered may be limited by gastrointestinal side effects and reduced absorption.[59-61]

Several intravenous formulations appropriate for patients receiving dialysis can also be used for patients not receiving dialysis. These include iron dextran (the low-molecular-weight form), ferric gluconate, iron sucrose, ferumoxytol, iron isomaltoside, and ferric carboxymaltose. Each has its own approved dosing and administration instructions, with most requiring multiple infusions over many days.[62,63] The safety profiles of these formulations also vary, with some requiring a test dose to monitor for rare anaphylactic reactions before giving a full dose.[59,62,63] (Chapter 7 provides more information on the treatment of iron deficiency.)

# Copper

Copper status changes throughout the course of CKD. In earlier stages of CKD, increased levels of copper due to the decrease in filtration have been reported. This accumulation of copper has been considered a potential risk factor for worsening kidney function. However, in critical illness, when CRRT is required, copper is lost because of increased filtration. Observational studies have consistently highlighted a high prevalence of copper deficiency during CRRT in patients with critical illness.[7,64] In addition to the challenges posed by a changing copper status as kidney function declines, the fact that copper is an acute-phase reactant also presents challenges to assessment of copper deficiency during critical illness (Chapter 4). Because more than 94% of copper is bound to ceruloplasmin, ceruloplasmin remains the most reported measure of copper status in patients with critical illness.

## Treatment Strategies

Experts recommend that patients with CKD meet the Dietary Reference Intake for copper based on their age and sex. Excellent food sources of copper include shellfish, meat, legumes, nuts, and cheese. Otherwise, the copper assessment and treatment strategies presented in Chapter 8 should be considered for use.

# Summary of Micronutrient Assessment and Treatment in Chronic Kidney Disease

Box 10.4 summarizes the assessment and treatment of micronutrient deficiencies in patients with CKD.[5,6,18,19,56,57,59,65]

---

**BOX 10.4  Micronutrient Assessment and Treatment in Patients With Chronic Kidney Disease**[5,6,18,19,56,57,59,65]

### B Vitamins

**Laboratory values of importance**
Serum, plasma, or red blood cell folate
Serum vitamin B12

**Management strategy**
In chronic kidney disease (CKD) stages 3 through 5D or post-transplant with hyperhomocysteinemia associated with kidney disease, do not routinely supplement folate with or without vitamin B complex due to lack of evidence for reduction in adverse cardiovascular outcomes.

Prescribe a multivitamin supplement according to the nutrient assessment.

Supplement folate, vitamin B12, or vitamin B complex to correct for folate or vitamin B12 deficiency or insufficiency according to dietary intake, clinical signs, and symptoms.

### Vitamin C

**Laboratory values of importance**
Serum or plasma vitamin C

**Management strategy**
Vitamin C is safe to supplement at 75 to 90 mg/d. In adults with CKD stages 1 through 5D, it is reasonable to supplement at least 90 mg/d for males and 75 mg/d for females. Use caution with high dosages due to the risk of oxalate nephrolithiasis.[a]

*Continued on next page*

**BOX 10.4 Micronutrient Assessment and Treatment in Patients With Chronic Kidney Disease[5,6,18,19,56,57,59,65] (cont.)**

## Vitamins A, E, and K

| | |
|---|---|
| Laboratory values of importance | Retinol |
| | α-Tocopherol |
| | Serum vitamin K, prothrombin time and international normalized ration (INR) |
| Management strategy | Avoid supplementation of vitamins A and E in patients with CKD. |
| | Consider up to 10 mcg vitamin K if the patient has low dietary intake or long-term antibiotic use. |
| | Do not provide vitamin K supplementation to patients receiving anticoagulant medicines. |

## Vitamin D

| | |
|---|---|
| Laboratory values of importance | Serum 25-hydroxyvitamin D |
| Management strategy | Supplement vitamin D2, 50 mcg/d (2,000 IU/d) for insufficiency and 100 to 200 mcg/d (4,000-8,000 IU/d) for deficiency, to reach a serum level of 30 ng/mL or greater. |
| | Calcitriol may be prescribed at an initial dose of 0.25 mcg/d in stage 5 CKD. |

## Calcium

| | |
|---|---|
| Laboratory values of importance | Serum total calcium, *or* |
| | Corrected calcium, *or* |
| | Serum ionized calcium |
| Management strategy | Daily calcium needs (1,000–1,200 mg for adults) should be met through a combination of dietary calcium intake and, if needed, supplemental calcium. |
| | In patients with hypercalcemia, individualize treatment based on serum values and prescribed vitamin D analogues in stage 5D CKD. The starting dose for cinacalcet is 30 mg, by mouth (PO), twice daily; for etelcalcetide dosing is 5 mg intravenous three times weekly. |

**BOX 10.4  Micronutrient Assessment and Treatment in Patients With Chronic Kidney Disease[5,6,18,19,56,57,59,65] (cont.)**

## Copper

| | |
|---|---|
| Laboratory values of importance | Ceruloplasmin |
| Management strategy | Supplement copper to the Dietary Reference Intakes based on patient's age and sex. |

## Iron

| | |
|---|---|
| Laboratory values of importance | Serum ferritin<br>Transferrin saturation |
| Management strategy | **Oral dosing[b]**<br>Ferrous sulfate: 65 mg tablet, one to three times daily<br>Ferrous gluconate: 35 mg, one to three times daily<br>**Intravenous dosing[c]**<br>Iron sucrose: 100 mg over the course of 10 sequential dialysis sessions (for those on hemodialysis); five doses of 200 mg over the course of 14 days (nondialysis-dependent)<br>Ferric gluconate in sucrose complex: Eight doses of 125 mg over the course of eight sequential dialysis sessions<br>Ferric carboxymaltose: 15 mg per kg of body weight (maximum 750 mg per dose), repeat 7 days later if necessary<br>Iron dextran: Based on iron deficit[b] |

## Sodium

| | |
|---|---|
| Laboratory values of importance | Serum sodium |
| Management strategy | Limit sodium intake to less than 2,300 mg/d to reduce blood pressure and assist in the management of fluid retention. |

*Continued on next page*

Chronic Kidney Disease

Chronic Kidney
Disease

**BOX 10.4  Micronutrient Assessment and Treatment in Patients With Chronic Kidney Disease[5,6,18,19,56,57,59,65] (cont.)**

### Potassium

| | |
|---|---|
| Laboratory values of importance | Serum potassium |
| Management strategy | Adjust dietary potassium to maintain the serum level within the normal range. Base treatment on individual patient needs. |
| | Hyperkalemia may be treated with potassium binders with doses titrated to maintain a normal serum potassium level. |

### Phosphorus

| | |
|---|---|
| Laboratory values of importance | Serum phosphorus |
| Management strategy | Base treatment on the individual patient's serum level. |
| | Treat a high serum level with a diet moderate in phosphorus and with phosphate binders titrated to maintain serum levels within normal laboratory ranges (3.0–4.5 mg/dL). |

[a] Recommendations for transgender people were not provided.

[b] The efficacy of oral iron supplements in patients with CKD is limited because of diminished gastrointestinal absorption due to increased serum levels of hepcidin.

[c] Based on iron deficit. Iron deficit is estimated by several different equations. Preferred equations may vary between products and institutions.

# References

1. Mann JF, Sheridan P, McQueen MJ, et al. Homocysteine lowering with folic acid and B vitamins in people with chronic kidney disease—results of the renal Hope-2 study. *Nephrol Dial Transplant.* 2008;23(2):645-653. doi:10.1093/ndt/gfm485

2. Brady CB, Gaziano JM, Cxypoliski RA, et al. Homocysteine lowering and cognition in CKD: the Veterans Affairs homocysteine study. *Am J Kidney Dis.* 2009;54(3):440-449. doi:10.1053/j.ajkd.2009.05.013

3. Badri S, Vahdat S, Seirafian S, Pourfarzam M, Gholipur-Shahraki T, Ataei S. Homocysteine-lowering interventions in chronic kidney disease. *J Res Pharm Pract*. 2021;10(3):114-124. doi:10.4103/jrpp.jrpp_75_21

4. Cappuccilli M, Bergamini C, Giacomelli FA, et al. Vitamin B supplementation and nutritional intake of methyl donors in patients with chronic kidney disease: a critical review of the impact on epigenetic machinery. *Nutrients*. 2020;12(5):1234. doi:10.3390/nu12051234

5. Chazot C, Steiber A, Kopple JD. Vitamin needs and treatment for chronic kidney disease patients. *J Ren Nutr*. Published online September 28, 2022. doi:10.1053/j.jrn.2022.09.008

6. NKF KDOQI clinical practice guidelines. National Kidney Foundation. Accessed April 15, 2023. www.kidney.org/professionals/guidelines

7. Fah M, Van Althuis LE, Ohnuma T, et al. Micronutrient deficiencies in critically ill patients receiving continuous renal replacement therapy. *Clin Nutr ESPEN*. 2022;50:247-254. doi:10.1016/j.clnesp.2022.05.008

8. KDIGO guidelines. Kidney Disease: Improving Global Outcomes (KDIGO). Accessed April 15, 2023. https://kdigo.org/guidelines

9. Ikizler TA, Burrowes JD, Byham-Gray LD, et al. KDOQI clinical practice guideline for nutrition in CKD: 2020 update. *Am J Kidney Dis*. 2020;76 (3 suppl 1):S1-S107. doi:10.1053/j.ajkd.2020.05.006

10. Kidney Disease: Improving Global Outcomes (KDIGO) Glomerular Diseases Work Group. KDIGO 2021 clinical practice guideline for the management of glomerular diseases. *Kidney Int*. 2021;100(4S):S1-S276. doi:10.1016/j.kint.2021.05.021

11. Renal caps prescribing information. Drugs.com. Updated March 27, 2023. Accessed April 15, 2023. www.drugs.com/pro/renal-caps.html

12. Nephro-Vite RX tablets. Package insert. Allergan; March 2016. Accessed April 15, 2023. www.rxabbvie.com/pdf/nephro-vite-rx_pi.pdf

13. Centrum Adults Multivitamin/Multimineral Supplement. Supplement Facts panel. Accessed April 15, 2023. www.centrum.com/products/multivitamins/centrum-adults

14. Saka Y, Naruse T, Kato A, et al. Thiamine status in end-stage chronic kidney disease patients: a single-center study. *Int Urol Nephrol*. 2018;50(10):1913-1918. doi:10.1007/s11255-018-1974-y

15. Moradi H, Said HM. Functional thiamine deficiency in end-stage renal disease: malnutrition despite ample nutrients. *Kidney Int*. 2016;90(2): 252-254. doi:10.1016/j.kint.2016.04.017

16. Doshida Y, Itabashi M, Takei T, et al. Reduced plasma ascorbate and increased proportion of dehydroascorbic acid levels in patients undergoing hemodialysis. *Life (Basel)*. 2021;11(10):1023. doi:10.3390/life11101023

17. Honore PM, Spapen HD, Marik P, Boer W, Oudemans-van Straaten H. Dosing vitamin C in critically ill patients with special attention to renal replacement therapy: a narrative review. *Ann Intensive Care.* 2020;10(1):23. doi:10.1186/s13613-020-0640-6

18. Lin WV, Turin CG, McCormick DW, Haas C, Constantine G. Ascorbic acid-induced oxalate nephropathy: a case report and discussion of pathologic mechanisms. *CEN Case Rep.* 2019;8(1):67-70. doi:10.1007/s13730-018-0366-6

19. Lumlertgul N, Siribamrungwong M, Jaber BL, Susantitaphong P. Secondary oxalate nephropathy: a systematic review. *Kidney Int Rep.* 2018;3(6):1363-1372. doi:10.1016/j.ekir.2018.07.020

20. Boaz M, Smetana S, Weinstein T, et al. Secondary prevention with antioxidants of cardiovascular disease in endstage renal disease (SPACE): randomised placebo-controlled trial. *Lancet.* 2000;356(9237):1213-1218. doi:10.1016/s0140-6736(00)02783-5

21. Lonn E, Bosch J, Yusuf S, et al. Effects of long-term vitamin E supplementation on cardiovascular events and cancer: a randomized controlled trial. *JAMA.* 2005;293(11):1338-1347. doi:10.1001/jama.293.11.1338

22. Vitamin E: fact sheet for health professionals. Office of Dietary Supplements, National Institutes of Health. Updated March 26, 2021. Accessed March 19, 2023. https://ods.od.nih.gov/factsheets/VitaminE-HealthProfessional

23. Holden RM, Morton AR, Garland JS, Pavlov A, Day AG, Booth SL. Vitamins K and D status in stages 3-5 chronic kidney disease. *Clin J Am Soc Nephrol.* 2010;5(4):590-597. doi:10.2215/CJN.06420909

24. Cranenburg EC, Schurgers LJ, Uiterwijk HH, et al. Vitamin K intake and status are low in hemodialysis patients. *Kidney Int.* 2012;82(5):605-610. doi:10.1038/ki.2012.191

25. Cozzolino M, Mangano M, Galassi A, Ciceri P, Messa P, Nigwekar S. Vitamin K in chronic kidney disease. *Nutrients.* 2019;11(1):168. doi:10.3390/nu11010168

26. Neradova A, Schumacher SP, Hubeek I, Lux P, Schurgers LJ, Vervloet MG. Phosphate binders affect vitamin K concentration by undesired binding, an in vitro study. *BMC Nephrol.* 2017;18(1):149. doi:10.1186/s12882-017-0560-3

27. Jankowska M, Szupryczyńska N, Dębska-Ślizień A, et al. Dietary intake of vitamins in different options of treatment in chronic kidney disease: is there a deficiency? *Transplant Proc.* 2016;48(5):1427-1430. doi:10.1016/j.transproceed.2015.11.039

28.    Westenfeld R, Krueger T, Schlieper G, et al. Effect of vitamin K2 supplementation on functional vitamin K deficiency in hemodialysis patients: a randomized trial. *Am J Kidney Dis.* 2012;59(2):186-195. doi:10 .1053/j.ajkd.2011.10.041

29.    Lin PC, Chou CL, Ou SH, Fang TC, Chen JS. Systematic review of nutrition supplements in chronic kidney diseases: a GRADE approach. *Nutrients.* 2021;13(2):469. doi:10.3390/nu13020469

30.    Jean G, Souberbielle JC, Chazot C. Vitamin D in chronic kidney disease and dialysis patients. *Nutrients.* 2017;9(4):328. doi:10.3390/nu9040328

31.    Negrea L. Active vitamin D in chronic kidney disease: getting right back where we started from? *Kidney Dis (Basel).* 2019;5(2):59-68. doi:10.1159 /000495138

32.    Xu Y, Evans M, Soro M, Barany P, Carrero JJ. Secondary hyperparathyroidism and adverse health outcomes in adults with chronic kidney disease. *Clin Kidney J.* 2021;14(10):2213-2220. doi:10.1093 /ckj/sfab006

33.    Sprague SM, Coyne D. Control of secondary hyperparathyroidism by vitamin D receptor agonists in chronic kidney disease. *Clin J Am Soc Nephrol.* 2010;5(3):512-518. doi:10.2215/CJN.03850609

34.    Jean G, Vanel T, Terrat JC, Chazot C. Prevention of secondary hyperparathyroidism in hemodialysis patients: the key role of native vitamin D supplementation. *Hemodial Int.* 2010;14(4):486-491. doi:10.1111 /j.1542-4758.2010.00472.x

35.    Hill Gallant KM, Spiegel DM. Calcium balance in chronic kidney disease. *Curr Osteoporos Rep.* 2017;15(3):214-221. doi:10.1007/s11914-017 -0368-x

36.    Bargagli M, Ferraro PM, Vittori M, Lombardi G, Gambaro G, Somani B. Calcium and vitamin D supplementation and their association with kidney stone disease: a narrative review. *Nutrients.* 2021;13(12):4363. doi:10.3390/nu13124363

37.    Hill KM, Martin BR, Wastney ME, et al. Oral calcium carbonate affects calcium but not phosphorus balance in stage 3-4 chronic kidney disease. *Kidney Int.* 2013;83(5):959-966. doi:10.1038/ki.2012.403

38.    Institute of Medicine (US) Committee to Review Dietary Reference Intakes for Vitamin D and Calcium; Ross AC, Taylor CL, Yaktine AL, Del Valle HB, eds. *Dietary Reference Intakes for Calcium and Vitamin D.* National Academies Press; 2011.

39.    Label: Sensipar—cinacalcet hydrochloride tablet, coated. DailyMed, National Library of Medicine. Updated June 8, 2010. Accessed April 6, 2022. https://dailymed.nlm.nih.gov/dailymed/drugInfo.cfm?setid =8f390187-1071-4000-b778-1d21c518cc9c

40. Label: Parsabiv—etelcalcetide injection, solution. DailyMed, National Library of Medicine. Updated February 17, 2021. Accessed April 6, 2022. https://dailymed.nlm.nih.gov/dailymed/drugInfo.cfm?setid=cd270093 -c6a8-4596-a4ab-e6aa0a2c8a0c

41. Block GA, Klassen PS, Lazarus JM, Ofsthun N, Lowrie EG, Chertow GM. Mineral metabolism, mortality, and morbidity in maintenance hemodialysis. *J Am Soc Nephrol.* 2004;15(8):2208-2218. doi:10.1097/01 .ASN.0000133041.27682.A2

42. Kovesdy CP, Kalantar-Zadeh K. Bone and mineral disorders in pre-dialysis CKD. *Int Urol Nephrol.* 2008;40(2):427-440. doi:10.1007/s11255 -008-9346-7

43. Isaka Y, Hamano T, Fujii H, et al. Optimal phosphate control related to coronary artery calcification in dialysis patients. *J Am Soc Nephrol.* 2021;32(3):723-735. doi:10.1681/ASN.2020050598

44. Lopes MB, Karaboyas A, Bieber B, et al. Impact of longer term phosphorus control on cardiovascular mortality in hemodialysis patients using an area under the curve approach: results from the DOPPS. *Nephrol Dial Transplant.* 2020;35(10):1794-1801. doi:10.1093/ndt /gfaa054

45. Stremke ER, Hill Gallant KM. Intestinal phosphorus absorption in chronic kidney disease. *Nutrients.* 2018;10(10):1364. doi:10.3390 /nu10101364

46. Kidney Disease: Improving Global Outcomes (KDIGO) CKD-MBD Update Work Group. KDIGO 2017 clinical practice guideline update for the diagnosis, evaluation, prevention, and treatment of chronic kidney disease-mineral and bone disorder (CKD-MBD). *Kidney Int Suppl.* 2017;7(3):e1. doi:10.1016/j.kisu.2017.10.001

47. Rastogi A, Bhatt N, Rossetti S, Beto J. Management of hyperphosphatemia in end-stage renal disease: a new paradigm. *J Ren Nutr.* 2021;31(1):21-34. doi:10.1053/j.jrn.2020.02.003

48. Clase CM, Carrero JJ, Ellison DH, et al. Potassium homeostasis and management of dyskalemia in kidney diseases: conclusions from a Kidney Disease: Improving Global Outcomes (KDIGO) Controversies Conference. *Kidney Int.* 2020;97(1):42-61. doi:10.1016/j.kint.2019.09.018

49. Kovesdy CP, Matsushita K, Sang Y, et al. Serum potassium and adverse outcomes across the range of kidney function: a CKD Prognosis Consortium meta-analysis. *Eur Heart J.* 2018;39(17):1535-1542. doi:10 .1093/eurheartj/ehy100

50. Kloner RA, Gross C, Yuan J, Conrad A, Pergola PE. Effect of patiromer in hyperkalemic patients taking and not taking RAAS inhibitors. *J Cardiovasc Pharmacol Ther.* 2018;23(6):524-531. doi:10.1177 /1074248418788334

51. Palmer BF, Clegg DJ. Treatment of abnormalities of potassium homeostasis in CKD. *Adv Chronic Kidney Dis.* 2017;24(5):319-324. doi:10.1053/j.ackd.2017.06.001

52. Gilligan S, Raphael KL. Hyperkalemia and hypokalemia in CKD: prevalence, risk factors, and clinical outcomes. *Adv Chronic Kidney Dis.* 2017;24(5):315-318. doi:10.1053/j.ackd.2017.06.004

53. Palmer BF, Carrero JJ, Clegg DJ, et al. Clinical management of hyperkalemia. *Mayo Clin Proc.* 2021;96(3):744-762. doi:10.1016/j.mayocp.2020.06.014

54. Picard K. Potassium additives and bioavailability: are we missing something in hyperkalemia management? *J Ren Nutr.* 2019;29(4): 350-353. doi:10.1053/j.jrn.2018.10.003

55. Kidney Disease: Improving Global Outcomes (KDIGO) CKD Work Group. KDIGO 2012 clinical practice guideline for the evaluation and management of chronic kidney disease. *Kidney Int Suppl.* 2013;3(1):1-150.

56. Camaschella C. Iron-deficiency anemia. *N Engl J Med.* 2015;372(19): 1832-1843. doi:10.1056/NEJMra1401038

57. Batchelor EK, Kapitsinou P, Pergola PE, Kovesdy CP, Jalal DI. Iron deficiency in chronic kidney disease: updates on pathophysiology, diagnosis, and treatment. *J Am Soc Nephrol.* 2020;31(3):456-468. doi:10.1681/ASN.2019020213

58. Hutson PR. Hematology: red and white blood cell tests. In: Lee M, ed. *Basic Skills in Interpreting Laboratory Data.* 3rd ed. ASHP; 2004:441-467.

59. Gutiérrez OM. Treatment of iron deficiency anemia in CKD and end-stage kidney disease. *Kidney Int Rep.* 2021;6(9):2261-2269. doi:10.1016/j.ekir.2021.05.020

60. Anderson GJ, Frazer DM, McLaren GD. Iron absorption and metabolism. *Curr Opin Gastroenterol.* 2009;25(2):129-135. doi:10.1097/MOG.0b013e32831ef1f7

61. Kidney Disease: Improving Global Outcomes (KDIGO) Anemia Work Group. KDIGO clinical practice guideline for anemia in chronic kidney disease. *Kidney Int Suppl.* 2012;2(4):279-335.

62. Kumpf VJ. Update on parenteral iron therapy. *Nutr Clin Pract.* 2003;18(4):318-326. doi:10.1177/0115426503018004318

63. Hampson K, Nguyen T. A review of intravenous iron replacement medications for nurse practitioners. *J Nurs Pract.* 2020;16(3):224-227.

64. Kamel AY, Dave NJ, Zhao VM, Griffith DP, Connor MJ Jr, Ziegler TR. Micronutrient alterations during continuous renal replacement therapy in critically ill adults: a retrospective study. *Nutr Clin Pract.* 2018;33(3):439-446. doi:10.1177/0884533617716618

65. Venofer. Package insert. American Regent; 2018. Accessed March 7, 2024. https://americanregent.com/media/1836/venofer-prescribing-information.pdf

# CHAPTER 11

# Wound Healing

Nancy Munoz, DCN, MHA, RDN, FAND;
Nancy Storms Walsh, RDN; and
Emanuele Cereda, MD, PhD

## Introduction

Poor nutritional status and disease-related malnutrition are linked to increased risk for many complications, including skin breakdown and reduced healing rates. This is likely caused by impaired immune function, reduced collagen synthesis, and diminished tensile strength during the wound healing process.[1] The Academy of Nutrition and Dietetics and the American Society for Parenteral and Enteral Nutrition supported the release of the 2012 diagnostic criteria for malnutrition, which include six criteria for determining nutritional status.[2] One of these criteria, inadequate oral intake, increases the risk of micronutrient deficiency; this point is essential to understanding the literature on pressure injuries and wounds. Current wound care guidelines do not suggest the need for routine micronutrient supplementation unless inadequate intake is suspected or confirmed.[1] However, these same guidelines do support the need for oral nutritional supplements when a patient experiences inadequate oral intake or weight loss, as these supplements include protein and many micronutrients that are essential for optimal wound healing. The assessment and optimization of nutritional status in individuals with wounds should incorporate a comprehensive treatment plan that includes meeting micronutrient needs.

Pressure injuries can occur at any juncture along the continuum of care. A lack of nutrients is more relevant than an excess, and there is substantial evidence supporting the importance of good nutrition in sustaining tissue viability and promoting the healing process. Optimizing protein energy intake is essential for promoting positive outcomes in individuals with pressure injuries.

This chapter reviews the putative and evidence-based benefits of individual micronutrients in the healing of wounds, specifically pressure injuries and diabetic ulcers, in patients with wounds other than burns. (Micronutrient deficiencies in patients with burn wounds are addressed in Chapter 15.) Where data are lacking for specific dosing strategies for patients with wounds, refer to Chapters 5 through 8 for standard dosing recommendations. Although it is common practice to supplement micronutrients when wounds are present, it is important to recognize that supplementation is only indicated in the presence of a suspected or confirmed deficiency.

# Vitamins

## Vitamin A

Vitamin A plays an active role in all stages of wound healing, primarily functioning as a hormone. By stimulating epithelial and fibroblast mitosis and growth, vitamin A enhances cellular differentiation, epithelialization, granulation, angiogenesis, collagen (both synthesis and cross-linking of newly formed collagen), and extracellular matrix formation. Furthermore, vitamin A contributes to controlling immune cell development and differentiation in response to various stimuli. Carotenoids (beta carotene, lutein, and zeaxanthin), some of which are converted to vitamin A, also work as valuable antioxidants. Because of this, the nutrition management of pressure injuries often includes initiation of vitamin A, despite the lack of evidence-based studies supporting this practice.[3] In patients with conditions that cause inflammation (eg, wounds), catabolic status impairs vitamin A availability secondary to depletion of retinol-binding protein, and assessment of vitamin A deficiency is warranted.[4,5] Concomitant assessment of zinc and iron status is warranted, as zinc contributes to the formation of retinol-binding protein and iron is required to mobilize hepatic vitamin A stores.

Retinoids are used in dermatology, and evidence for their use in primary or secondary vitamin A deficiency is available and recognized enough to promote their use for optimizing serum levels.[6] Limited data regarding diabetic ulcers or pressure injuries have suggested benefits for vitamin A treatment topically or as part of a multinutrient treatment approach in the form of an oral nutritional supplement.[7,8] However, other research has found a lack of efficacy of vitamin A treatments in patients with pressure injuries and has highlighted concerns for potential toxicity.[3] The data are inconclusive regarding the effectiveness of routine vitamin A supplementation to support wound healing in patients with nonburn wounds.

The dosing strategies for vitamin A discussed in Chapter 5 are recommended for hypovitaminosis in patients with wounds, but clinicians should be cognizant of the impact that inflammation has on serum vitamin A levels. In addition to conducting a serum retinol assessment, the clinician should order serum or plasma zinc and iron studies, as these are also essential to interpretation and determining an optimal treatment strategy.

# B Vitamins

Most B vitamins function as coenzymes that facilitate the essential metabolic processes required to meet the increased nutrient needs of patients with skin injuries. The contributions of the B vitamins to wound healing include the following:

- Thiamin acts as a coenzyme in carbohydrate metabolism, energy production, and modulation of the immune response.[9,10]

- Riboflavin acts as a coenzyme in carbohydrate metabolism and energy production. It also functions as an immune modulator of mucosal-associated invariant T cells, which aid in destroying bacteria or inhibiting bacteria growth, restoring tissue, and modulating graft-vs-host disease.[11-13] Riboflavin is required in iron metabolism. It also serves as a coenzyme in the maintenance of homocysteine homeostasis and may potentially reduce inflammation.

- Niacin functions in many enzymatic and nonenzymatic reactions throughout the body, providing intermediaries for the biosynthesis of more than 400 compounds.[10] It is a precursor to adenosine diphosphate ribose, which is a key transcriptional regulator of various cells, including immune cells. Immune cells have niacin receptors distributed peripherally to modulate inflammatory cascades. Niacin has antioxidant effects and also helps transform nutrients into energy, create cholesterol and fats, and create and repair DNA.[14]

- Pantothenic acid is a substrate for coenzyme A; as such, it promotes energy production and protein and fat utilization, interacting with approximately 4% of all enzymes.[10] Pantothenic acid repletion has not been proven effective for many broad health claims related to energy level, hair loss, acne, arthritis, adrenal support, antiaging, and wound healing.

- Vitamin B6 is essential for protein metabolism, acting as a critical coenzyme in the functioning of more than 140 different ubiquitous enzymes.[10] It is involved with collagen production and in the synthesis of hemoglobin, affecting the oxygen-carrying capacity of the blood.[13] Vitamin B6 supports immune function by contributing to the production of leukocytes and interleukin-2, and it supports the maintenance of normal homocysteine levels in the blood, potentially limiting inflammation.

- Biotin acts as a coenzyme in carbohydrate, fatty acid, and amino acid metabolism, as well as energy production, all of which promote healing.[10]

- Folate is a cofactor in synthesizing amino acids, DNA, and RNA, which are critical for rapid cell division. It promotes the production and maturation of red blood cells and serves in inflammation modulation in homocysteine reactions.

- Vitamin B12 supports the formation of healthy red blood cells, aids in collagen production, and plays an immunomodulating role in lymphocyte production.[13] Vitamin B12 is needed for inflammation modulation in homocysteine reactions, and it facilitates the metabolism of DNA, RNA, proteins, and lipids.

Each B vitamin, as part of a balanced and complete diet, provides critical support for wound healing, although there is a paucity of evidence supporting individual B vitamin supplementation. Folate appears to hold the most promise. As a single-nutrient intervention, folate has shown some benefit in the treatment of diabetic ulcer wounds (5 mg/d over 4 weeks) and venous ulcer wounds (1.2 mg/d for 12 months).[15,16] Meeting the Dietary Reference Intakes (DRIs) for the B vitamins, including folate, is necessary for optimal wound healing. Oral nutritional supplements should be considered when oral intake is inadequate to support meeting the DRIs. In the case of inadequate oral intake or hypovitaminosis, clinicians should use the dosing strategies discussed in Chapter 6 when biochemical levels are depleted.

# Vitamin C

Vitamin C is a crucial nutrient for connective tissue and skin health. It is essential for collagen synthesis (particularly in the cross-linking of newly formed collagen, enabling the hydroxylation of lysine) and fibroblast maturation. Low serum levels result in defective collagen formation, reduced resistance to tensile stress, and increased risk of wound dehiscence.[17,18] During wound healing, the activation of macrophages as part of the immune response produces reactive oxygen species and vitamin C controls cell damage to maintain cell integrity.

Current nutrition practice includes giving vitamin C to patients with pressure injuries, despite limited evidence that it plays an independent role in wound healing.[3] Conflicting study findings may be secondary to poor blood glucose optimization, which was a confounding factor in earlier studies of the role of vitamin C in pressure injuries. One trial from 1974 conducted in an acute care setting showed benefits with 1 month of vitamin C repletion (500 mg/d by mouth) in patients with pressure injuries.[19] A 1995 study reported that vitamin C supplementation did not affect wound healing rate or wound healing per se.[20] A literature review published in 2021 reported that patients with pressure injuries receiving vitamin C and zinc had improved outcomes.[21] However, this review included many older references that might not reflect the state of the science today. Because of this, the fundamental independent contribution of vitamin C to wound healing cannot be fully established.

There is good-quality evidence from randomized trials on the use of formula enriched with vitamin C, zinc, and other micronutrients to treat patients with pressure injuries.[22,23] The patient should be assessed for a biochemical deficiency using leukocyte or plasma vitamin C values, in addition to a C-reactive protein test and a complete blood count to rule out anemia. In the setting of poor wound healing and biochemical deficiency, vitamin C replacement as outlined in Chapter 6 is warranted. In patients with inadequate oral intake, the use of oral nutritional supplements should be considered when the patient is unable to increase oral intake through diet alone. In individuals at high risk for deficiency (as seen during inflammation and ischemia reperfusion), a dose higher than the recommended DRI for vitamin C may be needed.[24]

# Vitamin D

Vitamin D receptors are present in the nuclei of many tissue cells. Activated vitamin D (calcitriol) plays numerous roles in wound healing.[25,26] It recruits monocytes in the inflammatory phase of healing, which help fight infection and activate T cells. The T cells then reduce cytokines and growth factors to promote the proliferation of fibroblasts and synthesis of collagen. Activated vitamin D also supports the presence of macrophages in the inflammatory response, which help defend the host; detect, engulf, and destroy pathogens and cell debris; support the advancement and conclusion of inflammation; and support cell reproduction and tissue repair after the injury.

Nevertheless, there is a lack of evidence to support individual vitamin D treatments for wound healing. A review published in 2021 reported positive outcomes in patients with diabetic foot ulcers who received vitamin D, although results were neutral in those with venous ulcers or hypertrophic scars.[21] Specifically, one randomized, double-blind, placebo-controlled trial found that 50,000 IU vitamin D administered every 2 weeks for 12 weeks resulted in improved healing of diabetic foot ulcers compared to placebo.[27] However, the data suggest that the placebo and treatment groups contained a high number of participants who were already deficient in vitamin D. This is of importance because vitamin D status, along with the status of many other vitamins discussed in this chapter, affects wound healing when a deficiency is present, thus warranting supplementation. It is not surprising, then, that vitamin D treatment substantially improved wound healing compared to placebo in the study. Because vitamin D deficiency is common in the United States, assessing a patient's 25-hydroxyvitamin D status and C-reactive protein level is warranted. If status is suboptimal, the clinician should use the dosing strategies for vitamin D presented in Chapter 5, as data specific to patients with wounds are lacking.

# Vitamin E

During wound healing, the activation of macrophages produces reactive oxygen species. Controlling the oxidative state produced by the release of reactive oxygen species and the inflammatory response is essential for wound healing and tissue repair. Vitamin E deficiency (and vitamin and mineral deficiency in general) prolongs cell migration and proliferation, thus affecting wound healing.[28]

Few studies have investigated vitamin E treatment in wound management, and among those reported in the literature, results are mixed.[21] A randomized, double-blind, placebo-controlled trial that provided oral vitamin E to patients with diabetic ulcers noted improvements in ulcer dimensions with treatment vs placebo.[29] In another study, topical delivery of vitamin E had positive results vs oral delivery.[30] It is important to understand the difference in clinical findings between oral treatment and topical treatment. Furthermore, when determining a patient's need for vitamin E treatment, the clinician should also assess -tocopherol and lipid levels. Chapter 5 provides vitamin E dosing strategies when a biochemical deficiency is present.

# Vitamin K

Achieving hemostasis is the first goal of the wound-healing process. Although vitamin K contributes very little to wound healing, vitamin

K deficiency contributes to decreased coagulation, impairing hemostasis and the inflammatory phase of wound healing. The tissue trauma succeeding skin injury causes hemorrhage. Platelets aggregate and degranulate to trigger factor XII to promote clot formation and hemostasis.[31]

When there is concern for possible vitamin K deficiency, practitioners can assess prothrombin time in addition to serum vitamin K and triglyceride levels to determine if biochemical deficiency is present (Chapter 5). No specific recommendations are available for vitamin K treatment in patients with nonburn wounds who are at high risk for vitamin K deficiency.

# Minerals

## Copper

Copper contributes to the synthesis and stabilization of proteins in the skin's extracellular matrix and to angiogenesis. As such, it is an indispensable nutrient in supporting skin strength, blood vessels, and epithelial and connective tissue throughout the body.[31]

In the skin, copper fuels dermal fibroblasts and collagen production; it stabilizes the extracellular matrix (once formed) and promotes cross-linking collagen and elastin matrixes. It is also a cofactor of superoxide dismutase, an antioxidant enzyme, and it inhibits oxidative processes such as membrane damage and lipid peroxidation.[32]

Clinical practice guidelines for the prevention and treatment of pressure ulcers and injuries suggest that there is growing evidence to support the use of high-energy, high-protein oral nutritional supplements containing arginine, zinc, and antioxidants (including copper). These supplements are linked to substantial improvements in measures of pressure injury healing and are more effective than high-energy, high-protein oral supplements that lack optimal dosing of these nutrients.[1,33] The role of copper appears to be clearer in patients with burns than in patients with nonburn chronic wounds.[21] In individuals with a suspected or confirmed copper deficiency, a multivitamin providing

100% of the DRI is the recommended intervention.[33] Practitioners should exercise caution when administering high-dose zinc treatment, as it can lead to copper deficiency. Chapter 8 provides assessment and dosing strategies for patients with suboptimal serum or plasma copper, ceruloplasmin, and complete blood count values.

# Iron

Iron is essential for tissue perfusion, as it transports oxygen to all body tissues. Iron is required for collagen synthesis and new cell regeneration.[31] Therefore, iron deficiency has been linked to skin-related disorders such as pallor, pruritus, brittle hair and nails, and increased risk for bacterial and fungal skin infections.[34]

Practitioners should take care not to exceed dietary iron requirements, as consuming excessive amounts of iron can contribute to skin changes such as hemosiderin staining and lipodermatosclerosis.[35] Excessive iron can also affect the response of macrophage cells, causing an uncontrolled proinflammatory cell activation that can have a potential impact on wound healing.[34] In patients with nonburn wounds who are at high risk for iron deficiency, supplementation should be considered. Chapter 7 includes a thorough overview of the assessment and treatment strategies for patients with suboptimal iron levels.

# Zinc

Zinc-containing proteins serve an important function in the body and are highly relevant to tissue viability and wound healing. Zinc exerts anti-inflammatory and antimicrobial effects and is necessary for tissue granulation and re-epithelialization (cellular growth and proliferation), angiogenesis, collagen synthesis, and connective-tissue remodeling (extracellular matrix) as a cofactor of matrix metalloproteinases.[36]

The independent role of zinc status in wound healing is closely related to deficiency status.[36] However, zinc status is not routinely assessed in every health care setting, which creates challenges to understanding current practices and outcomes. As with many of the micronutrients discussed in this chapter, there is good-quality evidence from randomized trials to support the use of oral nutritional supplements, including those enriched with zinc, in patients with pressure injuries.[23,37] Benefits—namely, reduced infectious complications—can also be observed in critically ill patients, including those with severe burn injuries.[38] However, the independent role of zinc is not fully established. Evidence on supplementation in the absence of deficiency is limited and relies on small studies. A Cochrane meta-analysis reported no improvement in patients with vascular ulcers, and only one small trial reported a benefit in parameters of ulcer size and metabolic profiles in patients with diabetic foot ulcers.[39,40] The European Pressure Ulcer Advisory Panel (EPUAP), National Pressure Injury Advisory Panel (NPIAP), and Pan Pacific Pressure Injury Alliance (PPPIA) all support the use of "high-calorie, high-protein, arginine, zinc, and antioxidant-rich oral nutritional supplements or enteral formula for adults with a stage 2 or greater pressure injury who are malnourished or at risk of malnutrition."[23]

Although the data are insufficient to suggest the routine supplementation of zinc to support wound healing in patients with nonburn wounds, clinicians should use the zinc dosing strategies discussed in Chapter 8 when biochemical levels are depleted.

# Amino Acids

The literature has shown that the amino acids arginine and glutamine increase the rate of skin healing; this increase is due to several actions, including the effect these substances have on immune-cell proliferation.

## Arginine

Arginine promotes nitrogen balance; it is an important building block for collagen synthesis and enhances hydroxyproline content in wound tissues through the arginine-proline pathway, increasing the tensile strength of wound tissues. Arginine also contributes to nitric oxide synthesis by vascular endothelial cells, which increases local blood flow and stimulates new blood vessel formation by favoring the release of endothelial progenitor cells from the bone marrow. Several animal-model and human studies have shown the efficacy of isolated arginine treatments in improving healing processes in incisional wounds (collagen synthesis, hydroxyproline deposition, and healing rate).[41,42] Furthermore, there is good-quality evidence from randomized trials on the use of formula enriched with arginine and other micronutrients to treat pressure injuries.[22,23] The independent role of arginine in the healing of chronic wounds such as pressure injuries cannot be fully established, though the provision of about 9 g/d is safe and likely beneficial.[23] The provision of a nutritional formula enriched in immunonutrients (arginine, nucleotides, and n-3 fatty acids) for at least 5 days prior to surgery may help reduce wound infections and anastomotic leakage.[7,43-45]

# Glutamine

Fibroblasts utilize glutamine more than they do any other amino acid. Glutamine enhances wound healing, in part because it increases the concentration of arginine and citrulline, thus enabling the production of nitric oxide in the absence of extracellular arginine. Although glutamine is recognized mainly for improving immunologic function, another important role is its capacity to modulate protective and resistance responses to injuries (antioxidant and cytoprotective effects), and in the expression of heat shock proteins. Unlike with arginine, there is limited evidence to support the use of glutamine to treat pressure injuries, as most research has focused on burns. Repletion of glutamine has been associated with faster wound healing rates, but indirect positive effects include the maintenance of mucosal integrity and a reduction in infection rates, which could reduce length of hospital stay and mortality. Studies show that decreased mucosal damage results in benefits such as reduced painful mucosal symptoms and ulceration associated with chemotherapy and radiation in the head and neck regions, esophagus, stomach, and small intestine (mucositis, stomatitis, pharyngitis, esophagitis, and enteritis).[43,44,46-48]

# Arginine and Glutamine Deficiencies

Arginine and glutamine are semi-essential, or conditionally essential, amino acids. True deficiency is rare, and manifestations of deficiency symptoms are hard to establish and likely the consequence of stress conditions (cancer, sepsis, infection, surgery, and trauma). Therefore, consequences of deficiency may include impaired healing and immune function, resulting in increased infection rates and mortality. More severe chemoradiotherapy-related mucositis can also occur.

# Recommended Intakes

There are no specific Recommended Dietary Allowances for arginine and glutamine. A balanced diet provides enough amino acids for homeostasis, growth, and health maintenance. However, repletion studies indicate that a benefit in stress conditions can be seen with the provision of 9 g arginine daily and 15 g (0.3–0.5 g per kilogram of body weight) glutamine daily.[7,43,44] In addition, the EPUAP/NPIAP/PPPIA guidelines support the use of "high-calorie, high-protein, arginine, zinc, and antioxidant-rich oral nutritional supplements or enteral formula for adults with a stage 2 or greater pressure injury who are malnourished or at risk of malnutrition."[23]

# Treatment Summary

Chronic wounds may require micronutrient support beyond the DRIs. The clinician should review dietary intake data in conjunction with conducting a thorough assessment of wound healing to determine the need for biochemical assessment or the establishment of a micronutrient treatment strategy. In patients with poor dietary intake or an inability to meet nutrient requirements by diet alone, the use of a reputable multivitamin/mineral supplement or initiation of a high-energy, high-protein oral nutritional supplement should be considered.[23,49] The EPUAP/NPIAP/PPPIA recommendations for optimizing micronutrient intake are summarized in Table 11.1 on page 234.[23]

**TABLE 11.1 Selected Recommendations for Micronutrient Optimization in the Prevention and Treatment of Nonburn Wounds[23]**

| Recommendation | Strength of evidence[a] | Strength of recommendation[b] | Good practice statement[c] |
|---|---|---|---|
| Offer high-energy, high-protein fortified foods and/or nutritional supplements in addition to the usual diet for adults who are at risk of developing a pressure injury and who are also malnourished or at risk of malnutrition, if nutritional requirements cannot be achieved by normal dietary intake. | C | ↑ | Not included |
| Offer high-energy, high-protein nutritional supplements in addition to the usual diet for adults with a pressure injury who are malnourished or at risk of malnutrition, if nutritional requirements cannot be achieved by normal dietary intake. | B1 | ↑↑ | Not included |
| Provide high-energy, high-protein, arginine-, zinc-, and antioxidant-rich oral nutritional supplements or enteral formula for adults with a stage 2 or greater pressure injury who are malnourished or at risk of malnutrition. | B1 | ↑ | Not included |
| Discuss the benefits and harms of enteral or parenteral feeding to support overall health, in light of preferences and goals of care, with individuals at risk of pressure injuries who cannot meet their nutritional requirements through oral intake despite nutrition interventions. | Not included | Not included | Yes |
| Discuss the benefits and harms of enteral or parenteral feeding to support pressure injury treatment in light of preferences and goals of care for individuals with pressure injuries who cannot meet their nutritional requirements through oral intake despite nutrition interventions. | B1 | ↑ | Not included |
| For neonates and children with or at risk of pressure injuries who have inadequate oral intake, consider fortified foods, age-appropriate nutritional supplements, or enteral or parenteral support. | Not included | Not included | Yes |

[a] Strength of evidence is based on evidence quantity, levels, and consistency. B1 = level 1 studies of moderate/low quality providing direct evidence or level 2 studies of high/moderate quality providing direct evidence. C = level 5 studies (indirect evidence) or a body of evidence with inconsistencies that cannot be explained, reflecting uncertainty.

[b] The strength of a recommendation is the extent to which a health professional can be confident that adherence to the recommendation will do more good than harm.

↑ = probably do it; ↑↑ = definitely do it.

[c] Good practice statements are not supported by a body of evidence but are considered to be important for clinical practice.

# References

1.  Munoz N, Posthauer ME, Cereda E, Schols JMGA, Haesler E. The role of nutrition for pressure injury prevention and healing: the 2019 international clinical practice guideline recommendations. *Adv Skin Wound Care*. 2020;33(3):123-136. doi:10.1097/01.ASW.0000653144 .90739.ad

2.  White JV, Guenter P, Jensen G, et al. Consensus statement of the Academy of Nutrition and Dietetics/American Society for Parenteral and Enteral Nutrition: characteristics recommended for the identification and documentation of adult malnutrition (undernutrition). *J Acad Nutr Diet*. 2012;112(5):730-738. doi:10.1016/j.jand.2012.03.012

3.  Bafna K, Chen T, Simman R. Is treating patients with stage 4 pressure ulcers with vitamins A and C, zinc, and arginine justified? *Wounds*. 2021;33(3):77-80.

4.  Zinder R, Cooley R, Vlad LG, Molnar JA. Vitamin A and wound healing. *Nutr Clin Pract*. 2019;34(6):839-849. doi:10.1002/ncp.10420

5.  Polcz ME, Barbul A. The role of vitamin A in wound healing. *Nutr Clin Pract*. 2019;34(5):695-700. doi:10.1002/ncp.10376

6.  Mukherjee S, Date A, Patravale V, Korting HC, Roeder A, Weindl G. Retinoids in the treatment of skin aging: an overview of clinical efficacy and safety. *Clin Interv Aging*. 2006;1(4):327-348. doi:10.2147/ciia .2006.1.4.327

7.  van Anholt RD, Sobotka L, Meijer EP, et al. Specific nutritional support accelerates pressure ulcer healing and reduces wound care intensity in non-malnourished patients. *Nutrition*. 2010;26(9):867-872. doi:10.1016/j .nut.2010.05.009

8.  Tom WL, Peng DH, Allaei A, Hsu D, Hata TR. The effect of short-contact topical tretinoin therapy for foot ulcers in patients with diabetes. *Arch Dermatol*. 2005;141(11):1373-1377. doi:10.1001/archderm.141.11.1373

9.  Riyapa D, Rinchai D, Muangsombut V, et al. Transketolase and vitamin B1 influence on ROS-dependent neutrophil extracellular traps (NETs) formation. *PLoS One*. 2019;14(8):e0221016. doi:10.1371/journal.pone .0221016

10. Kennedy DO. B Vitamins and the brain: mechanisms, dose and efficacy—a review. *Nutrients*. 2016;8(2):68. doi:10.3390/nu8020068

11. Mak JYW, Liu L, Fairlie DP. Chemical modulators of mucosal associated invariant T cells. *Acc Chem Res*. 2021;54(17):3462-3475. doi:10.1021/acs .accounts.1c00359

12.  von Martels JZH, Bourgonje AR, Klaassen MAY, et al. Riboflavin supplementation in patients with Crohn's disease [the RISE-UP study]. *J Crohns Colitis.* 2020;14(5):595-607. doi:10.1093/ecco-jcc/jjz208

13.  Thompson C, Fuhrman MP. Nutrients and wound healing: still searching for the magic bullet. *Nutr Clin Pract.* 2005;20(3):331-347. doi:10.1177/0115426505020003331

14.  Makarov MV, Trammell SAJ, Migaud ME. The chemistry of the vitamin B3 metabolome. *Biochem Soc Trans.* 2019;47(1):131-147. doi:10.1042/BST20180420

15.  Boykin JV Jr, Hoke GD, Driscoll CR, Dharmaraj BS. High-dose folic acid and its effect on early stage diabetic foot ulcer wound healing. *Wound Repair Regen.* 2020;28(4):517-525. doi:10.1111/wrr.12804

16.  de Franciscis S, De Sarro G, Longo P, et al. Hyperhomocysteinaemia and chronic venous ulcers. *Int Wound J.* 2015;12(1):22-26. doi:10.1111/iwj.12042

17.  Palmieri B, Vadalà M, Laurino C. Nutrition in wound healing: investigation of the molecular mechanisms, a narrative review. *J Wound Care.* 2019;28(10):683-693. doi:10.12968/jowc.2019.28.10.683

18.  Pullar JM, Carr AC, Vissers MCM. The roles of vitamin C in skin health. *Nutrients.* 2017;9(8):866. doi:10.3390/nu9080866

19.  Taylor TV, Rimmer S, Day B, Butcher J, Dymock IW. Ascorbic acid supplementation in the treatment of pressure-sores. *Lancet.* 1974;2(7880):544-546. doi:10.1016/s0140-6736(74)91874-1

20.  ter Riet G, Kessels AG, Knipschild PG. Randomized clinical trial of ascorbic acid in the treatment of pressure ulcers. *J Clin Epidemiol.* 1995;48(12):1453-1460. doi:10.1016/0895-4356(95)00053-4

21.  Saeg F, Orazi R, Bowers GM, Janis JE. Evidence-based nutritional interventions in wound care. *Plast Reconstr Surg.* 2021;148(1):226-238. doi:10.1097/PRS.0000000000008061

22.  Cereda E, Neyens JCL, Caccialanza R, Rondanelli M, Schols JMGA. Efficacy of a disease-specific nutritional support for pressure ulcer healing: a systematic review and meta-analysis. *J Nutr Health Aging.* 2017;21(6):655-661. doi:10.1007/s12603-016-0822-y

23.  European Pressure Ulcer Advisory Panel, National Pressure Injury Advisory Panel, and Pan Pacific Pressure Injury Alliance. *Prevention and Treatment of Pressure Ulcers/Injuries: Quick Reference Guide.* Haesler E, ed. 3rd ed. EPUAP/NPIAP/PPPIA; 2019.

24.  Berger MM, Shenkin A, Schweinlin A, et al. ESPEN micronutrient guideline. *Clin Nutr.* 2022;41(6):1357-1424. doi:10.1016/j.clnu.2022.02.015

Wound Healing

25.    Toninello P, Montanari A, Bassetto F, Vindigni V, Paoli A. Nutritional support for bariatric surgery patients: the skin beyond the fat. *Nutrients*. 2021;13(5):1565. doi:10.3390/nu13051565

26.    Gushiken LFS, Beserra FP, Bastos JK, Jackson CJ, Pellizzon CH. Cutaneous wound healing: an update from physiopathology to current therapies. *Life (Basel)*. 2021;11(7):665. doi:10.3390/life11070665

27.    Razzaghi R, Pourbagheri H, Momen-Heravi M, et al. The effects of vitamin D supplementation on wound healing and metabolic status in patients with diabetic foot ulcer: a randomized, double-blind, placebo-controlled trial. *J Diabetes Complications*. 2017;31(4):766-772. doi:10.1016/j.jdiacomp.2016.06.017

28.    Posthauer ME, Dorner B, Collins N. Nutrition: a critical component of wound healing. *Adv Skin Wound Care*. 2010;23(12):560-574. doi:10.1097/01.ASW.0000391185.81963.e5

29.    Afzali H, Jafari Kashi AH, Momen-Heravi M, et al. The effects of magnesium and vitamin E co-supplementation on wound healing and metabolic status in patients with diabetic foot ulcer: a randomized, double-blind, placebo-controlled trial. *Wound Repair Regen*. 2019;27(3):277-284. doi:10.1111/wrr.12701

30.    Fiori G, Galluccio F, Braschi F, et al. Vitamin E gel reduces time of healing of digital ulcers in systemic sclerosis. *Clin Exp Rheumatol*. 2009;27(3 suppl 54):51-54.

31.    Baranoski S, Sibbald G, Levine JM. Skin: an essential organ. In: *Wound Care Essentials: Practice Principles*. 5th ed. Wolters Kluwer Health; 2020.

32.    Borkow G. Using copper to improve the well-being of the skin. *Curr Chem Biol*. 2014;8(2):89-102. doi:10.2174/2212796809666150227223857

33.    Kottner J, Cuddigan J, Carville K, et al. Prevention and treatment of pressure ulcers/injuries: the protocol for the second update of the international Clinical Practice Guideline 2019. *J Tissue Viability*. 2019;28(2):51-58. doi:10.1016/j.jtv.2019.01.001

34.    Wright JA, Richards T, Srai SK. The role of iron in the skin and cutaneous wound healing. *Front Pharmacol*. 2014;5:156. doi:10.3389/fphar.2014.00156

35.    Caggiati A, Rosi C, Casini A, et al. Skin iron deposition characterises lipodermatosclerosis and leg ulcer. *Eur J Vasc Endovasc Surg*. 2010;40(6):777-782. doi:10.1016/j.ejvs.2010.08.015

36.    Lin PH, Sermersheim M, Li H, Lee PHU, Steinberg SM, Ma J. Zinc in wound healing modulation. *Nutrients*. 2017;10(1):16. doi:10.3390/nu10010016

37. Cereda E, Neyens JCL, Caccialanza R, Rondanelli M, Schols JMGA. Efficacy of a disease-specific nutritional support for pressure ulcer healing: a systematic review and meta-analysis. *J Nutr Health Aging.* 2017;21(6):655-661. doi:10.1007/s12603-016-0822-y

38. Kurmis R, Greenwood J, Aromataris E. Trace element supplementation following severe burn injury: a systematic review and meta-analysis. *J Burn Care Res.* 2016;37(3):143-159. doi:10.1097/BCR.0000000000000259

39. Wilkinson EA, Hawke CI. Oral zinc for arterial and venous leg ulcers. *Cochrane Database Syst Rev.* 2000;(2):CD001273. doi:10.1002/14651858.CD001273

40. Momen-Heravi M, Barahimi E, Razzaghi R, Bahmani F, Gilasi HR, Asemi Z. The effects of zinc supplementation on wound healing and metabolic status in patients with diabetic foot ulcer: a randomized, double-blind, placebo-controlled trial. *Wound Repair Regen.* 2017;25(3):512-520. doi:10.1111/wrr.12537

41. Arribas-López E, Zand N, Ojo O, Snowden MJ, Kochhar T. The effect of amino acids on wound healing: a systematic review and meta-analysis on arginine and glutamine. *Nutrients.* 2021;13(8):2498. doi:10.3390/nu13082498

42. Stechmiller JK, Childress B, Cowan L. Arginine supplementation and wound healing. *Nutr Clin Pract.* 2005;20(1):52-61. doi:10.1177/011542650502000152

43. Cereda E, Gini A, Pedrolli C, Vanotti A. Disease-specific, versus standard, nutritional support for the treatment of pressure ulcers in institutionalized older adults: a randomized controlled trial. *J Am Geriatr Soc.* 2009;57(8):1395-1402. doi:10.1111/j.1532-5415.2009.02351.x

44. Banks MD, Graves N, Bauer JD, Ash S. Cost effectiveness of nutrition support in the prevention of pressure ulcer in hospitals. *Eur J Clin Nutr.* 2013;67(1):42-46. doi:10.1038/ejcn.2012.140

45. Shils ME, Shike M, Ross AC, Caballero B, Cousins RJ, eds. *Modern Nutrition in Health and Disease.* 10th ed. Lippincott Williams and Wilkins; 2006.

46. Neyens JCL, Cereda E, Meijer EP, Lindholm C, Schols JMGA. Arginine-enriched oral nutritional supplementation in the treatment of pressure ulcers: a literature review. *Wound Medicine.* 2017;16:46-51. doi:10.1016/j.wndm.2016.07.002

47. Tuffaha HW, Roberts S, Chaboyer W, Gordon LG, Scuffham PA. Cost-effectiveness analysis of nutritional support for the prevention of pressure ulcers in high-risk hospitalized patients. *Adv Skin Wound Care.* 2016;29(6):261-267. doi:10.1097/01.ASW.0000482992.87682.4c

48. Arinzon Z, Peisakh A, Berner YN. Evaluation of the benefits of enteral nutrition in long-term care elderly patients. *J Am Med Dir Assoc.* 2008;9(9):657-662. doi:10.1016/j.jamda.2008.06.002

49. Academy of Nutrition and Dietetics. Surgical and chronic wounds. Nutrition Care Manual. Accessed June 28, 2023. www.nutritioncaremanual.org/topic.cfm?ncm_toc_id=255665&ncm_category_id=1&lvl=255665&ncm_heading=Nutrition%20Care

# CHAPTER 12

# Preterm Neonates

Mary Petrea Cober, PharmD, BCNSP, BCPPS, FASPEN; and
Jane Ziegler, DCN, RDN, LDN

## Introduction

Micronutrient requirements are not well defined for healthy preterm infants and preterm infants with acute medical complications. Preterm infants have lower body stores of nutrients and immature body systems and organs, and they accumulate greater postnatal nutritional deficits. All of these factors increase their risk for developing malnutrition, nutrient depletions or deficiencies, and postnatal growth restriction. Ensuring appropriate repletion and supplementation of micronutrients helps prevent deficiencies, improves outcomes, and allows for growth and development. With modern medicine, survival rates for preterm neonates continue to improve, even at progressively lower gestational ages and birthweights.[1,2]

Nutritional deficits, even if short-term, can lead to negative health consequences over time.[2] Nutritional challenges for preterm infants are caused by a disruption in either the maternal transfer of micronutrients or the fetal accretion of micronutrients, or both. Premature infants may also be unable to synthesize adequate amounts of essential nutrients and digestive enzymes. Despite the paucity of published research to guide nutrition management, clinicians should continuously review the evidence regarding the estimated micronutrient needs of this population.[1-4]

Appropriate nutrition management helps optimize neurodevelopmental outcomes and reduce the risk of comorbidities such as sepsis, metabolic bone disease, and retinopathy of prematurity, among others.[2]

Box 12.1 on page 242 defines the neonatal terminology used throughout this chapter.[5,6]

# Developmental Physiology, Digestion, and Absorption

The second and third trimesters of pregnancy are critical time periods for both the anatomical and functional development of the gastrointestinal (GI) system in the fetus. Premature birth results in immaturity of the digestive and absorptive capacities, along with motility issues of the GI system. Development of the fetal GI tract begins at approximately 3 to 4 weeks. The fetus can ingest the amniotic fluid that assists in the development of the GI system as early as 12 to 13 weeks. The GI tract continues to develop throughout the third trimester, which is a critical time for micronutrient accretion. Preterm birth increases the risk of nutritional complications caused by an underdeveloped GI system, which increases the risk of inadequate nutrient delivery to the infant. Infants at the highest risk are those born at earlier gestational ages.

Digestion and absorption of nutrients by the preterm infant intestine can occur at approximately 24 weeks' gestation, with select digestive enzymes being available even earlier. Digestion and absorption markedly improve as the infant matures and enteral feeding is initiated.[1,7,8] GI motor activity is slower to develop, which limits the ability of the infant to tolerate enteral feeds and increases the risk of necrotizing enterocolitis. In early fetal life, maturation of the GI tract is accompanied by the development of different digestive enzymes. Digestive enzymes, including gastric pepsin and brush-border enzymes, develop in parallel, but their concentrations are low in the premature infant.[3] Micronutrients support adequate growth and neurodevelopment, and attention should be given to their use and monitoring in preterm infants. Of particular concern in this population are the requirements for calcium, phosphorus, magnesium, vitamin D, iron, zinc, copper, and selenium.[4]

## BOX 12.1  Neonatal Terminology[5,6]

| Term | Definition or criteria |
| --- | --- |
| Neonate | First 28 days of life |
| Infant | First year of life |
| Gestational age | Elapsed time in weeks from start of mother's last menstrual period to birth of infant |
| Chronological age | Elapsed time since birth |
| Term infant | Gestational age 37 weeks or more |
| Preterm infant | Gestational age less than 37 weeks |
| Late preterm infant | Gestational age of 34 through 36 weeks |
| Moderate preterm infant | Gestational age of 32 through 34 weeks |
| Very preterm infant | Gestational age less than 32 weeks |
| Extremely preterm infant | Gestational age less then 25 weeks |
| Low birthweight (LBW) | Weight less than 2,500 g at birth |
| Very low birthweight (VLBW) | Weight less than 1,500 g at birth |
| Extremely low birthweight (ELBW) | Weight less than 1,000 g at birth |
| Intrauterine growth restriction (IUGR) | Deviation or reduction in expected fetal growth rate |
| Small for gestational age (SGA) | Less than 10th percentile for gestational age per population growth chart |
| Appropriate for gestational age (AGA) | 10th through 90th percentile for gestational age per population growth chart |
| Large for gestational age (LGA) | Greater than 90th percentile for gestational age per population growth chart |

Preterm
Neonates

# Micronutrients of Concern

Table 12.1 lists the enteral requirements for the micronutrients addressed in this chapter.[9,10]

| TABLE 12.1 Enteral Requirements for Select Nutrients in Preterm Infants[9,10] | |
|---|---|
| **Nutrient** | **Requirement[a]** |
| Calcium | 100-220 mg/kg/d |
| Copper | 120-230 mcg/kg/d |
| Iron | 2-3 mg/kg/d |
| Magnesium | 8-15 mg/kg/d |
| Phosphorus | 70-120 mg/kg/d |
| Selenium | 7-10 mcg/kg/d |
| Vitamin D | 10-25 mcg/d (400-1,000 IU/d) |
| Zinc | 2-3 mg/kg/d |

[a] Requirements may vary by infant weight categories

## Calcium

During the third trimester, fetal mineral accretion occurs exponentially. The full-term infant has the advantage of having peak calcium accretion during this last trimester, which is obtained through active transfer of calcium across the placenta. Both this transport of calcium and bone remodeling require parathyroid hormone (PTH), PTH-related peptide, and 25-hydroxyvitamin D.[1] Preterm infants, infants with low birthweight, and infants with intrauterine growth restriction have lower calcium and phosphorus stores compared to term infants. In addition, low calcium content in the body at birth is worsened by a limited or inadequate calcium supply from the infant's diet, resulting in poor calcium balance.[1,9] Transient hypoparathyroidism and the use of medications, including diuretics and other calciuric drugs, also contribute to poor calcium balance.[1,11] A positive calcium balance is necessary for bone mineralization during the postnatal period. Calcium absorption through transcellular calcium pathways in the early neonatal period occurs primarily in the jejunum and ileum and contributes to a positive calcium balance.[2] The transport of calcium is dependent on other nutrients, particularly lactose and fatty acids.

The highest bone calcium deposition rate occurs in infancy and is a direct function of intestinal absorption. Intestinal absorption of calcium and subsequent bone accretion in preterm infants can be influenced by several factors, including the supply of calcium and phosphorus, vitamin D dose, regulation of mineral homeostasis and bone mineralization, prolonged parenteral nutrition (PN), immobilization, and select medications, including diuretics and theophylline. Calcium is not well absorbed in the form of calcium phosphate; calcium chloride, calcium citrate, and calcium carbonate have higher solubilities and are more readily absorbed. Calcium gluconate and glycerophosphate are also more soluble and more readily absorbed.[11]

# Phosphorus

High accretion of phosphorus in the fetus occurs in the third trimester, with the highest accretion of most mineral deposition occurring from around 24 weeks until term. Along with calcium, phosphorus is necessary for skeletal development, and both play important roles in cellular metabolism. Preterm birth is associated with metabolic bone disease, or rickets of prematurity, which is inversely related to degree of prematurity.[9] Phosphorus absorption is linked to the retention of both calcium and nitrogen. Intestinal absorption of phosphorus (approximately 90%) is considered efficient in the premature infant, regardless of whether the infant is fed human milk or formula, which allows for sufficient accretion when calcium and nitrogen retention meet the needs of the growing infant. Phosphorus absorption occurs primarily in the jejunum by active and passive transport.[9,11]

# Vitamin D

Vitamin D is critical, as it is involved in bone mineralization and other metabolic functions. Vitamin D status in the neonate is directly related to maternal vitamin D status and may reflect maternal supplementation and birth season (related to maternal sun exposure).[2,9] Maternal vitamin D deficiency is associated with preterm birth, neonatal respiratory distress syndrome, and acute infections (respiratory or GI). Most bone mineralization occurs in the last trimester of pregnancy; therefore, preterm infants have a lower bone mineral content.[2,9,11,12] Vitamin D requirements for preterm infants are thought to be higher than those for term infants because they experience prolonged hospitalizations and have limited sunlight exposure. In addition, since vitamin D is primarily transferred to the fetus in the third trimester of pregnancy, preterm infants are at risk for low vitamin D levels.

Low vitamin D status is common in neonates who are fed formula or human milk. Preterm infants of extremely low birthweight are at risk for metabolic bone disease, with those born before the third trimester being the most at risk. Other factors that increase the risk for metabolic bone disease include difficulty achieving adequate enteral intake of calcium, phosphorus, and vitamin D; immobility; use of long-term PN; use of unfortified human milk; delayed enteral fortification of feeds; and adverse effects of medications such as diuretics, steroids, and antiseizure medications (eg, phenobarbital).[2]

# Iron

Iron is involved in hemoglobin synthesis and oxygen transport, and it is vital to many enzymatic processes, including energy production. Adequate iron intake is important for brain development, as iron deficiency is associated with adverse neurodevelopmental outcomes. Preterm infants absorb 25% to 40% of iron from supplements, 11% to 27% from iron-fortified formulas, and up to 50% from human milk. This exceeds absorption rates seen in term infants.[2] Both preterm and low-birth-weight infants are at an elevated risk for iron deficiency owing to their low iron stores at birth and rapid growth that increases iron requirements. Iron

Preterm
Neonates

storage is accumulated in the third trimester of pregnancy—a result of active transport across the placenta—and premature birth ceases this placental transfer. Iron stores may be further decreased secondary to maternal iron deficiency anemia, hypertension, or diabetes; blood draws; and intrauterine growth restriction. Multiple pregnancies and maternal obesity may also cause decreased iron stores in the infant. These maternal conditions may lead to placental insufficiency, resulting in decreased prenatal iron transfer.[2,10]

Alternatively, iron has a pro-oxidative effect and can be a substrate for pathogens; thus, excessive iron intake should be avoided. Ferritin monitoring is recommended in preterm infants receiving multiple rounds of blood transfusions.[13]

# Zinc

Zinc has a role in catalytic, structural, and regulatory functions within the cell and is an essential cofactor for several hundred enzymes. Zinc is required for tissue integrity, especially in the GI and respiratory tracts. It plays a role in immunomodulation, bone development, growth hormone regulation, taste, and appetite, and is essential for growth and tissue differentiation. Zinc deficiency has been related to stunted growth, skin rashes, increased risk for infection, and poor neurodevelopment.[10] Individuals with large GI losses, diarrhea, exudative skin conditions, or hypermetabolism have a higher need for zinc due to substantial losses or limited stores.[15] Zinc accretion in utero occurs primarily in the third trimester; therefore, premature infants are at higher risk for deficiency.[1,2,14] Serum zinc level may not be a reliable indicator of zinc status in infants, but it is a widely used and available indicator of zinc deficiency risk. Excessive intake of zinc can alter the absorption of copper.[10,15,16]

# Copper

Copper is essential in several important enzyme processes, some of which involve connective tissue synthesis and collagen cross-linking. Copper is also necessary for regulation of the electron transport systems, energy metabolism, and iron metabolism, and it is a vital component of superoxide dismutase, an antioxidant and scavenger of free radicals. Preterm infants have lower hepatic stores of copper compared to term infants, as is the case with most micronutrients that accumulate in the last trimester of pregnancy. As a result, preterm infants have higher copper needs but are also at risk for biliary stasis. These increased requirements, along with limited stores and the potential for high GI losses, should be balanced against a reduced excretion of copper via bile. Cholestasis may result when there is excessive copper accumulation, leading to liver disease.[10,16]

## Selenium

Selenium, a trace element, performs various physiological functions in the form of selenoproteins, including selenium-dependent glutathione peroxidase, selenoprotein P, and iodothyronine-5'-deiodinase. These proteins are essential to antioxidant defense and help scavenge free radicals. They also support thyroid function, as they are responsible for the catalyzation of thyroxine to triiodothyronine.[10] Preterm infants are at an increased risk of poor selenium status due to insufficient stores at birth, increased requirements during rapid growth, and rapid uptake of selenium during periods of inflammation.[17] Studies have shown an association between low selenium status and bronchopulmonary dysplasia.[18,19] In contrast, improved selenium status has been linked to reduced risk of sepsis and fewer days spent on ventilation.[20-22]

Preterm
Neonates

# Micronutrient Assessment and Monitoring

Assessment of micronutrient deficiencies or toxicities is especially challenging in the neonatal population. Monitoring requires drawing blood volumes that are often considered excessive in both quantity and frequency.

The most common electrolytes requiring monitoring and supplementation for appropriate growth are calcium and phosphorus, but this can prove difficult in neonates. Calcium is frequently measured via basic metabolic panels. These do not include a test for ionized calcium, which is the bioavailable form used to interpret calcium status. Therefore, total serum calcium levels are used. However, total serum calcium levels must be adjusted for hypoalbuminemia when present. Total calcium levels vary, depending on the parameters of a given laboratory standard.[9] For phosphorus, accepted target levels for neonates are higher than those recommended for older infants and pediatric patients.[9,23]

As iron deficiency anemia adversely affects brain development, neonatal iron status is frequently monitored.[23] Iron needs can be highly variable, depending on the amount of blood loss and frequency of transfusions. Routine monitoring of hemoglobin and ferritin is recommended.[10,23] For neonates fed via PN, iron is not typically added to the solution (unlike other trace minerals routinely added, such as zinc, copper, and selenium) unless long-term PN is required, as in the case of intestinal failure; this is because iron may be incompatible with lipid injectable emulsions that are often coinfused with the PN solution.

Vitamin D is also frequently monitored in neonates. Maternal vitamin D deficiency is prevalent, and because infants only have 50% to 75% of the 25-hydroxyvitamin D level of their mothers, many preterm infants are deficient at birth.[9]

Other micronutrients, such as zinc, copper, and selenium, are typically monitored only in patients with increased losses or suspected deficiencies or toxicities (eg, patients with intestinal failure, high ostomy outputs, wounds, diarrhea, cholestasis, or long-term PN use). Deficiencies of these micronutrients are far more common, whereas toxicities are more infrequent. Unfortunately, zinc, copper, and selenium are difficult to accurately monitor with currently available laboratory tests.[23] For example, although zinc deficiency is particularly concerning in preterm infants, use of either serum or plasma zinc levels is not a sensitive indicator for deficiency.[23,24] Monitoring zinc in this population is, therefore, reserved only for those with increased losses who are at the greatest risk for deficiencies.

Copper status can be assessed by measuring plasma concentrations of copper or ceruloplasmin, the main copper-binding protein in plasma.[25] Poor sensitivity with marginal copper deficiency makes assessment difficult, and levels can be falsely elevated with inflammation.[26] Because copper is eliminated via the biliary tract, patients with PN-associated cholestasis are at risk for elevated levels and should have their doses reduced in this circumstance.

Selenium status is monitored by measuring serum or plasma concentrations of selenium or the activity of glutathione peroxidase in plasma or red blood cells. However, some studies have shown that hypoalbuminemia, seen with systemic inflammation, may alter selenium levels.[17,23,27] Unfortunately, glutathione peroxidase activity is not appropriate for the monitoring of selenium status in preterm infants because their levels are affected by immaturity and oxygen exposure.[28] Serum levels reflect recent intake, whereas red blood cell concentrations reflect more remote intake. Therefore, monitoring of selenium in premature infants is reserved only for those with known or suspected malabsorption (as in short bowel syndrome or intestinal failure).

Box 12.2 on page 250 summarizes the micronutrient assessment and monitoring recommendations for preterm infants as covered in this chapter.[9,10,23-25,28-34]

# Daily Intake and Repletion

Human milk is the preferred source of nutrients for infants. However, for preterm infants born with low micronutrient stores, human milk should be fortified with either human milk–based or cow's milk–based fortifiers to meet most recommended intake levels for macronutrients and micronutrients. Preterm neonates who are born with inadequate stores and who may further develop nutritional deficiencies during their stay in the neonatal intensive care unit may require additional supplementation. This section reviews the recommendations for supplementing calcium, phosphorus, iron, vitamin D, zinc, copper, and selenium. The recommendations are summarized in Table 12.2 on page 254.[9,10,23,27,29,35-41]

## Calcium and Phosphorus

Calcium and phosphorus intake and repletion should be considered throughout the preterm neonate's stay in intensive care, first parenterally for very-low-birthweight infants and then enterally for all premature infants. For parenteral administration, the calcium-to-phosphorus molar

## BOX 12.2 Laboratory Assessment and Monitoring Considerations for Micronutrient Status in Preterm Infants[9,10,23-25,28-34]

### *Calcium, total serum*

| | |
|---|---|
| Normal range[a] | Aged 0 to 12 months: 8.5 to 11.0 mg/dL |
| Target | 8.8 mg/dL |

**Monitoring considerations[b]**

| | |
|---|---|
| Initial | Daily |
| Chronic | Every 1 to 4 weeks |

Monitor at least once when patient is receiving full enteral nutrition (EN), preferably at age 4 to 6 weeks.

Monitor more frequently if patient is receiving parenteral nutrition (PN) or critically ill.

If concern for metabolic bone disease,[c,d] monitor at age 4 to 6 weeks and then every 1 to 2 weeks if abnormal, or every 2 to 4 weeks for 3 months if normal.

### *Calcium, ionized*

| | |
|---|---|
| Normal range[a] | Aged 0 to 31 days: 3.9 to 6.0 mg/dL |
| | Aged 1 to 6 months: 3.7 to 5.9 mg/dL |

**Monitoring considerations[b]**

| | |
|---|---|
| Initial | Daily |
| Chronic | Every 1 to 4 weeks |

Monitor at least once when patient is receiving full EN, preferably at age 4 to 6 weeks.

Monitor more frequently if patient is receiving PN or critically ill.

If concern for metabolic bone disease,[c,d] consider monitoring at age 4 to 6 weeks and then every 1 to 2 weeks if abnormal, or every 2 to 4 weeks for 3 months if normal.

### *Phosphorus, serum*

| | |
|---|---|
| Normal range[a] | Aged 0 to 14 days: 5.6 to 10.5 mg/dL |
| | Aged 15 days to 12 months: 4.8 to 8.4 mg/dL |
| Target | Minimum of 4 mg/dL, improved bone mineralization if maintained at 5.6 mg/dL (1.8 mmol/L) |

**BOX 12.2 Laboratory Assessment and Monitoring Considerations for Micronutrient Status in Preterm Infants[9,10,23-25,28-34] (cont.)**

**Monitoring considerations[b]**

Initial          Daily

Chronic          Every 1 to 4 weeks

Monitor at least once when patient is receiving full EN, preferably at age 4 to 6 weeks.

Monitor more frequently if patient is receiving PN, critically ill, small for gestational age (SGA), or intrauterine growth restricted (IUGR).

If concern for metabolic bone disease,[c,d] monitor at age 4 to 6 weeks and then every 1 to 2 weeks if abnormal, or every 2 to 4 weeks for 3 months if normal.

Levels at age 2 to 3 weeks are predictive of bone mineral content at discharge.

## *Iron*

**Hemoglobin**

Normal range[a]          Neonates: 13.4 to 16.6 g/L; anemic if less than 13.5 g/L

**Serum ferritin**

Normal range[a]          Males: 24 to 336 ng/mL

          Females: 11 to 307 ng/mL

          Neonates:

- Iron deficient if less than 35 ng/mL
- Discontinue iron therapy if greater than 300 ng/mL

**Monitoring considerations[b]**

Monitor hemoglobin if patient has an increased need for oxygen therapy or known malabsorptive state (ie, short bowel syndrome or intestinal failure).

Monitor serum ferritin if patient is anemic or receiving iron supplementation. Typically monitor by age 1 month and then monthly thereafter while patient is receiving supplementation or if concerns for deficiency increase.

*Continued on next page*

> **BOX 12.2  Laboratory Assessment and Monitoring Considerations for Micronutrient Status in Preterm Infants[9,10,23-25,28-34] (cont.)**

## Vitamin D (25-hydroxyvitamin D)

Normal range[a]   Less than 10 ng/mL: severe deficiency
10 to 19 ng/mL: mild to moderate deficiency
20 to 50 ng/mL: optimal level
51 to 80 ng/mL: increased risk of hypercalciuria
Greater than 80 ng/mL: toxicity possible
Neonates: deficient if <20 ng/dL (<50 mmol/L)

**Monitoring considerations[b]**

Monitor if concern for metabolic bone disease, if unable to provide 10 to 25 mcg/d (400 to 1,000 IU/d) due to limited EN intake, or if calcium or phosphorus values are abnormal. Typically monitor by age 4 to 6 weeks along with calcium and phosphorus levels, and then monthly thereafter while patient is receiving supplementation or if concerns for deficiency increase.

## Zinc, serum

Normal range[a]   Aged 0 to 10 y: 60 to 120 mcg/dL

**Monitoring considerations[b]**

Not a sensitive indicator for mild to moderate deficiency

Monitor in patients with greatest risk for deficiencies (those with wounds, high ostomy outputs, or excessive diarrhea as seen with short bowel syndrome or malabsorption states). Typically monitor at the time of initial concern and then every 2 to 4 weeks while patient is receiving supplementation or if concerns for deficiency are ongoing.

## Copper

**Serum copper**

Normal range[a]   Aged 0 to 2 months: 40 to 140 mcg/dL
Aged 3 to 6 months: 40 to 160 mcg/dL

**Serum ceruloplasmin**

Normal range[a]   Aged 0 to 8 weeks: 7.4 to 23.7 mg/dL
Aged 9 weeks to 5 months: 13.5 to 32.9 mg/dL

**BOX 12.2  Laboratory Assessment and Monitoring Considerations for Micronutrient Status in Preterm Infants[9,10,23-25,28-34] (cont.)**

**Monitoring considerations[b]**

Not a sensitive indicator for mild deficiency

Monitor if malabsorption is known or suspected (as with short bowel syndrome or intestinal failure). Typically monitor at the time of initial concern and then every 1 to 3 months while patient is receiving supplementation or if concerns for deficiency or toxicity exist.

## Selenium, serum

Normal range[a]      Aged 0 to 2 months: 45 to 90 mcg/L

Aged 3 to 6 months: 50 to 120 mcg/L

**Monitoring considerations[b]**

Not a sensitive indicator for deficiency

Monitor if malabsorption is known or suspected (as with short bowel syndrome or intestinal failure) or if patient is receiving long-term PN. Typically monitor at the time of initial concern and then every 1 to 3 months while patient is receiving supplementation or if concerns for deficiency are ongoing.

[a] Laboratory reference ranges are dependent on the test used and vary slightly between laboratories. Use the reference ranges for the specific laboratory that processed the sample.
[b] Monitoring of micronutrients in preterm neonates is extremely difficult, given concerns for blood volume requirements and the lack of sensitivity of available biochemical assessment measurements to determine deficiencies. This leads many clinicians to monitor only when deficiency is suspected.
[c] Concern for metabolic bone disease exists with any of the following: birthweight < 1500 g, gestational age < 28 weeks, long-term (>4 weeks) PN, difficulty reaching full fortified feeds, short bowel syndrome/intestinal failure, elevated parathyroid hormone, malabsorption, or prolonged use of medications that impair bone (diuretics, corticosteroids, phenobarbital).
[d] When concern for metabolic bone disease exists, the following laboratory values should be obtained in addition to calcium, ionized calcium, and phosphorus: alkaline phosphatase (including consideration for alkaline phosphatase isoenzymes to distinguish elevated values as related to either liver or bone), parathyroid hormone, 25-hydroxyvitamin D, kidney tubular resorption of phosphate, and urinary calcium-to-creatinine ratio. Alkaline phosphatase and kidney tubular resorption of phosphate should be screened at age 4 to 6 weeks and then periodically if normal but concern for metabolic bone disease continues. If abnormal, monitor parathyroid hormone and 25-hydroxyvitamin D. If normal, monitor metabolic bone laboratory values every 2 to 4 weeks for 3 months. If abnormal, start treatment dosing and monitor metabolic bone laboratory values every 1 to 2 weeks with urinary calcium-to-creatinine ratio.

TABLE 12.2 Micronutrient Intake and Repletion Strategies for Preterm Neonates [9,10,23,27,29,35-41]

| Nutrient | Routine daily intake to maintain physiologically normal level | | Repletion dosing if deficient | |
| | PN | EN | PN | EN |
| --- | --- | --- | --- | --- |
| Calcium | 1.25-2.00 mmol/kg (50-80 mg/kg) Ca:P = 1.0-1.3 to 1 | 3.0-5.5 mmol/kg (120-220 mg/kg) Ca:P = 2:1 | Ca:P = 0.8-1.0 to 1 | |
| Phosphorus | 1.25-3.00 mmol/kg (39-93 mg/kg) Ca:P = 1.0-1.3 to 1 | 2.3-3.9 mmol/kg (70-120 mg/kg) Ca:P = 2:1 | Ca:P = 0.8-1.0 to 1 | |
| Iron | N/A | Elemental iron, 2 mg/kg Recommend time of initiation based on birthweight:<br>• <1.5 kg at age 2 wk<br>• 1.5-2.0 kg at age 2-4 wk<br>• 2.0-2.5 kg at age 4-6 wk | 0.20-0.25 mg/kg/d or 1.5 mg/kg/dose once weekly Use iron dextran or iron sucrose | Elemental iron, 3-4 mg/kg/d (up to 6 mg/kg/d with erythropoietin) |

*Continued on next page*

254

| | | | | |
|---|---|---|---|---|
| Vitamin D | 10 mcg (400 IU)[a] | 10 mcg (400 IU)[b] | Single vitamin product unavailable. Consider increasing dose by increasing multivitamin product in the solution if other fat-soluble vitamins are deficient or within normal range. | AAP recommends 15-25 mcg/d (600-1,000 IU/d) ESPGHAN recommends 20-25 mcg/d (800-1,000 IU/d). |
| Zinc | 400-500 mcg/kg | Elemental zinc, 2-3 mg/kg | Increase dose from baseline daily intake based on deficiency and subsequent monitoring. | |
| Copper | 40 mcg/kg | 120-230 mcg/kg Zn:Cu not to exceed 20:1 to ensure adequate intestinal absorption of copper | Increase dose from baseline daily intake based on deficiency and subsequent monitoring. | |
| Selenium | 7 mcg/kg | 7-10 mcg/kg | Increase dose from baseline daily intake based on deficiency and subsequent monitoring. | |

Abbreviations: AAP, American Academy of Pediatrics; Ca, calcium; Cu, copper; EN, enteral nutrition; ESPGHAN, European Society for Paediatric Gastroenterology, Hepatology and Nutrition; kg, kilogram of body weight; NA, not applicable; P, phosphorus; PN, parenteral nutrition; Zn, zinc.

[a] Pediatric PN multivitamin products contain 400 IU (10 mcg) vitamin D per 5 mL. Not all neonatal patients receive the entire 5 mL of this product daily and are, therefore, at a greater risk for deficiencies.

[b] The AAP recommends providing 400 IU (10 mcg) vitamin D per day to all neonates and infants who are exclusively fed human milk. If a neonate or infant is not consuming at least 1,000 mL of standard infant formula per day, they will not receive 400 IU (10 mcg) vitamin D per day and may require an additional enteral source.

Preterm
Neonates

ratio must be considered. After the first few days of life, the optimal ratio for bone mineralization and other metabolic functions is 1–1.3:1.[9] This equates to a calcium provision of 1.25 to 2 mmol per kilogram of body weight per day (50–80 mg per kilogram of body weight per day) and a phosphorus provision of 1.25 to 3 mmol/kg/d (39–93 mg/kg/d) for patients receiving PN.[9] However, in preterm neonates at risk for hypophosphatemia due to neonatal refeeding syndrome, the initial PN requirements immediately after birth indicate the need for a lower ratio of 0.8–1:1.[35,36] (A complete discussion of the PN management of neonatal refeeding syndrome is beyond the scope of this chapter.)

For daily enteral intake to maintain physiological normal levels of calcium and phosphorus, higher amounts are needed to account for intestinal absorption. Whereas intestinal phosphorus absorption appears to be approximately 90% of intake, calcium absorption in preterm neonates is lower, at 50% to 65%.[9] To account for the increased needs and decreased absorption in this population, the European Society for Paediatric Gastroenterology, Hepatology and Nutrition (ESPGHAN)[37] and the American Academy of Pediatrics (AAP)[42] recommend the enteral provision of calcium and phosphorus as described in Table 12.2 on page 256. Although the use of human milk is the gold standard for enteral nutrition in all infants, to achieve the recommended intake of calcium and phosphorus, use of human-milk fortifier is required.[12]

# Iron

Enteral iron is one of the most common micronutrients given to neonates. Whereas infant formulas are fortified with iron, human milk contains only 0.5 mg elemental iron per liter.[43] For this reason, the AAP recommends providing 2 mg elemental iron per kilogram of body weight per day as either a separate enteral dose or a combination of an enteral dose and infant formula (see Table 12.2).[38] The most common enteral iron supplement used in the neonatal population is ferrous sulfate. Dosing of ferrous sulfate is based on the elemental iron component of the salt form, which is 20% for ferrous sulfate (ie, 15 mg elemental iron in 75 mg ferrous sulfate). Recommended initial dosing of elemental iron for prevention of iron deficiency anemia is 2 to 3 mg/kg/d. Doses as high as 6 mg/kg/d may be needed for infants receiving erythropoietin therapy.[43] If ferritin levels remain low and are less than 35 to 70 ng/mL, then the dose of elemental iron should be increased to 3 to 4 mg/kg/d.[10] For patients who cannot receive enteral doses for required daily intake or for repletion, an intravenous preparation of iron may be administered; either iron dextran or iron sucrose can be used. Parenteral iron formulations may be administered in lipid injectable emulsion–free PN solutions (ie, 2-in-1 PN admixture) or as a separate intravenous infusion. Typical dosing for parenteral iron replacement is provided in Table 12.2.[43] This dose may be given daily or as a combined dose for several days in less frequent intervals.

# Vitamin D

Vitamin D commonly requires intake and repletion in states of deficiency. Human milk does not provide adequate daily intake amounts of vitamin D for repletion or even to prevent deficiency. For this reason, vitamin D supplementation is recommended for all infants receiving human milk or less than 1,000 mL of infant formula per day.[44]

Enteral vitamin D is primarily supplied as either ergocalciferol (D2) or cholecalciferol (D3). Cholecalciferol is the preferred agent for its better absorption and more appropriate concentration for the doses required by neonates (400 IU/mL or 10 mcg/mL). The AAP[42] and ESPGHAN[37] recommendations for vitamin D for premature infants are provided in Table 12.2. The higher dosing range should be used for infants with known deficiencies or with increased needs stemming from the use of other medications (eg, furosemide, phenobarbital, steroids).

# Zinc, Copper, and Selenium

Other micronutrients requiring repletion in neonates, particularly in patients with absorption issues, include zinc, copper, and selenium. These three trace elements are provided in PN either as individual components or as part of a multi–trace element combination product. Intravenous dosing recommendations from ESPGHAN and the American Society for Parenteral and Enteral Nutrition (ASPEN) are based on the neonatal patient's age and weight and are provided in Table 12.2.[39,40] For patients who continue to need enteral trace element repletion, the doses for zinc, copper, and selenium are provided in Table 12.2.

# *References*

1.  BhatiaJ, Griffin I, Anderson D, Kler N, Domellöf M. Selected macro/
    micronutrient needs of the routine preterm infant. *J Pediatr.* 2013;162
    (3 suppl):S48-S55. doi:10.1016/j.jpeds.2012.11.053

2.  Ilardi L, Proto A, Ceroni F, et al. Overview of important micronutrients
    supplementation in preterm infants after discharge: a call for consensus.
    *Life (Basel).* 2021;11(4):331. doi:10.3390/life11040331

3.  Tudehope D, Fewtrell M, Kashyap S, Udaeta E. Nutritional needs of the
    micropreterm infant. *J Pediatr.* 2013;162(3 suppl):S72-S80. doi:10.1016/j
    .jpeds.2012.11.056

4.  Raiten DJ, Steiber AL, Carlson SE, et al. Working group reports:
    evaluation of the evidence to support practice guidelines for
    nutritional care of preterm infants—the Pre-B Project. *Am J Clin Nutr.*
    2016;103(2):648S-678S. doi:10.3945/ajcn.115.117309

5.  Engle WA; American Academy of Pediatrics Committee on Fetus and
    Newborn. Age terminology during the perinatal period. *Pediatrics.*
    2004;114(5):1362-1364. doi:10.1542/peds.2004-1915

6.  Sharma D, Shastri S, Sharma P. Intrauterine growth restriction:
    antenatal and postnatal aspects. *Clin Med Insights Pediatr.* 2016;10:67-83.
    doi:10.4137/CMPed.S40070

7.  Indrio F, Neu J, Pettoello-Mantovani M, et al. Development of the
    gastrointestinal tract in newborns as a challenge for an appropriate
    nutrition: a narrative review. *Nutrients.* 2022;14(7):1405. doi:10.3390
    /nu14071405

8.  Rogido M, Griffin I. Macronutrient digestion and absorption in the
    preterm infant. *Neoreviews.* 2019;20(1):e25-e36. doi:10.1542/neo.20-1-e25

9.  Taylor SN. Calcium, magnesium, phosphorus, and vitamin D.
    In: Koletzko B, Cheah F, Domellof M, Poindexter BB, Vain N, van
    Goudoever JB, eds. *Nutritional Care of Preterm Infants: Scientific Basis and
    Practical Guidelines.* 2nd ed. Karger; 2021:122-139.

10. Domellöf M. Microminerals: iron, zinc, copper, selenium, manganese,
    iodine, chromium and molybdenum. In: Koletzko B, Cheah F, Domellof
    M, Poindexter BB, Vain N, van Goudoever JB, eds. *Nutritional Care of
    Preterm Infants: Scientific Basis and Practical Guidelines.* 2nd ed. Karger;
    2021:140-148.

11. Beggs MR, Lee JJ, Busch K, et al. TRPV6 and Ca$_v$1.3 mediate distal small
    intestine calcium absorption before weaning. *Cell Mol Gastroenterol
    Hepatol.* 2019;8(4):625-642. doi:10.1016/j.jcmgh.2019.07.005

12. Greer FR. Calcium and phosphorus and the preterm infant. *NeoReviews.*
    2016;17(4):e195-e202.

13. Rao R, Georgieff MK. Iron therapy for preterm infants. *Clin Perinatol.* 2009;36(1):27-42. doi:10.1016/j.clp.2008.09.013

14. Brion LP, Heyne R, Lair CS. Role of zinc in neonatal growth and brain growth: review and scoping review. *Pediatr Res.* 2021;89(7):1627-1640. doi:10.1038/s41390-020-01181-z

15. Dumrongwongsiri O, Winichagoon P, Chongviriyaphan N, Suthutvoravut U, Grote V, Koletzko B. Zinc and iron adequacy and relative importance of zinc/iron storage and intakes among breastfed infants. *Matern Child Nutr.* 2022;18(1):e13268. doi:10.1111/mcn.13268

16. Zemrani B, McCallum Z, Bines JE. Trace element provision in parenteral nutrition in children: one size does not fit all. *Nutrients.* 2018;10(11):1819. doi:10.3390/nu10111819

17. Rao A, Jericho H, Patton T, et al. Factors affecting selenium status in infants on parenteral nutrition therapy. *J Pediatr Gastroenterol Nutr.* 2021;73(3):e73-e78. doi:10.1097/MPG.0000000000003174

18. Tindell R, Tipple T. Selenium: implications for outcomes in extremely preterm infants. *J Perinatol.* 2018;38(3):197-202. doi:10.1038/s41372-017-0033-3

19. Darlow BA, Austin NC. Selenium supplementation to prevent short-term morbidity in preterm neonates. *Cochrane Database Syst Rev.* 2003;2003(4):CD003312. doi:10.1002/14651858.CD003312

20. Leite HP, Nogueira PC, Iglesias SB, de Oliveira SV, Sarni RO. Increased plasma selenium is associated with better outcomes in children with systemic inflammation. *Nutrition.* 2015;31(3):485-490. doi:10.1016/j.nut.2014.09.008

21. Aggarwal R, Gathwala G, Yadav S, Kumar P. Selenium supplementation for prevention of late-onset sepsis in very low birth weight preterm neonates. *J Trop Pediatr.* 2016;62(3):185-193. doi:10.1093/tropej/fmv096

22. Bayliss PA, Buchanan BE, Hancock RG, Zlotkin SH. Tissue selenium accretion in premature and full-term human infants and children. *Biol Trace Elem Res.* 1985;7(1):55-61. doi:10.1007/BF02916547

23. Domellöf M. Nutritional care of premature infants: microminerals. In: Koletzko B, Poindexter B, Uauy R, eds. *Nutritional Care of Preterm Infants: Scientific Basis and Practical Guidelines.* Karger; 2014:121-139.

24. Jen M, Yan AC. Syndromes associated with nutritional deficiency and excess. *Clin Dermatol.* 2010;28(6):669-685. doi:10.1016/j.clindermatol.2010.03.029

25. Rükgauer M, Klein J, Kruse-Jarres JD. Reference values for the trace elements copper, manganese, selenium, and zinc in the serum/plasma of children, adolescents, and adults. *J Trace Elem Med Biol.* 1997;11(2):92-98. doi:10.1016/S0946-672X(97)80032-6

26. MacKay M, Mulroy CW, Street J, et al. Assessing copper status in pediatric patients receiving parenteral nutrition. *Nutr Clin Pract.* 2015;30(1):117-121. doi:10.1177/0884533614538457

27. Selenium. Lexicomp Toxicology (database). Wolters Kluwer. 2022. Accessed December 30, 2022.

28. Loui A, Raab A, Braetter P, Obladen M, de Braetter VN. Selenium status in term and preterm infants during the first months of life. *Eur J Clin Nutr.* 2008;62(3):349-355. doi:10.1038/sj.ejcn.1602715

29. Domellöf M, Braegger C, Campoy C, et al. Iron requirements of infants and toddlers. *J Pediatr Gastroenterol Nutr.* 2014;58(1):119-129. doi:10.1097/MPG.0000000000000206

30. Backström MC, Kouri T, Kuusela AL, et al. Bone isoenzyme of serum alkaline phosphatase and serum inorganic phosphate in metabolic bone disease of prematurity. *Acta Paediatr.* 2000;89(7):867-873.

31. Laboratory reference range values. In: Soghier L, Fratantoni K, Reyes C, Mullins K, eds. *Reference Range Values for Pediatric Care.* 2nd ed. American Academy of Pediatrics; 2019:69-108.

32. Test catalog. Mayo Clinic Laboratories. Accessed December 30, 2022. www.mayocliniclabs.com/test-catalog

33. Szeszycki E, Cruse W, Beitezel M. Evaluation and monitoring of pediatric patients receiving specialized nutrition support. In: Corkins M, ed. *The A.S.P.E.N. Pediatric Nutrition Support Core Curriculum.* 2nd ed. American Society for Parenteral and Enteral Nutrition; 2015:615-640.

34. Faienza MF, D'Amato E, Natale MP, et al. Metabolic bone disease of prematurity: diagnosis and management. *Front Pediatr.* 2019;7:143. doi:10.3389/fped.2019.00143

35. Hair AB, Chetta KE, Bruno AM, Hawthorne KM, Abrams SA. Delayed introduction of parenteral phosphorus is associated with hypercalcemia in extremely preterm infants. *J Nutr.* 2016;146(6):1212-1216. doi:10.3945/jn.115.228254

36. Senterre T, Abu Zahirah I, Pieltain C, de Halleux V, Rigo J. Electrolyte and mineral homeostasis after optimizing early macronutrient intakes in VLBW infants on parenteral nutrition. *J Pediatr Gastroenterol Nutr.* 2015;61(4):491-498. doi:10.1097/MPG.0000000000000854

37. Agostoni C, Buonocore G, Carnielli VP, et al. Enteral nutrient supply for preterm infants: commentary from the European Society of Paediatric Gastroenterology, Hepatology and Nutrition Committee on Nutrition. *J Pediatr Gastroenterol Nutr.* 2010;50(1):85-91. doi:10.1097/MPG.0b013e3181adaee0

38. Baker RD, Greer FR; Committee on Nutrition, American Academy of Pediatrics. Diagnosis and prevention of iron deficiency and iron-deficiency anemia in infants and young children (0-3 years of age). *Pediatrics*. 2010;126(5):1040-1050. doi:10.1542/peds.2010-2576

39. Domellöf M, Szitanyi P, Simchowitz V, Franz A, Mimouni F; ESPGHAN/ESPEN/ESPR/CSPEN working group on pediatric parenteral nutrition. ESPGHAN/ESPEN/ESPR/CSPEN guidelines on pediatric parenteral nutrition: iron and trace minerals. *Clin Nutr*. 2018;37(6 pt B):2354-2359. doi:10.1016/j.clnu.2018.06.949

40. Vanek VW, Borum P, Buchman A, et al. A.S.P.E.N. position paper: recommendations for changes in commercially available parenteral multivitamin and multi-trace element products. *Nutr Clin Pract*. 2012;27(4):440-491. doi:10.1177/0884533612446706

41. Darlow BA, Winterbourn CC, Inder TE, et al. The effect of selenium supplementation on outcome in very low birth weight infants: a randomized controlled trial. The New Zealand Neonatal Study Group. *J Pediatr*. 2000;136(4):473-480. doi:10.1016/s0022-3476(00)90010-6

42. American Academy of Pediatrics Committee on Nutrition. Nutritional needs of the preterm infant. In: Kleinman RE, Greer FR, eds. *Pediatric Nutrition*. 8th ed. American Academy of Pediatrics; 2019:113-162.

43. Mills RJ, Davies MW. Enteral iron supplementation in preterm and low birth weight infants. *Cochrane Database Syst Rev*. 2012;(3):CD005095. doi:10.1002/14651858.CD005095.pub2

44. Wagner CL, Greer FR; American Academy of Pediatrics Section on Breastfeeding; American Academy of Pediatrics Committee on Nutrition. Prevention of rickets and vitamin D deficiency in infants, children, and adolescents. *Pediatrics*. 2008;122(5):1142-1152. doi:10.1542/peds.2008-1862

# CHAPTER 13

# Critical Care

Michelle L. Kozeniecki Schneider, MS, RDN, CNSC, CCTD, FASPEN, and Jayshil J. Patel, MD

## Introduction

Micronutrients affect virtually every enzyme system in the body and are essential for the metabolism and utilization of macronutrients.[1] Patients who are critically ill often have preexisting or acquired risk factors for malnutrition, such as decreased nutrient intake and excessive utilization and loss of nutrients, and they are at risk for developing micronutrient deficiencies. In addition, conditions that define critical illness, such as sepsis, respiratory failure, trauma, and burns, activate inflammatory pathways that increase oxidative stress and, therefore, increase the body's demand for antioxidants. Accumulative micronutrient deficiencies are associated with increased infections and organ dysfunction. This chapter (1) reviews the risk factors for micronutrient deficiency in critical illness, (2) identifies and outlines the signs and symptoms of deficiency seen in clinical practice, (3) describes micronutrient administration strategies for critically ill patients, and (4) identifies and describes the rationale for using individual micronutrients as therapies in critically ill patients.

# Risk Factors for Micronutrient Deficiency in Critical Illness

A patient's preexisting comorbidities and nutritional status prior to admission to the intensive care unit (ICU) can place the critically ill patient at risk for micronutrient deficiencies. A thorough evaluation of the patient's medical and surgical histories, dietary intake, and recent weight changes can provide clues to the mechanisms for preexisting micronutrient deficiencies. The mechanisms for micronutrient deficiencies acquired during critical illness (during the ICU stay) can be grouped into three categories: increased micronutrient losses, inadequate intake or assimilation, and increased systemic requirements. An appraisal of conditions that define critical illness and ICU interventions can identify the mechanisms for acquired micronutrient deficiencies.

## Presence of Comorbid Conditions Prior to Intensive Care

Many patients who are admitted to the ICU for an acute illness or injury have one or more comorbid conditions. Certain preexisting illnesses—such as cancer, diabetes, and heart, kidney, and liver diseases—are risk factors for both ICU admission and micronutrient deficiencies that may exist prior to ICU admission. From a mechanistic standpoint, diminished oral intake in patients with a history of anorexia-inducing conditions, such as cirrhosis, respiratory failure, and heart failure, can contribute to various micronutrient deficiencies. Malabsorptive conditions, including chronic pancreatitis and inflammatory bowel disease, can promote micronutrient deficiencies despite adequate intake. Chronic inflammatory conditions generate oxidative stress and increase micronutrient (antioxidant) utilization.

# Increased Micronutrient Losses

## Diarrhea

In healthy individuals, micronutrient loss through urine and stool is minimal. Critical illness–related conditions and therapies can contribute to increased micronutrient loss. Diarrhea has been reported in up to 78% of critically ill patients[2] and may be related to the underlying disease process (eg, clostridial colitis) or even micronutrient (niacin) deficiency. Although not standardized, the most common definitions of diarrhea are the following: three or more loose or watery bowel movements in a 24-hour period, or stool output (by weight) of more than 200 g/d.[3] Identifying the precipitating factor for diarrhea is crucial for both predicting specific micronutrient deficiencies and guiding treatment.[4] Osmotic diarrhea, for example, is related to medications that contain nonabsorbable ions or sugars and may resolve when the offending medication is discontinued.[5] Regardless of the cause, diarrhea is associated with increased losses of zinc, potassium, and magnesium, all of which should be monitored and repleted. Decreased small bowel transit time diminishes nutrient absorption of micronutrients such as copper, zinc, and iron. Steatorrhea may indicate loss of fat-soluble vitamins (A, D, E, K).

## Wounds

Because of risk factors such as immobilization and surgery, wounds are common during critical care. Exudate from wounds contains water, electrolytes, nutrients, inflammatory mediators, white blood cells, and waste products. Chronic venous ulceration, dehisced surgical wounds, burns, inflammatory ulcers, and skin-donor sites can produce a large amount of exudate, and micronutrient losses can occur. Open-abdomen wounds may result in more micronutrient loss than nonabdomen wounds. In a prospective observational study that evaluated the micronutrient content of wound exudate from 17 patients undergoing negative-pressure wound therapy, the 24-hour exudate volume and micronutrient loss was greater in patients with open-abdomen wounds compared to those with soft-tissue wounds.[4] In the open-abdomen group, average exudate loss was 900 mL/d; mean 24-hour losses of vitamins A, C, and E were

0.31 mg, 2.5 mg, and 10 mg, respectively; and 24-hour losses of zinc, iron, and copper were 0.5 mg, 0.4 mg, and 0.25 mg, respectively.[6] Exudate from chronic wounds may be a major source of micronutrient loss. (Chapter 11 provides more information on wounds.)

## Diuretics and Renal Replacement Therapy

Renal losses can also contribute to micronutrient deficiencies. Critically ill patients (without kidney failure) may receive diuretic therapy, and the use of loop or thiazide diuretics has been associated with increased urinary excretion of calcium, magnesium, potassium, zinc, and thiamin.[7,8] Kidney failure is common in patients in the ICU. For patients with acute kidney failure without renal replacement therapy, recovering from conditions such as acute tubular necrosis can induce polyuria with increased micronutrient loss.[9] Continuous renal replacement therapy (CRRT), a form of renal replacement therapy used in hemodynamically unstable patients, allows for the clearance of small molecules, providing control of blood urea nitrogen, creatinine, and other toxins.[10] Small solutes such as vitamins, trace minerals, and other nutrients are lost in the process. Several studies have measured serum micronutrient levels in critically ill patients requiring CRRT; others have measured the micronutrient content of CRRT effluent. In one study, low serum levels of water-soluble vitamins, zinc, selenium, and copper were identified, with the nutrients being lost in effluent.[11] A 2021 scoping review of micronutrient losses in CRRT summarized 35 publications and found thiamin, vitamin C, copper, and selenium deficiencies as a result of effluent losses.[12] The likelihood of micronutrient deficiency is highest in patients undergoing CRRT for more than 7 days.

# Inadequate Micronutrient Intake or Assimilation

## Inadequate Intake

Anorexia, nausea, vomiting, diarrhea, and pain are risk factors for poor volitional intake, and critically ill patients often receive enteral nutrition

(EN) therapy to help meet their needs. Most commercially available EN formulas provide the Dietary Reference Intakes (DRIs) for vitamins and minerals in volumes of 900 to 1,500 mL, depending on the energy density. Patients who are prescribed and receive enteral volumes sufficient to meet their full energy and protein needs are also likely receiving adequate micronutrients; however, enteral feeding intolerance, malabsorption, or decreased gut transit time can contribute to increased micronutrient loss, despite adequate EN prescription. In addition, several factors can result in critically ill patients not meeting their EN prescriptions:

- Multiple studies have demonstrated incomplete delivery of prescribed enteral formula volumes, often due to patient-related, provider-related, and system-related barriers; in such cases, critically ill patients receive approximately 50% of prescribed volumes.[13-15]

- Critically ill patients receiving EN are often placed on "nothing by mouth" status because of real or perceived gastrointestinal dysfunction or as a prerequisite for a test or procedure.

- EN dose recommendations during the acute phase of critical illness (eg, the first week of ICU admission) have shifted from a full-energy target prescription to restricted feeding progression, whatever the route.[16,17]

Current guidelines for critical care nutrition recommend feeding critically ill patients between 12 and 25 kcal per kilogram of body weight per day during the first 7 to 10 days.[17] Prolonged intentional and unintentional restricted feeding may be a risk factor for acquired micronutrient deficiencies.

## Inadequate Assimilation

For patients who are critically ill and receiving EN in amounts sufficient to provide the DRIs for vitamins and minerals, improper route or timing of medication delivery may prevent the assimilation needed for absorption and digestion. For example, the timing of pancreatic enzyme replacement or bile acid therapy for conditions such as exocrine pancreatic insufficiency or hepatobiliary diseases, respectively, should be in accordance with the EN schedule to maximize the potential for fat and fat-soluble vitamin absorption. Similarly, medications known to impair vitamin and mineral absorption need to be reviewed for appropriate administration with EN and multivitamin/mineral administration (refer to Box 13.1).[18,19] Finally, familiarity with micronutrient bioavailability is important in determining whether enteral or parenteral administration will meet patient's needs. Enteral thiamin, for example, yields poor rate-limited bioavailability, such that healthy individuals can assimilate a maximum of only 4.5 mg from a dose of 30 mg or higher. Thiamin administered parenterally guarantees better bioavailability in instances of severe deficiency states, such as refeeding syndrome, severe alcoholism, and conditions limiting gut thiamin absorption.[20,21]

| BOX 13.1 Common Medications That Interact With Micronutrients[18,19] | |
|---|---|
| *Medication* | *Potential drug-micronutrient interactions* |
| Carbamazepine | Lowers biotin status |
| | May impair absorption of folate, riboflavin, and vitamins B6 and B12 |
| Fluoroquinolones (eg, ciprofloxacin, levofloxacin) | Drug absorption or bioavailability is reduced by antacids, supplements, or enteral nutrition formulas that contain multivalent cations (eg, calcium, iron, magnesium, zinc). |
| Isoniazid | Impairs vitamin B6 status |
| Metformin | May impair absorption and concentration of thiamin and vitamin B12 |
| Phenytoin | May interfere with folate, carnitine, and vitamin D absorption or metabolism |
| | Drug toxicity may increase with carnitine deficiency. |
| Warfarin | Drug bioavailability is compromised by vitamin C supplementation. |
| | Drug effects are counteracted by vitamin K. |

*Critical Care*

## Increased Micronutrient Requirements Due to Systemic Inflammatory Response

A systemic inflammatory response is common in sepsis, burns, and trauma. Plasma concentrations of vitamins and minerals generally decrease in the presence of inflammation and oxidative stress as a result of vitamin or mineral sequestration, redistribution, capillary leakage, protein binding, and utilization as antioxidants (Chapter 4).[1,22] Micronutrient needs may increase during the acute phase of critical illness to support the biochemical and enzymatic functions required for resolving organ failure and regaining metabolic homeostasis. Critical illness induces mitochondrial dysfunction and oxidative stress, which generates high quantities of free radicals. Micronutrients with antioxidant properties, such as vitamin C, zinc, vitamin D, and selenium, may be rapidly utilized. Beyond their nutritional purpose, these micronutrients may have a potential role as therapies to attenuate or reverse inflammation-induced complications such as organ dysfunction (see Micronutrients as Therapy later in this chapter).

### Summary of Risk Factors

Box 13.2 summarizes the ICU-related risk factors for micronutrient deficiency.

# Micronutrient Assessment and Monitoring

Practices for monitoring critically ill patients for micronutrient deficiencies vary among clinicians. In a survey of 334 clinicians, 96% of whom were physicians, only 24.3% of respondents reported monitoring for deficiencies through clinical signs or laboratory abnormalities.[23]

Monitoring for micronutrient deficiencies includes recognizing both the risk factors that generate deficiency and the clinical phenotypes of deficiencies. Clinical manifestations of deficiency are likely indicative

## BOX 13.2 Intensive Care Unit–Related Risk Factors for Micronutrient Deficiency

| *Risk factors* | *Micronutrients of concern* |
|---|---|
| **Comorbid conditions** | |
| Pancreatitis | Fat-soluble vitamins (A, D, E, and K) |
| Inflammatory bowel disease | All (depending on extent and location of inflammation) |
| Cirrhosis | Vitamin A, vitamin D, thiamin, folate, zinc |
| End-stage renal disease | Vitamin D, calcium, iron, folate, vitamin B12 |
| **Increased micronutrient losses** | |
| Increased urine output | Thiamin, zinc |
| Diarrhea | Zinc |
| Wounds and drains | Zinc |
| Renal replacement therapy | Vitamin B6, vitamin B12, vitamin C, thiamin, copper, selenium, zinc |
| Chyle leak | Selenium |
| **Inadequate intake or assimilation of micronutrients** | |
| Inadequate intake | All |
| Alcohol abuse | Thiamin, folate, vitamin B6, vitamin B12, vitamin C, zinc |
| Bariatric surgery | Fat-soluble vitamins (A, D, E, and K), thiamin, vitamin B6, vitamin B12, iron, copper, zinc |
| **Increased micronutrient requirements** | |
| Systemic inflammatory response | Vitamin A, vitamin B6, vitamin C, vitamin D, thiamin, iron, selenium, zinc |

of severe or prolonged micronutrient depletion and require prompt treatment.

# Physical, Neurological, and Cardiac Assessments

While much focus is given to the examination of fat and muscle stores during a nutrition focused physical exam, an equal amount of attention to the hair, eyes, mouth, nails, and skin can assist in identifying micronutrient deficiencies. Skin changes, such as erythema and poor wound healing, are often evaluated in the context of infection or pressure injury prevention, with interventions aimed at treating or eliminating the cause. In the VITA-TRACE survey, only 13.8% of respondents reported monitoring skin lesions (dermatitis; dry, fragile skin; delayed wound healing) as potential indicators of micronutrient deficiency.[23] Because conditions that define critical illness and interventions can induce skin changes similar to those caused by micronutrient deficiencies, vitamin and mineral deficiencies (specifically vitamin A, the B vitamins, vitamin C, copper, and zinc) may go unrecognized and untreated. For example, although hair loss can have multiple etiologies, including being a side effect of β-blockers medications, deficiencies in zinc, iron, and biotin can also contribute to hair loss.[24]

Optimal functioning of the nervous system is dependent on thiamin, niacin, vitamin B6, folate, vitamin B12, vitamin E, and copper. Neurologic symptoms are common in critically ill patients and may have many causes. Micronutrient deficiencies should be considered when symptoms such as confusion, memory deficits, neuropathy, myelopathy, and progressive weakness are present and remain unexplained.[25] Vitamin B12 deficiency is known to cause peripheral neuropathy and has multiple etiologies, including a vegan diet, use of medications (eg, metformin and pantoprazole), gastric bypass surgery, and autoimmune conditions. When B12 deficiency is severe, it can cause subacute combined degeneration with progressive degeneration of the spinal cord, which can manifest with symptoms of peripheral neuropathy and loss of proprioception.[26]

Thiamin deficiency has been observed in patients who abuse alcohol, patients who have had gastric bypass surgery, patients with refeeding syndrome, and populations with a diet that consists mainly of polished rice or milled white cereals.[27] Thiamin deficiency causes two clinical phenotypes: Wernicke-Korsakoff syndrome and beriberi. Wernicke-Korsakoff syndrome consists of two syndromes that represent different neurologic stages of thiamin deficiency. Wernicke syndrome is acute and is marked by encephalopathy, ophthalmoplegia, and gait disturbances; Korsakoff syndrome is a chronic neurologic condition characterized by impaired short-term memory and confabulation.[28] In a necropsy study of 131 cases that resulted in diagnoses of Wernicke encephalopathy and Korsakoff syndrome, 20% of patients had been diagnosed with thiamin deficiency prior to death.[29]

Adult beriberi occurs in dry and wet forms. Dry beriberi is peripheral neuropathy characterized by both motor and sensory abnormalities; wet beriberi is high-output heart failure.[30] A diagnosis of high-output heart failure is made based on a combination of clinical history with identification of risk factors, physical examination, and imaging, including echocardiography and invasive testing. Both wet and dry beriberi may be difficult to distinguish from conditions that define critical illness (heart failure) and acquired conditions (critical illness–related polyneuropathy). Empiric therapy for patients at risk for thiamin deficiency may be warranted.

# Laboratory Assessment

To help identify and treat deficiencies before clinical manifestations develop, clinicians may choose to monitor micronutrient status by evaluating laboratory and biochemical markers when risk factors are present. The clinician must first recognize the limitations of measuring micronutrient levels in critical illness. Inflammation and micronutrient redistribution affect the concentration of micronutrients in the body, and measuring levels may be unreliable. For example, during inflammation, serum levels of vitamins A, C, D, and E, as well as iron, zinc, thiamin, and selenium, decrease. Copper and chromium levels increase in response to inflammation. For these reasons, and because an elevated

Critical Care

C-reactive protein (CRP) level is a marker of inflammation, experts suggest that reliable clinical interpretations of plasma micronutrient levels can be made as follows: the zinc level is interpretable when the CRP level is less than 2 mg/dL; selenium and vitamin A and D levels are interpretable when CRP is less than 1 mg/dL; and vitamin B6 and C levels are interpretable when CRP is less than 0.5 mg/dL.[31]

Measuring serum lactic acid may be beneficial in identifying thiamin deficiency. Lactic acid is an end product of anaerobic metabolism, and lactic acidosis is the most common cause of an elevated-anion-gap metabolic acidosis in hospitalized patients. Thiamin pyrophosphate is a cofactor in pyruvate dehydrogenase, which converts pyruvate to acetyl coenzyme A, a precursor for the Krebs cycle. Thiamin deficiency can impair the conversion of pyruvate to acetyl coenzyme A; when this happens, the pyruvate is converted to lactic acid instead.[32] In critically ill patients with risk factors for thiamin deficiency who are found to have a noncirculatory shock-related (type A) lactic acidosis, it may be reasonable to administer thiamin empirically before dextrose, and to deliver doses of 100 to 200 mg/d during the first 3 to 5 days, combined with multimicronutrients, especially while ramping up the enteral feeding.[32,33]

# Treatment Strategies

Researchers have studied the provision of exogenous vitamins and minerals during the acute-phase response to stress for decades. Although the daily intake requirements for vitamins and minerals are established for healthy individuals, defining "adequate" intake in critical illness remains difficult.

When a patient's basal micronutrient needs are not met through oral, EN, or parenteral nutrition (PN) therapy, delivery of the remaining amount is called *complementation*.[1,21] Patients whose daily micronutrient needs are not being met through an oral diet or EN therapy should receive either a single-component product or multivitamin/mineral product to complement their intake.

When a patient has deficiencies or increased micronutrient losses, the provision of micronutrients to restore a normal status is called *repletion*.[1,21] For patients with increased losses of nutrients through urine, stool, chyle, or renal replacement therapy, it is reasonable to provide additional amounts of those vitamins and trace minerals to compensate for losses.[22] Patients receiving PN with the standard daily amount of multiple-vitamin infusion and multiple-trace-element products may require additional amounts of individual micronutrients, although not all micronutrients may be compatible with the PN solution and may need to be given separately. If the clinician is unsure of the amount lost, it may be possible to collect 24-hour samples of fluids such as effluent or chyle and analyze them for micronutrient content.

# Micronutrients as Therapy

In general, during homeostasis, there is a balance in the body between the availability of oxidants and the production of antioxidants. *Oxidative stress* is the disturbance in the balance between the production of pro-oxidants—namely, reactive oxygen species (ROS) and reactive nitrogen species (RNS)—and antioxidants. ROS involve superoxide anion, hydroxyl radical, and hydrogen peroxide. The most common RNS are nitric oxide and peroxynitrite. An *antioxidant* is any substance that prevents the transfer of electrons to and from molecular oxygen and organic molecules, stabilizes organic radicals (such as ROS and RNS), and terminates organic radical reactions. Vitamins, enzyme cofactors, and endogenous compounds all serve as antioxidants.[34]

Conditions that define critical illness in adults, such as sepsis, acute respiratory distress syndrome (ARDS), and ischemia-reperfusion injury, create oxidative stress whereby pro-oxidant production exceeds antioxidant capacity. Pro-oxidants such as ROS and RNS contain unpaired electrons that have an affinity for other atoms and molecules, creating cellular damage, which perpetuates oxidative stress.[34] Furthermore, oxidative stress can (1) impair microcirculatory blood flow, (2) alter coagulation, and (3) promote endothelial cell dysfunction, all of which serve to perpetuate oxidative stress.[35] Critical illness increases antioxidant utilization, loss, and redistribution, and critically ill patients have been found to have low levels of antioxidants, including vitamin D, vitamin C, zinc, and selenium, a finding that has been associated with worse clinical outcomes.[22] Thus, over the past 10 years, the experimental practice of metabolic resuscitation has emerged, whereby supraphysiologic doses of micronutrients have been tested as forms of therapy in critically ill patients with various oxidative stress–inducing disease processes, including sepsis, septic shock, and ARDS. In the most remedial sense, the basis for supplementation with supraphysiologic doses is to increase antioxidant concentration and activity to rebalance the body toward oxidative homeostasis. Numerous micronutrients have been tested alone and in combination as therapies in critically ill patients. This section focuses on zinc, selenium, vitamin C (with and without thiamin), and vitamin D.

# Zinc

Zinc is a divalent cation. More than 250 proteins contain zinc, including enzymes involved in antioxidant pathways, lipid and glucose metabolism, tissue repair, wound healing, and immune responses to infection.[36] These properties make it a suitable candidate for testing in critically ill patients.

Four randomized controlled trials (RCTs) have tested intravenous zinc in critically ill patients.[37,38] The largest trial included 68 patients and found no statistically significant difference in mortality between the zinc-supplemented group and the control group (odds ratio [OR], 0.47; 95% CI, 0.16–1.38).[39] When the data from the four trials were aggregated in a meta-analysis, no difference in mortality was seen with intravenous zinc (OR, 1.54; 95% CI, 0.23–1.44; $P$ = .24).[37] The trials included a small number of patients and mainly included patients with burns and head trauma. There was substantial heterogeneity in the methods of zinc delivery. For instance, zinc dose varied between trials and three of the four studies provided other micronutrients along with zinc, limiting the ability to interpret which micronutrient had an effect (if any). Further high-quality RCTs, to test various doses of zinc monotherapy and combination therapy in subgroups of critically ill patients, are warranted. Even though it is safe (human beings tolerate zinc in doses as high as 100 mg/d), zinc monotherapy or in combination with other micronutrients has not been endorsed by major critical care guidelines for routine use in critically ill patients.

# Selenium

Selenium is present in more than 30 selenoproteins.[40] Four forms of selenoproteins are important in antioxidant defenses.[40,41] Several observational studies have shown that the systemic inflammatory response in critically ill patients is associated with a reduction in plasma selenium concentration and plasma glutathione peroxidase activity and correlates inversely with the severity of illness and clinical outcomes.[42] In an RCT that included 40 critically ill patients with ARDS, patients who received sodium selenite had higher serum selenium levels and lower inflammatory markers, as well as meaningful differences in airway resistance and lung compliance, compared to patients receiving placebo, suggesting that selenium modulates inflammatory responses and improves lung mechanics.[43]

To date, 22 RCTs with different study designs have tested the efficacy of intravenous selenium in critically ill patients. Twelve of them tested intravenous selenium vs placebo, five tested higher vs lower doses (ranging from 500 to 4,000 mcg/d), and five evaluated selenium vs other antioxidants.[44] When data were aggregated in a meta-analysis of 19 trials that included 3,341 critically ill patients (1,694 receiving intravenous selenium and 1,647 control subjects), intravenous selenium was found to have no effect on 28-day mortality (relative risk [RR], 0.96; 95% CI, 0.85–1.09; $P$ = .54) or length of ICU stay.[45] For patients with sepsis and septic shock, the two largest trials (which randomly assigned patients to 1,000 mcg intravenous sodium selenite followed by 1,000 mcg over a 24-hour infusion) found no difference in 28-day mortality.[46,47] Selenium may have benefits in other critically ill patient populations, including those undergoing cardiothoracic surgery, for whom observational data have shown low blood levels of selenium.[22] The Sodium Selenite Administration in Cardiac Surgery (SUSTAIN CSX) trial will be the largest RCT to evaluate the effect of high-dose perioperative selenium in patients undergoing high-risk cardiac surgery.[48]

Critical Care

# Vitamin D

Although vitamin D is most appreciated for its role in calcium regulation, absorption, and metabolism, vitamin D receptors are present in every tissue of the body, suggesting that this micronutrient has a wide range of biochemical properties and plays many roles, including in optimally functioning innate and immune systems. Nuclear vitamin D receptors are found on macrophages, B cells, and T cells, and research has shown that the binding of the nuclear vitamin D receptor increases antimicrobial peptides and anti-inflammatory defensins, as well as augment barrier function through cell membrane stabilization.[49] These properties have led to increased interest in studying the impact of vitamin D deficiency and repletion on critically ill patients. Vitamin D deficiency is prevalent in this population, and deficiency has been associated with worse clinical outcomes, including longer duration of mechanical ventilation, longer ICU stay, and greater severity of lung injury.[50]

In 2017, a meta-analysis of seven RCTs that included more than 700 patients found that vitamin D administration in critically ill patients vs placebo was associated with a statistically significant lower risk for mortality (OR, 0.70; 95% CI, 0.50–0.98; $P$ = .04).[51] Most of the studies were small trials, with the largest one including 475 patients.[52] In 2019, the Vitamin D to Improve Outcomes by Leveraging Early Treatment (VIOLET) study became the largest RCT to compare vitamin D to placebo in critically ill patients.[53] VIOLET researchers randomly assigned critically ill patients with vitamin D levels of less than 20 ng/mL to receive either a single enteral dose of 540,000 IU vitamin D or placebo within 2 hours of assignment to test the primary outcome of 90-day mortality. All patients had a mean vitamin D level of 11 ng/mL (±4.7). By day 3, the vitamin D group raised its mean level to nearly 47 ng/mL, whereas mean level in the placebo group remained at 11 ng/mL. Despite increasing blood vitamin D levels, the single-dose of enteral vitamin D did not lead to a difference in 90-day mortality, number of ventilator-free days, or development of new ARDS, compared to placebo. In 2020, an updated meta-analysis found that vitamin D supplementation was not associated with reduced all-cause mortality, length of ICU stay, hospital stay, or mechanical ventilation.[54] More than 20 ongoing studies are testing vitamin D in critical illness, including the VITDAL-IZE trial, which randomly assigns critically ill patients to either vitamin D plus medium-chain triglyceride (MCT) or MCT alone, with a primary outcome of 28-day mortality; it is the largest trial testing vitamin D in critically ill patients.[55] For now, the results of the well-designed VIOLET study suggest that single, high-dose, enteral vitamin D supplementation should not be routinely provided to patients with critical illness.

# Vitamin C

Vitamin C, or ascorbic acid, is an essential micronutrient, and deficiency is associated with both altered immune and inflammatory responses and worse clinical outcomes. Multiple animal models have demonstrated that vitamin C restores vascular responsiveness to vasoactive agents, ameliorates microcirculatory blood flow, preserves endothelial barriers, prevents apoptosis, and augments bacterial defense systems.[56,57] Due to vitamin C's antioxidant properties and role in multiple biochemical and biologic processes, its use in critically ill patients has gained substantial interest in recent years.

Building on data showing low plasma vitamin C concentrations (<0.41 mg/dL) in human patients with sepsis and acute lung injury, coupled with data showing improved outcomes with intravenous vitamin C administration in animals with these same conditions, a phase 1 trial investigated and confirmed the safety of intravenous vitamin C infusion in critically ill patients.[58] A subsequent study, a retrospective before-and-after study, showed that patients who received HAT therapy—combination hydrocortisone (a glucocorticoid), ascorbic acid (intravenous vitamin C), and thiamin—had improved hospital mortality rates compared to historical subjects who did not receive HAT therapy.[59] Researchers postulated that the addition of hydrocortisone to intravenous vitamin C has a synergistic effect on improving outcomes; thiamin is added to prevent hyperoxalosis from intravenous vitamin C administration, but it may also have synergistic effects. Since the publication of these two studies (in 2014 and 2017, respectively), multiple RCTs have compared intravenous vitamin C, with and without combined thiamin and hydrocortisone, to placebo in critically ill patients.[60]

Critical Care

In 2021, four systematic reviews with meta-analyses were published; they included between eight and 43 RCTs that evaluated intravenous vitamin C use in patients with sepsis or septic shock or patients in the general ICU. There were substantial differences among the RCTs with respect to inclusion criteria (and thus patient populations studied), methodology, and intervention (eg, intravenous vitamin C monotherapy vs HAT therapy). Nonetheless, all the reviews found no positive effect of intravenous vitamin C on 28-day or 1-year mortality.[61] One review that included subgroup analyses based on intravenous vitamin C dose (high vs low) suggested lower mortality in patients who received a higher dose. Another review found a direct signal of benefit with intravenous vitamin C monotherapy.[60] More recently, the Lessening Organ Dysfunction With Vitamin C (LOVIT) trial investigators randomly assigned 872 patients with sepsis (receiving vasopressor therapy) to intravenous vitamin C (50 mg per kilogram of body weight) or placebo across multiple sites and found that patients who received intravenous vitamin C had a higher risk of death at day 28 compared to patients who received placebo (RR, 1.17; 95% CI, 0.98–1.40).[62] Overall, current guidelines for the management of sepsis and septic shock do not endorse intravenous vitamin C as a standard-of-care therapy. The weak but hypothesis-generating signal of benefit for high-dose intravenous monotherapy suggests further RCTs are warranted to test the effect of different doses in specific subgroups of critically ill patients.[61]

# Multimicronutrient Clinical Trials

On the basis of the physiological rationale that combination micronutrients exert pleiotropic and synergistic antioxidant, immune, and metabolic effects, multimicronutrient therapies such as the following have been tested in patients with critical illness.

- **Patients with burns**—A meta-analysis of eight studies comparing selenium, copper, and zinc alone or in combination vs placebo found that therapy with combined parenteral micronutrients was associated with a statistically significant decrease in infectious episodes. However, the meta-analysis was limited by the inclusion of nonrandomized experimental trials and patients ranging in age from 6 to 67 years, which suggests substantial heterogeneity in treatment effect.[63] (Chapter 15 provides more information on burns.)

- **Trauma and cardiac surgical patients**—A double-blind, placebo-controlled, single-center trial of parenteral antioxidants (selenium, zinc, vitamin C, and thiamin) found that the antioxidant intervention, vs placebo, did not reduce early organ dysfunction.[64]
- **Critically ill surgical patients**—A randomized, prospective trial randomly assigned 595 patients to an antioxidant combination of vitamins E and C or placebo and found that early combination antioxidant administration, vs placebo, reduced the risk of multiple organ failure (RR, 0.43; 95% CI, 0.19–0.96).[65]

A systematic review and meta-analysis of 25 studies reporting mortality in critically ill patients found that antioxidant supplementation was associated with a statistically significant reduction in overall mortality (RR, 0.88; 95% CI, 0.78–1.00; $P$ = .04). Among subgroups, the 17 studies that delivered intravenous antioxidants reported no difference in overall mortality. The aggregate of 12 studies that reported infectious complications found that antioxidant supplementation was associated with a trend toward reduction in overall infections (RR, 0.94; 95% CI, 0.88–1.02; $P$ = .14). An aggregate of eight studies reporting duration of mechanical ventilation found that antioxidants, vs placebo, were associated with a statistically significant reduction in duration of ventilation (weighted mean difference, –2.27 days; 95% CI, –4.46 to –0.09; $P$ = .04). There were no differences in ICU or hospital length of stay.[66]

Among the 28 trials testing the efficacy of combination antioxidants in critically ill patients, there was heterogeneity in the patient population (eg, medical, surgical, trauma, burn), intervention (eg, type, combination, and route of antioxidant delivery), and outcomes reported, all of which limit the generalizability of results.

# References

1. Berger MM, Shenkin A, Schweinlin A, et al. ESPEN micronutrient guideline. *Clin Nutr.* 2022;41(6):1357-1424. doi:10.1016/j.clnu.2022.02.015

2. Hay T, Bellomo R, Rechnitzer T, et al. Constipation, diarrhea, and prophylactic laxative bowel regimens in the critically ill: a systematic review and meta-analysis. *J Crit Care.* 2019;52:242-250. doi:10.1016/j.jcrc.2019.01.004

3. World Health Organization. The treatment of diarrhoea: a manual for physicians and other senior health workers. 2006. Accessed February 22, 2024. https://apps.who.int/iris/bitstream/handle/10665/43209/9241593180.pdf

4. Blaser AR, Starkopf J, Kirsimägi Ü, Deane AM. Definition, prevalence, and outcome of feeding intolerance in intensive care: a systematic review and meta-analysis. *Acta Anaesthesiol Scand.* 2014;58(8):914-922. doi:10.1111/aas.12302

5. Sweetser S. Evaluating the patient with diarrhea: a case-based approach. *Mayo Clin Proc.* 2012;87(6):596-602. doi:10.1016/j.mayocp.2012.02.015

6. Hourigan LA, Omaye ST, Keen CL, Jones JA, Dubick MA. Vitamin and trace element loss from negative-pressure wound therapy. *Adv Skin Wound Care.* 2016;29(1):20-25. doi:10.1097/01.ASW.0000473680.06666.6a

7. Brater DC. Diuretic therapy. *N Engl J Med.* 1998;339(6):387-395. doi:10.1056/NEJM199808063390607

8. Drug-induced nutrient depletions. NatMed (Therapeutic Research Center). Accessed February 19, 2022. https://naturalmedicines.therapeuticresearch.com/tools/charts/drug-induced-nutrient-depletions.aspx

9. Singbartl K, Kellum JA. AKI in the ICU: definition, epidemiology, risk stratification, and outcomes. *Kidney Int.* 2012;81(9):819-825. doi:10.1038/ki.2011.339

10. Kamel AY, Dave NJ, Zhao VM, Griffith DP, Connor MJ Jr, Ziegler TR. Micronutrient alterations during continuous renal replacement therapy in critically ill adults: a retrospective study. *Nutr Clin Pract.* 2018;33(3):439-446. doi:10.1177/0884533617716618

11. Ostermann M, Summers J, Lei K, et al. Micronutrients in critically ill patients with severe acute kidney injury—a prospective study. *Sci Rep.* 2020;10(1):1505. doi:10.1038/s41598-020-58115-2

12. Berger MM, Broman M, Forni L, Ostermann M, De Waele E, Wischmeyer PE. Nutrients and micronutrients at risk during renal replacement therapy: a scoping review. *Curr Opin Crit Care.* 2021;27(4):367-377. doi:10.1097/MCC.0000000000000851

13. O'Meara D, Mireles-Cabodevila E, Frame F, et al. Evaluation of delivery of enteral nutrition in critically ill patients receiving mechanical ventilation. *Am J Crit Care*. 2008;17(1):53-61.

14. Kozeniecki M, McAndrew N, Patel JJ. Process-related barriers to optimizing enteral nutrition in a tertiary medical intensive care unit. *Nutr Clin Pract*. 2016;31(1):80-85. doi:10.1177/0884533615611845

15. Alberda C, Gramlich L, Jones N, et al. The relationship between nutritional intake and clinical outcomes in critically ill patients: results of an international multicenter observational study. *Intensive Care Med*. 2009;35(10):1728-1737. doi:10.1007/s00134-009-1567-4

16. Singer P, Blaser AR, Berger MM, et al. ESPEN guideline on clinical nutrition in the intensive care unit. *Clin Nutr*. 2019;38(1):48-79. doi:10.1016/j.clnu.2018.08.037

17. Compher C, Bingham AL, McCall M, et al. Guidelines for the provision of nutrition support therapy in the adult critically ill patient: the American Society for Parenteral and Enteral Nutrition. *JPEN J Parenter Enteral Nutr*. 2022;46(1):12-41. doi:10.1002/jpen.2267

18. Boullata J, ed. *Guidebook on Enteral Medication Administration*. American Society of Parenteral and Enteral Nutrition; 2019.

19. Apeland T, Froyland ES, Kristensen O, Strandjord RE, Mansoor MA. Drug-induced pertubation of the aminothiol redox-status in patients with epilepsy: improvement by B-vitamins. *Epilepsy Res*. 2008;82(1):1-6. doi:10.1016/j.eplepsyres.2008.06.003

20. Flannery AH, Adkins DA, Cook AM. Unpeeling the evidence for the banana bag: evidence-based recommendations for the management of alcohol-associated vitamin and electrolyte deficiencies in the ICU. *Crit Care Med*. 2016;44(8):1545-1552. doi:10.1097/CCM.0000000000001659

21. Blaauw R, Osland E, Sriram K, et al. Parenteral provision of micronutrients to adult patients: an expert consensus paper. *JPEN J Parenter Enteral Nutr*. 2019;43(suppl 1):S5-S23. doi:10.1002/jpen.1525

22. Berger MM, Manzanares W. Micronutrients early in critical illness, selective or generous, enteral or intravenous? *Curr Opin Clin Nutr Metab Care*. 2021;24(2):165-175. doi:10.1097/MCO.0000000000000724

23. Vankrunkelsven W, Gunst J, Amrein K, et al. Monitoring and parenteral administration of micronutrients, phosphate and magnesium in critically ill patients: the VITA-TRACE survey. *Clin Nutr*. 2021;40(2):590-599. doi:10.1016/j.clnu.2020.06.005

24. Esper DH. Utilization of nutrition-focused physical assessment in identifying micronutrient deficiencies. *Nutr Clin Pract*. 2015;30(2):194-202. doi:10.1177/0884533615573054

25. Kumar N. Neurologic presentations of nutritional deficiencies. *Neurol Clin*. 2010;28(1):107-170. doi:10.1016/j.ncl.2009.09.006

26. Stabler SP. Vitamin B12 deficiency. *N Engl J Med*. 2013;368(21):2041-2042. doi:10.1056/NEJMcl304350

27. Sriram K, Manzanares W, Joseph K. Thiamine in nutrition therapy. *Nutr Clin Pract*. 2012;27(1):41-50. doi:10.1177/0884533611426149

28. Halverson JD. Micronutrient deficiencies after gastric bypass for morbid obesity. *Am Surg*. 1986;52(11):594-598.

29. Harper CG, Giles M, Finlay-Jones R. Clinical signs in the Wernicke-Korsakoff complex: a retrospective analysis of 131 cases diagnosed at necropsy. *J Neurol Neurosurg Psychiatry*. 1986;49(4):341-345. doi:10.1136/jnnp.49.4.341

30. Wiley KD, Gupta M. Vitamin B1 (Thiamine) Deficiency. In: StatPearls (online). StatPearls Publishing; 2023. NCBI Bookshelf. Accessed April 2, 2024. www.ncbi.nlm.nih.gov/books/NBK537204/#article-18223.s8

31. Duncan A, Talwar D, McMillan DC, Stefanowicz F, O'Reilly DS. Quantitative data on the magnitude of the systemic inflammatory response and its effect on micronutrient status based on plasma measurements. *Am J Clin Nutr*. 2012;95(1):64-71. doi:10.3945/ajcn.111.023812

32. Robinson CL, Patel JJ. B minus: Wernicke's encephalopathy. *Am J Med*. 2018;131(11):1321-1323. doi:10.1016/j.amjmed.2018.07.037

33. Preiser JC, Arabi YM, Berger MM, et al. A guide to enteral nutrition in intensive care units: 10 expert tips for the daily practice. *Crit Care*. 2021;25(1):424. doi:10.1186/s13054-021-03847-4

34. Koekkoek WA, van Zanten AR. Antioxidant vitamins and trace elements in critical illness. *Nutr Clin Pract*. 2016;31(4):457-474. doi:10.1177/0884533616653832

35. Infusino F, Marazzato M, Mancone M, et al. Diet supplementation, probiotics, and nutraceuticals in SARS-CoV-2 infection: a scoping review. *Nutrients*. 2020;12(6):1718. doi:10.3390/nu12061718

36. Olechnowicz J, Tinkov A, Skalny A, Suliburska J. Zinc status is associated with inflammation, oxidative stress, lipid, and glucose metabolism. *J Physiol Sci*. 2018;68(1):19-31. doi:10.1007/s12576-017-0571-7

37. Heyland DK, Jones N, Cvijanovich NZ, Wong H. Zinc supplementation in critically ill patients: a key pharmaconutrient? *JPEN J Parenter Enteral Nutr*. 2008;32(5):509-519. doi:10.1177/0148607108322402

38. Critical Care Nutrition systematic reviews. Critical Care Nutrition. Accessed March 16, 2022. www.criticalcarenutrition.com/ccn-systematic-review

39. Young B, Ott L, Kasarskis E, et al. Zinc supplementation is associated with improved neurologic recovery rate and visceral protein levels of patients with severe closed head injury. *J Neurotrauma*. 1996;13(1):25-34. doi:10.1089/neu.1996.13.25

40. Holben DH, Smith AM. The diverse role of selenium within selenoproteins: a review. *J Am Diet Assoc.* 1999;99(7):836-843. doi:10.1016/S0002-8223(99)00198-4

41. Labunskyy VM, Hatfield DL, Gladyshev VN. Selenoproteins: molecular pathways and physiological roles. *Physiol Rev.* 2014;94(3):739-777. doi:10.1152/physrev.00039.2013

42. Manzanares W, Langlois PL, Heyland DK. Pharmaconutrition with selenium in critically ill patients: what do we know? *Nutr Clin Pract.* 2015;30(1):34-43. doi:10.1177/0884533614561794

43. Mahmoodpoor A, Hamishehkar H, Shadvar K, et al. The effect of intravenous selenium on oxidative stress in critically ill patients with acute respiratory distress syndrome. *Immunol Invest.* 2019;48(2):147-159. doi:10.1080/08820139.2018.1496098

44. Heyland DK, Lee ZY, Lew CCH, Ortiz LA, Patel J, Stoppe C. Parenteral selenium (alone or in combination). Critical Care Nutrition. February 2022. Accessed November 15, 2022. www.criticalcarenutrition.com/ccn-systematic-review

45. Zhao Y, Yang M, Mao Z, et al. The clinical outcomes of selenium supplementation on critically ill patients: a meta-analysis of randomized controlled trials. *Medicine (Baltimore).* 2019;98(20):e15473. doi:10.1097/MD.0000000000015473

46. Bloos F, Trips E, Nierhaus A, et al. Effect of sodium selenite administration and procalcitonin-guided therapy on mortality in patients with severe sepsis or septic shock: a randomized clinical trial. *JAMA Intern Med.* 2016;176(9):1266-1276. doi:10.1001/jamainternmed.2016.2514

47. Angstwurm MW, Engelmann L, Zimmermann T, et al. Selenium in Intensive Care (SIC): results of a prospective randomized, placebo-controlled, multiple-center study in patients with severe systemic inflammatory response syndrome, sepsis, and septic shock. *Crit Care Med.* 2007;35(1):118-126. doi:10.1097/01.CCM.0000251124.83436.0E

48. SodiUm SeleniTe Adminstration IN Cardiac Surgery (SUSTAIN CSX®-Trial). ClinicalTrials.gov identifier: NCT02002247. Updated June 1, 2021. Accessed November 1, 2023. https://clinicaltrials.gov/study/NCT02002247

49. McKinney TJ, Patel JJ, Benns MV, Nash NA, Miller KR. Vitamin D status and supplementation in the critically ill. *Curr Gastroenterol Rep.* 2016;18(4):18. doi:10.1007/s11894-016-0492-2

50. Patel JJ, McClave SA. Use of vitamin D in critical illness: a concept for whom the bell tolls. *JPEN J Parenter Enteral Nutr.* 2021;45(1):9-11. doi:10.1002/jpen.1946

51. Putzu A, Belletti A, Cassina T, et al. Vitamin D and outcomes in adult critically ill patients. A systematic review and meta-analysis of randomized trials. *J Crit Care.* 2017;38:109-114. doi:10.1016/j.jcrc.2016.10.029

52. Amrein K, Schnedl C, Holl A, et al. Effect of high-dose vitamin D3 on hospital length of stay in critically ill patients with vitamin D deficiency: the VITdAL-ICU randomized clinical trial. *JAMA.* 2014;312(15):1520-1530. doi:10.1001/jama.2014.13204

53. National Heart, Lung, and Blood Institute PETAL Clinical Trials Network; Ginde AA, Brower RG, Caterino JM, et al. Early high-dose vitamin D3 for critically ill, vitamin D-deficient patients. *N Engl J Med.* 2019;381(26):2529-2540. doi:10.1056/NEJMoa1911124

54. Peng L, Li L, Wang P, et al. Association between vitamin D supplementation and mortality in critically ill patients: a systematic review and meta-analysis of randomized clinical trials. *PLoS One.* 2020;15(12):e0243768. doi:10.1371/journal.pone.0243768

55. Amrein K, Parekh D, Westphal S, et al. Effect of high-dose vitamin D3 on 28-day mortality in adult critically ill patients with severe vitamin D deficiency: a study protocol of a multicentre, placebo-controlled double-blind phase III RCT (the VITDALIZE study). *BMJ Open.* 2019;9(11):e031083. doi:10.1136/bmjopen-2019-031083

56. Oudemans-van Straaten HM, Spoelstra-de Man AM, de Waard MC. Vitamin C revisited. *Crit Care.* 2014;18(4):460. doi:10.1186/s13054-014-0460-x

57. Carr AC. Vitamin C administration in the critically ill: a summary of recent meta-analyses. *Crit Care.* 2019;23(1):265. doi:10.1186/s13054-019-2538-y

58. Fowler AA III, Syed AA, Knowlson S, et al. Phase I safety trial of intravenous ascorbic acid in patients with severe sepsis. *J Transl Med.* 2014;12:32. doi:10.1186/1479-5876-12-32

59. Marik PE, Khangoora V, Rivera R, Hooper MH, Catravas J. Hydrocortisone, vitamin C, and thiamine for the treatment of severe sepsis and septic shock: a retrospective before-after study. *Chest.* 2017;151(6):1229-1238. doi:10.1016/j.chest.2016.11.036

60. Patel JJ, Ortiz-Reyes A, Dhaliwal R, et al. IV vitamin C in critically ill patients: a systematic review and meta-analysis. *Crit Care Med.* 2022;50(3):e304-e312. doi:10.1097/CCM.0000000000005320

61. Stoppe C, Lee ZY, Ortiz L, Heyland DK, Patel JJ. The potential role of intravenous vitamin C monotherapy in critical illness. *JPEN J Parenter Enteral Nutr.* 2022;46(5):972-976. doi:10.1002/jpen.2338

62.   Lamontagne F, Masse MH, Menard J, et al. Intravenous vitamin C in adults with sepsis in the intensive care unit. *N Engl J Med.* 2022;386(25):2387-2398. doi:10.1056/NEJMoa2200644

63.   Kurmis R, Greenwood J, Aromataris E. Trace element supplementation following severe burn injury: a systematic review and meta-analysis. *J Burn Care Res.* 2016;37(3):143-159. doi:10.1097/BCR .0000000000000259

64.   Berger MM, Soguel L, Shenkin A, et al. Influence of early antioxidant supplements on clinical evolution and organ function in critically ill cardiac surgery, major trauma, and subarachnoid hemorrhage patients. *Crit Care.* 2008;12(4):R101. doi:10.1186/cc6981

65.   Nathens AB, Neff MJ, Jurkovich GJ, et al. Randomized, prospective trial of antioxidant supplementation in critically ill surgical patients. *Ann Surg.* 2002;236(6):814-822. doi:10.1097/00000658-200212000-00014

66.   Heyland DK, Lee ZY, Lew CCH, Ortiz LA, Patel J, Stoppe C. Antioxidant nutrients: combined vitamins and trace elements. Critical Care Nutrition. March 2021. Accessed November 15, 2022. www .criticalcarenutrition.com/ccn-systematic-review

# CHAPTER 14

# Metabolic and Bariatric Surgery

Osman Mohamed Elfadil, MBBS;
Julie Parrott, MS, RDN; and
Manpreet S. Mundi, MD

## Introduction

The incidence of obesity, defined as a BMI of 30 or higher, continues to increase, with the overall prevalence in the United States now reaching close to 42%.[1] If current trends persist, by 2030 close to one in two adults (50%) in the United States will be obese, and 29 states will exceed 50%.[2] In addition, nearly 25% of American adults will have a BMI of 35, indicating advanced obesity that can negatively affect human health, associated with worse morbidity and outcomes.[2,3] These trends have important implications for health care, as obesity is associated with a number of comorbidities, including type 2 diabetes, hypertension, cardiovascular disease, and many types of cancer, as well as an increase in all-cause mortality.[4] Management of obesity and its associated comorbidities can result in direct and indirect medical costs that amount to hundreds of billions of dollars annually.[5] Fortunately, over the last two decades, the development of state-of-the-art treatment options for obesity have emerged, including robust lifestyle-modification programs, medications with a primary indication for treatment of obesity, and endoscopic procedures and bariatric surgeries. Bariatric surgery remains the most effective approach to long-term weight loss and improvement in obesity-related comorbidities, especially in individuals with class 3 obesity (BMI ≥40) or higher. Although advancements in surgical techniques have dramatically reduced the risks associated with bariatric surgery, including mortality, complications can still arise.[6] This chapter reviews the most common bariatric surgeries performed, as well as anatomical changes that contribute to complications, followed by a discussion of common micronutrient deficiencies and their diagnosis and treatment.

Of note, to maintain consistency in the use of terminology related to micronutrient treatments in bariatrics, in this chapter *supplementation* refers to giving higher-than-normal doses to maintain target nutrient levels, and *repletion* refers to giving higher-than-normal doses to achieve target nutrient levels.

# Risk Factors for Micronutrient Deficiency in Metabolic and Bariatric Surgery

The American Society for Metabolic and Bariatric Surgery (ASMBS) estimates that more than 256,000 surgeries for weight loss were performed in the United States in 2019.[7] The current indications for bariatric surgery include a BMI of 40 or higher without comorbidities or a BMI of 35 with medical comorbidities, including hypertension, type 2 diabetes, nonalcoholic fatty liver disease, obstructive sleep apnea, asthma, and obesity-hypoventilation syndrome. Data are emerging that describe metabolic benefits of bariatric surgery. Consequently, the term *metabolic* was added when referring to bariatric surgery, and the indications were expanded to include a BMI of 30 with difficult to control comorbidities, especially type 2 diabetes.[8] Large randomized controlled trials involving patients with type 2 diabetes have noted that bariatric surgery resulted in lower hemoglobin A1c levels, more sustained weight loss, less medication use, and a higher quality of life compared to medical management.[9]

# Metabolic and Bariatric Surgery Procedures

Metabolic and bariatric surgery (MBS) encompasses three main types of procedures: restrictive, malabsorptive, or a mixture of both. Restrictive procedures, which include laparoscopic gastric banding (refer to Figure 14.1) and sleeve gastrectomy (refer to Figure 14.2), typically reduce energy intake and produce early satiety through a reduction in the gastric reservoir capacity. Sleeve gastrectomy involves a metabolic component and can lead to favorable outcomes in metabolic syndrome, hepatic, renal, and inflammatory biomarkers.[10] These procedures can be associated with less weight loss compared to malabsorptive or mixed surgeries given that no changes are made to the intestines. The number of laparoscopic bands placed in patients in the United States has declined rapidly, and the sleeve gastrectomy is now the most popular procedure performed, accounting for more than 60% of all bariatric surgeries according to ASMBS.[7]

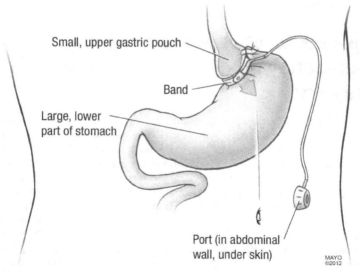

Small, upper gastric pouch

Band

Large, lower part of stomach

Port (in abdominal wall, under skin)

MAYO ©2012

FIGURE 14.1  Laparoscopic gastric banding

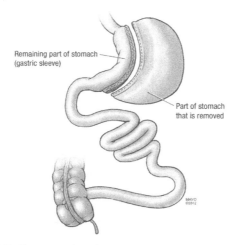

FIGURE 14.2 Sleeve gastrectomy

Purely malabsorptive procedures, such as the jejunoileal bypass, were first performed in the 1950s and remained popular into the early 1970s. They are no longer recommended, given the substantial associated complications, which include severe micronutrient deficiencies; however, clinicians may still encounter patients who have had malabsorptive procedures, as these patients may seek assistance with managing their resultant deficiencies or malnutrition.

Procedures that are mixed restrictive and malabsorptive include the Roux-en-Y gastric bypass (RYGB) (refer to Figure 14.3 on page 290) and the biliopancreatic diversion with duodenal switch (BPD-DS) (refer to Figure 14.4 on page 291). The RYGB starts with the creation of a small gastric pouch (typically with a volume of less than 30 mL) to which the jejunum is brought up and attached. At approximately 75 to 150 cm distal to the gastrojejunal anastomosis, the intestines are then joined through a jejunojejunal anastomosis. In some cases, the Roux limb, or the limb

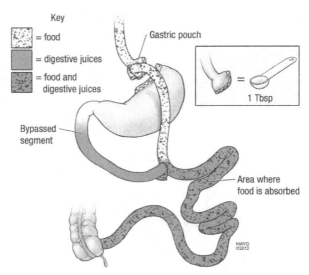

FIGURE 14.3  Roux-en-Y gastric bypass

from the gastrojejunal anastomosis and the jejunojejunal anastomosis, can be 200 cm or longer, creating a higher degree of malabsorption. The BPD-DS procedure starts with a sleeve gastrectomy along with a short common channel that is typically 100 to 150 cm in length. The length of the common channel determines the degree of malabsorption, with shorter common channels leading to more malabsorption and micronutrient deficiencies.

# Risk Factors for Micronutrient Deficiencies

When evaluating patients for micronutrient deficiencies following MBS, clinicians should keep in mind the anatomical changes made with each surgery, as well as the location of absorption for specific micronutrients (refer to Figure 9.1 on page 167). They should also recognize that

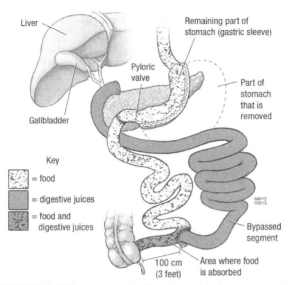

FIGURE 14.4  Biliopancreatic diversion with duodenal switch

obesity itself can be associated with micronutrient deficiencies, through expanded adipose tissue, greater volume of distribution, and low-grade inflammation that may cause increased oxidative stress, altered nutrient transporters, and increased utilization of antioxidant nutrients.[11] Other factors that can contribute to micronutrient deficiencies with bariatric surgery include the restrictive nature of both preoperative and postoperative diets.

Poor diet quality, including the consumption of too many ultraprocessed foods and beverages with refined sugars, predisposes individuals of all age groups to the development of obesity and micronutrient deficiencies.[12] Preoperatively, patients are often asked to lose weight, which may lead to further deficiencies. Those deficiencies are then carried over to the postoperative period[11] and can be compounded by the postoperative diet, which typically starts with clear liquids and progresses to blended foods, a soft diet, and regular-consistency meals by 3 months.[8] Energy intake also remains limited for quite some time after surgery; patients typically consume approximately 500 kcal/d initially and gradually increase to approximately 1,000 to 1,200 kcal/d by 6 months.[13,14]

Factors predisposing individuals to micronutrient deficiencies following MBS include:

- the amount of the stomach removed or bypassed
- the length of the common channel and the biliopancreatic limb
- the amount and availability of bile productions to mix with nutrients
- the preoperative diet and chronic obesity-induced inflammation
- the postoperative diet

Patients who undergo MBS are at risk of developing specific nutrient deficiencies unless appropriate supplementation is followed.[15,16] Oral, intramuscular, intravenous, or nasal routes can be used for micronutrient supplementation.[17]

# Assessment of Perioperative Micronutrient Deficiency

Research continues to report that MBS candidates often have at least one micronutrient deficiency at the time of surgery and that the deficiency increases in severity after surgery unless it is corrected.[11,16,18,19] Vitamin D deficiency is the most common deficiency after MBS, but the nutrient that presents the greatest risk of causing irreversible and permanent damage to the patient when deficient is thiamin (50% of patients have suboptimal levels after surgery).[19] Thiamin deficiency can develop quickly after MBS, and without proper treatment a patient's status can deteriorate quickly. If thiamin deficiency is suspected, experts recommend treatment before confirmation with laboratory results, and treatment should only be discontinued when symptoms resolve.[16,20] If symptoms are not identified and treated during the early phases of thiamin deficiency, Wernicke encephalopathy or Wernicke-Korsakoff syndrome may ensue.

Recognizing the symptoms of nutrient deficiencies and assessing the patient's dietary intake, along with obtaining available laboratory values, are essential steps to determining a patient's nutrient status. Patients with a deficiency that is not corrected before surgery are more likely to continue with that same deficiency and are at risk of developing others.[15,16] Micronutrient deficiencies may develop as a result of nutrient-nutrient or nutrient-drug interactions, reduced intake, or lack of appropriate vitamin and mineral supplementation.[15,21-23]

Some of the nutrient-nutrient interactions are known and are incorporated into patient education materials, such as the recommendation to avoid taking calcium and iron at the same time and to take them no less than 2 hours apart.[8,19,24] However, the impact of other nutrients affected by changes in gastric pH, oral contraceptives, and other medications may not be well known to clinicians and is not part of patient education materials. In fact, researchers have reported interactions with at least nine different categories of medications with all of the at-risk micronutrients in patients following MBS.[22] Thus, some nutrient-nutrient interactions may increase the likelihood of micronutrient deficiencies over time, even with recommended repletion and supplementation.[15,21-23]

Because micronutrient deficiencies do not improve after MBS without additional, higher doses of supplementation, clinicians are advised to:

- screen patients for micronutrient deficiencies preoperatively on the basis of both prevalence and risk;
- correct any micronutrient deficiencies before the patient undergoes MBS; and
- monitor patients to prevent and treat deficiencies postoperatively.

# Micronutrients of Concern

Malnutrition, macronutrient deficiencies, and micronutrient deficiencies are prevalent after MBS.[25-27] The mechanism leading to micronutrient deficiency is not fully understood.[25,27] In fact, a deficiency in fat-soluble vitamins measured solely by the absolute value of a laboratory assay or test may not reflect a "true deficiency" but rather an altered metabolism during inflammation or infection.[28] Thus, it is important to measure C-reactive protein, a marker of inflammation, when assessing serum levels of micronutrients. For example, retinol-binding protein is the carrier protein of vitamin A and a negative acute-phase protein, meaning that levels of retinol-binding protein and vitamin A will decrease during inflammation or infection and potentially after protein malabsorption, as has been reported in patients with RYGB and BPD-DS. If carrier proteins for micronutrients are altered due to malnutrition, inflammation, or infection, micronutrient supplementation could result in toxicity.[29] This is an emerging area of research and important to keep in mind when interpreting micronutrient deficiencies after MBS with malabsorption. (Refer to Chapters 4–8 for more information.)

Experts know that micronutrient deficiencies are present in MBS candidates both preoperatively and postoperatively.[19] For this reason, clinical practice guidelines recommend screening before surgery for most of the nutrients covered in this section and at frequent time intervals after surgery.[8,19] For more specific information on dietary sources, absorption, and metabolism of these nutrients, see the Appendix and Chapters 5 through 8.

# Fat-Soluble Vitamins

Deficiencies in the fat-soluble vitamins (vitamins A, D, E, and K) are common after bariatric surgery. However, due to a lack of epidemiological studies, estimated prevalence is based only on some smaller clinical observations and reviews.[26] Preoperative deficiency adds to the risk of developing postoperative deficiency.[30] Preoperative vitamin D deficiency is present in up to 95% of patients undergoing MBS.[8,19] Experts estimate that preoperative deficiencies of vitamins A and E are present in approximately 10% and less than 2% of patients undergoing MBS, respectively.[29]

## Vitamin A

Vitamin A deficiency is uncommon after RYGB, with deficiency occurring in 10% of patients 4 years after surgery.[11] However, deficiency is diagnosed in close to 70% of patients after a BPD-DS procedure in 4 years.[31] After MBS, repletion is required upon confirmation of clinical and laboratory diagnoses. In patients who have undergone BPD-DS, screening every 6 to 12 months is recommended.[32]

## Vitamin D

Although vitamin D deficiency can be associated with any MBS procedure, as many as 60% of patients who undergo malabsorptive procedures, such as BPD-DS, can become vitamin D deficient, owing to the shorter common channel and digestion disturbance. Dosing of vitamin D replacement therapy should be based on the patient's clinical presentation and serum 25-hydroxyvitamin D level.[33,34] Screening for metabolic bone diseases by bone density scan is recommend starting 2 years after surgery.[32]

## Vitamin E

Patients who undergo malabsorptive MBS procedures are at higher-than-normal risk of developing vitamin E deficiency. Theoretically, vitamin E deficiency can manifest as neurological deficits.[35] However, clinical deficiency is rarely documented in patients following MBS.[36] Thus, experts recommend screening in patients with symptoms.[19]

## Vitamin K

If vitamin K deficiency occurs, it almost always occurs postoperatively, with preoperative deficiency rarely documented.[37] Vitamin K deficiency is reportedly more common after BPD-DS than after nonmalabsorptive MBS procedures. This is because maldigestion and a short common channel cause reduced mixing of nutrients with biliopancreatic secretions.[11,37] Fat malabsorption may then occur, and, consequently, more than half of patients develop vitamin K deficiency within 3 to 4 years of malabsorptive procedures.[8] Although the exact prevalence of vitamin K deficiency in patients who have had nonmalabsorptive procedures is unknown, if a deficiency is clinically suspected after MBS, oral vitamin K replacement at a dose of 1 mg/d is recommended, with a target international normalized ratio of greater than 1.4.[37]

Metabolic &
Bariatric Surgery

# Water-Soluble Vitamins

## Thiamin

Thiamin is absorbed primarily through the duodenum and proximal jejunum. MBS procedures, especially BPD-DS and RYGB, bypass certain portions of the small intestine, causing malabsorption of thiamin.[38] Both excessive band tightness after gastric banding and stomal stenosis after RYGB, each of which can lead to intractable vomiting, can contribute to thiamin deficiency as soon as 2 weeks after surgery. Clinical manifestations of thiamin deficiency after MBS are typically documented at approximately 3 months postsurgery in patients with poor oral intake or vomiting, and in patients who abuse alcohol after surgery.[11] Although no large epidemiological studies have been conducted, experts estimate that thiamin deficiency develops in close to half of patients after MBS.[20] Thiamin deficiency was documented in one in five patients following RYGB in a prospectively studied post-RYGB cohort.[39] Treatment of a suspected thiamin deficiency should not be delayed.[8,19,40] Preoperative screening is recommended by some experts but is not universally accepted. Screening is recommended at 1, 3, and 6 months postoperatively for those who have had malabsorptive or restrictive MBS.[32]

## Folate

Since folate is absorbed over a large area, folate deficiency is relatively rare, including after bariatric surgery. Postoperative screening is recommended, particularly for females of childbearing age.[19]

## Vitamin B12

Vitamin B12 absorption typically occurs in the terminal ileum and is affected by several factors, including adequate intake, gastric acidity, gastric intrinsic factor, and pancreatic enzymes. MBS procedures may affect the anatomy or function of the stomach or terminal ileum and can affect vitamin B12 and intrinsic-factor receptors, leading to malabsorption.[41,42] Bariatric procedures reduce gastric acidity, the production of intrinsic factor, and the release of vitamin B12 from R-binders.[42] Vitamin B12 deficiency is common after MBS, occurring in approximately

20% of patients after BPD-DS and sleeve gastrectomy procedures, and in as many as 60% of patients after RYGB.[37,43] Routine postoperative screening is recommended every 3 months in the first year and annually thereafter.[19]

## Vitamin C

Vitamin C screening is not routinely performed in the bariatric setting, even though a substantial number (up to 43%) of cases of vitamin C deficiency have been reported in patients undergoing MBS.[11] With patients on severely restricted diets (such as in the early period following MBS), it is important to monitor for adherence to supplementation and the possible development of deficiency symptoms. Patients with concomitant iron deficiency after MBS should receive vitamin C supplementation, as it facilitates dietary iron absorption in the small intestine.[44]

# Trace Minerals

## Iron

Iron deficiency is the most commonly diagnosed micronutrient deficiency that can lead to anemia following MBS if left untreated.[11] The pathophysiological mechanisms involved in the development of iron deficiency after MBS include inadequate reduction of the ferric form of iron to the ferrous form due to reduced gastric acidity, anatomical changes leading to reduced surface area available for absorption (specifically in the RYGB procedure), and chronic gastrointestinal villi changes leading to reduced absorption. The prevalence of postoperative iron deficiency is reported to be between 18% and 50% for up to 11 years after surgery.[45]

Clinicians should assess the iron status of all patients both before and after surgery, using physiological signs and symptoms as well as laboratory results. Screening for iron deficiency before any MBS procedure is recommended. Within the first 3 months of any MBS procedure, clinicians should monitor for signs and symptoms of deficiency and obtain laboratory values, and then repeat this follow-up every 3 to 6 months until 1 year postprocedure, and then annually thereafter.[8,19]

*Metabolic &
Bariatric Surgery*

## Zinc

Zinc is typically absorbed in the duodenum and proximal jejunum; therefore, RYGB procedures are more likely to result in zinc deficiency than are other MBS procedures.[46] However, zinc deficiency after BPD-DS has been reported in as many as 50% of patients up to 4 years postoperatively.[31,47] Notably, zinc deficiency can often cause unexplained anemia and should be considered as a potential cause of microcytic anemia after RYGB if other causes of anemia are excluded.[46]

Although high doses of zinc may be required for severe deficiency, practitioners must recognize that these doses may unmask or worsen copper deficiency, as they may cause zinc to saturate a common binder, metallothionein, that is also needed for copper metabolism. Monitoring for symptoms of zinc deficiency is recommended, as blood zinc level may not correlate with the clinical picture.[37]

## Copper

Although copper deficiency is rare, researchers detected it in roughly 10% of patients in one study 2 years after RYGB.[48] The prevalence of copper deficiency after BPD-DS is substantially higher, developing in as many as seven in 10 patients after surgery.[49] Screening for copper deficiency after BPD-DS and RYGB is recommended frequently in the first 3 to 6 months, then annually or biannually after that.

# Prevention and Treatment Strategies

## Screening

Table 14.1 is a compilation of recommendations from micronutrient-focused clinical practice guidelines for preoperative and postoperative screening of patients for micronutrient deficiencies after MBS.[8,19]

**TABLE 14.1  Micronutrient Screening After Metabolic and Bariatric Surgery: Consensus Recommendations Based on Clinical Practice Guidelines[8,19]**

| Nutrient | Type of surgery | Preoperative screen | Postoperative screen |
|---|---|---|---|
| Thiamin | Malabsorptive[a] Sleeve gastrectomy | Yes[b] | Yes |
| Vitamin B12 and folate | Malabsorptive Sleeve gastrectomy | Yes | Yes |
| Iron | Malabsorptive Sleeve gastrectomy | Yes | Yes |
| Vitamin D and calcium | Malabsorptive Sleeve gastrectomy | Yes | Yes |
| Vitamin A | Malabsorptive | Yes[b] | Yes[bc] |
| Vitamins E and K | Malabsorptive | Yes[b] | Yes[bc] |
| Zinc and copper | Malabsorptive | Yes[b] | Yes[c] |

[a] Malabsorptive surgeries include Roux-en-Y gastric bypass, one-anastomosis gastric bypass, duodenal switch, and single-anastomosis duodenoileal with sleeve gastrectomy.
[b] When the patient has signs and symptoms of, or risk factors for, the deficiency.
[c] At least annually.

# Supplementation and Repletion

Table 14.2 on page 300 lists the micronutrient supplementation and repletion recommendations for patients who have undergone MBS, along with the symptoms of each deficiency and laboratory assays used to assess each deficiency.[8,19,24] The recommendations are based on current clinical practice guidelines, and the dosage amounts and blood levels are typically different from those advised for patients who have not had MBS. Repletion of micronutrient deficiencies requires higher doses and more frequent monitoring of laboratory results and clinical signs and symptoms.

Metabolic & Bariatric Surgery

**TABLE 14.2 Micronutrient Treatment After Metabolic and Bariatric Surgery: Consensus Recommendations Based on Clinical Practice Guidelines[8,19,24]**

| Nutrient | Common symptoms | Supplementation | Commonly used assays | Repletion |
|---|---|---|---|---|
| Thiamin | Muscle weakness, gait ataxia, edema in lower extremities, lactic acidosis | At least 12 mg/d<br>50-100 mg/d for at-risk[a] patients | Whole blood thiamin pyrophosphate: 2.5-7.5 mcg/dL (HPLC) or 74-222 nmol/L<br>Treat immediately if the patient has a prolonged episode of dysphagia, vomiting, poor dietary intake, or rapid weight loss. Do not wait for confirmation of deficiency by laboratory tests. | Oral: 100 mg two to three times daily until symptoms resolve<br>IV: 200 mg three times daily to 500 mg one to two times daily for 3-5 d, followed by 250 mg/d for 3-5 d or until symptoms resolve; then 100 mg/d orally, usually indefinitely or until risk factors have been resolved<br>IM: 250 mg/d for 3-5 d, or 100-250 mg/mo<br>Magnesium, potassium, and phosphorus should be repleted simultaneously in patients at risk for refeeding syndrome. |
| Vitamin B12 | Pallor, glossitis, peripheral neuropathy, conjunctival pallor | 350-500 mcg/d | Serum B12: <200 pg/mL, deficiency; <400 pg/mL, suboptimal<br>Serum methylmalonic acid: >0.376 mcmol/L, deficiency | Oral: 1,000 mcg/d<br>IM: 1,000 mcg/d until levels return to normal, then 1,000 mcg/mo |
| Folate | Pallor, glossitis, peripheral neuropathy, conjunctival pallor | 400-800 mcg/d<br>800-1,000 mcg/d in females of childbearing age | RBC folate: <305 nmol/L, deficiency; <227 nmol/L, anemia | Oral: 1,000 mcg/d<br>Check for vitamin B12 deficiency first. |

| | Signs/Symptoms | Dose | Lab Values | Management |
|---|---|---|---|---|
| Iron | Pallor, rough/dry skin patches, angular cheilitis, glossitis, decreased papillation, hair loss, koilonychia, dysgeusia, loss of appetite, dysphagia, pica, weakness, fatigue, poor body temperature regulation, dyspnea on exertion, difficulty with concentration | At least 18 mg/d for patients at low risk[a] 45-60 mg/d for patients at high risk[a] | One or more of the following (deficiency): Ferritin: <20 ng/mL TIBC: >450 mcg/dL Transferrin saturation: <20% | Oral: 150-300 mg elemental iron two to three times daily Should be taken separately from calcium supplements, acid-reducing medications, and foods rich in phytates or polyphenols. IV: Consult with a hematologist. |
| Calcium | Leg cramping, muscle weakness, hyperexcitability | 1,200-1,500 mg/d 1,800-2,400 mg/d for BPD-DS | Serum calcium: <9-10.5 mg/dL in patients without kidney disease, deficiency | Make sure vitamin D levels are sufficient. Check PTH level. Oral: Continue with 1,200-1,500 mg/d BPD-DS: 1,800-2,400 mg/d |
| Vitamin D | Bone pain, muscle weakness, steatorrhea | At least 75 mcg (3,000 IU/d) to maintain 25-hydroxyvitamin D level of 30 ng/mL | Serum vitamin D: 20-30 ng/mL (50-75 nmol/L), insufficiency <20 ng/mL (<50 nmol/L), deficiency | Oral: Vitamin D3, up to 150 mcg (6,000 IU/d); or vitamin D2, up to 1,250 mcg (50,000 IU) once or twice weekly |

Continued on next page

Metabolic &
Bariatric Surgery

TABLE 14.2 Micronutrient Treatment After Metabolic and Bariatric Surgery: Consensus Recommendations Based on Clinical Practice Guidelines[8,19,24] (cont.)

| Nutrient | Common symptoms | Supple-mentation | Commonly used assays | Repletion |
|---|---|---|---|---|
| Vitamin A | Hyperkerati-nization of the skin, Bitot spots, decreased visual acuity, xerophthal-mia, compromised immune function, hair casts, sym-metrical follicular papules with kera-tin plugs present on extensor surfaces | 5,000-10,000 IU/d (1,500-3,000 mcg/d) for vertical sleeve gastrectomy and RYGB >10,000 IU/d (>3,000 mcg/d) for BPD-DS | Plasma retinol: <10 mg/dL, deficiency | Oral: Without corneal changes: 10,000-25,000 IU/d (3,000-7,500 mcg/d) With corneal changes: 50,000-100,000 IU/d (15,000-30,000 mcg/d) |
| Vitamin E | Steatorrhea, neuromuscu-lar dysfunction, decreased visual acuity | 15 mg/d | Serum vitamin E (α-tocoph-erol concentration): <5 mg/mL, deficiency | Oral: varies, 100-400 IU/d |
| Vitamin K | Bleeding, hem-orrhage, bone demineralization, osteoporosis | 90-120 mcg/d | Serum phylloquinone: decreased with deficiency PT is not a sensitive measure of vitamin K status. Use PIV-KA-II if available | Oral: 1-2 mg/d IV: 10 mg/d |

| | | | |
|---|---|---|---|
| Zinc | Alopecia, acrodermatitis enteropathica, impaired wound healing, hypogeusia, dysgeusia, hyposmia, anorexia, diarrhea | 8-11 mg/d 16-22 mg/d for BPD-DS | Serum or plasma zinc: Females: <70 mcg/dL Males: <74 mcg/dL deficiency | Oral: 60 mg/d; should include added copper of 4-8 mg/d[a] |
| Copper | Depigmentation of hair, skin, nails; altered gait; peripheral neuropathy; vision loss | 1-2 mg/d 2 mg/d for BPD-DS | Serum or plasma copper: <12 mcmol/L or <75 mcg/dL deficiency | **Oral (for mild to moderate deficiency):** Copper gluconate or sulfate, 3-8 mg/d, until indices return to normal **IV (for severe deficiency):** Copper, 2-4 mg/d, for 6 d or until serum levels return to normal and neurologic symptoms resolve |

Abbreviations: BPD-DS, biliopancreatic diversion with duodenal switch; HPLC, high-performance liquid chromatography; IM, intramuscular; IV, intravenous; PIVKA-II, protein induced in vitamin K absence; PT, prothrombin time; PTH, parathyroid hormone; RBC, red blood cell; RYGB, Roux-en-Y gastric bypass; TIBC, total iron-binding capacity.

[a] For more information, see the supplementary materials in Parrott J, Frank L, Rabena R, Craggs-Dino L, Isom KA, Greiman L. American Society for Metabolic and Bariatric Surgery integrated health nutritional guidelines for the surgical weight loss patient 2016 update: micronutrients. *Surg Obes Relat Dis.* 2017;13(5):727-741. doi:10.1016/j.soard.2016.12.018.19

## Bariatric Multivitamin/Mineral Supplements

Patients who have had MBS and have no additional complications or risk factors for developing micronutrient deficiencies should take a bariatric-formulated multivitamin/mineral (MVM) supplement containing all of the micronutrients on the list that follows, ideally in one pill or chewable tablet, along with a separate calcium supplement, to achieve most clinical practice guideline recommendations.[50] Altogether, supplements taken by patients after MBS should provide the following nutrients:

- Thiamin: at least 12 mg/d
- Vitamin B12: 350 to 500 mcg/d
- Folate: 400 to 800 mcg/d
  - In females of childbearing age, 800 to 1,000 mcg/d
- Iron:
  - At least 18 mg/d for patients with low risk (nonmalabsorptive surgery and no history of iron deficiency)
  - At least 45 mg/d for other patients
- Vitamin D: 75 mcg/d (3,000 IU/d)
- Calcium: 1,200-1,500 mg/d
  - For BPD-DS, 1,800 to 2,400 mg/d
- Vitamin A: 5,000 to 10,000 IU/d (1,500 to 3,000 mcg/d)
- Vitamin E: 15 mg/d
- Vitamin K: 90 to 120 mcg/d
  - 300 mcg/d or higher for patients with duodenal switch and prior deficiencies
- Zinc: at least 8 to 11 mg/d (varies based on surgery); more for malabsorptive surgeries
- Copper: 1 mg for every 8 to 15 mg zinc/d

Patients who take supplements are not, however, immune to micronutrient deficiencies. There are a multitude of MVM supplements on the market that do not provide the specific nutrients needed following MBS. Some of these supplements are marketed to patients as providing a convenient quantity (only one or two pills per day instead of five or more) and method (chewable or capsule). Unfortunately, bariatric-formulated MVM supplements are not available from hospital pharmacies, nor by prescription in the United States and many other countries.[51] Thus, the patient has the following choices: (1) purchase an over-the-counter MVM designed for generally healthy people and make up the difference between what it provides and the recommended post-MBS amounts by taking the necessary vitamins and minerals separately; (2) choose an over-the-counter MVM with "bariatric" in the name of the product that meets the ASMBS recommendations (outlined above); or (3) choose a specialty (ie, purchased online) bariatric-formulated MVM. To further complicate matters, some bariatric supplement companies market specialty bariatric MVMs as "complete" without providing all the micronutrients recommended by clinical practice guidelines; this unknowingly leaves patients at an even greater risk for developing micronutrient deficiencies after MBS.[50,52]

## Adherence to Regimens and Guideline Recommendations

Research investigating the incorporation of clinical practice guideline recommendations into MBS programs and education has not shown very promising results. For instance, fewer than 25% of studies included in a 2021 systematic review and meta-analysis incorporated guideline recommendations for thiamin, vitamins B12, and vitamin D. This review looked only at sleeve gastrectomy and RYGB, finding that patients who had undergone RYGB demonstrated greater adherence to guideline supplementation recommendations than did patients with sleeve gastrectomy.[52]

In addition, patient adherence to micronutrient supplementation is reportedly poor. Reasons provided include forgetting to take the supplements, too many pills to take, adverse side effects, cost, not available by prescription, and not realizing it was important to take them.[53] The best supplementation strategy is to provide a regimen that is sustainable for the patient. The regimen may be based on the recommended micronutrient frequency, dose, strength, cost, accessibility, and patient tolerance. Supplementation regimens exist that meet all the clinical practice guideline recommendations and consist of a bariatric-formulated

MVM with an additional calcium supplement taken at a separate time.[50] Registered dietitian nutritionists should evaluate the MVM supplements being taken by the patient to ensure that all nutrient recommendations are being met. When assessing a patient's nutritional status and supplementation regimen, it is critical to ask patients about supplement dose, frequency, and form, and whether the MVM is being taken with foods, beverages, or other medications, and if so, which ones.[16,24]

Data indicate that research is needed to establish a better monitoring schedule for detecting micronutrient deficiencies after MBS.[52] Thus, screening at more frequent intervals (every 3 months), particularly in patients with a history of deficiencies, is recommended.[16,19,24]

# References

1. Stierman B, Afful J, Carroll MD, et al. *National Health and Nutrition Examination Survey 2017–March 2020 Pre-pandemic Data Files*. National Health Statistics Reports, no. 158. National Center for Health Statistics; 2021. doi:10.15620/cdc:106273

2. Ward ZJ, Bleich SN, Cradock AL, et al. Projected U.S. state-level prevalence of adult obesity and severe obesity. *N Engl J Med*. 2019;381(25):2440-2450. doi:10.1056/NEJMsa1909301

3. Djalalinia S, Qorbani M, Peykari N, Kelishadi R. Health impacts of obesity. *Pak J Med Sci*. 2015;31(1):239-242. doi:10.12669/pjms.311.7033

4. Hurt RT, Mundi MS, Ebbert JO. Challenging obesity, diabetes, and addiction: the potential of lorcaserin extended release. *Diabetes Metab Syndr Obes Targets Ther*. 2018;11:469-478. doi:10.2147/DMSO.S126855

5. Kim DD, Basu A. Estimating the medical care costs of obesity in the United States: systematic review, meta-analysis, and empirical analysis. *Value Health*. 2016;19(5):602-613. doi:10.1016/j.jval.2016.02.008

6. Arterburn DE, Telem DA, Kushner RF, Courcoulas AP. Benefits and risks of bariatric surgery in adults: a review. *JAMA*. 2020;324(9):879-887. doi:10.1001/jama.2020.12567

7. Estimate of bariatric surgery numbers, 2011-2019. American Society for Metabolic and Bariatric Surgery. Accessed June 6, 2022. https://asmbs.org/resources/estimate-of-bariatric-surgery-numbers

8.  Mechanick JI, Apovian C, Brethauer S, et al. Clinical practice guidelines for the perioperative nutrition, metabolic, and nonsurgical support of patients undergoing bariatric procedures—2019 update: cosponsored by American Association of Clinical Endocrinologists/American College of Endocrinology, The Obesity Society, American Society for Metabolic and Bariatric Surgery, Obesity Medicine Association, and American Society of Anesthesiologists. *Obes Silver Spring Md*. 2020;28(4):O1-O58. doi:10.1002/oby.22719

9.  Schauer PR, Bhatt DL, Kirwan JP, et al. Bariatric surgery versus intensive medical therapy for diabetes—5-year outcomes. *N Engl J Med*. 2017;376(7):641-651. doi:10.1056/NEJMoa1600869

10. Wojciak PA, Pawłuszewicz P, Diemieszczyk I, et al. Laparoscopic sleeve gastrectomy: a study of efficiency in treatment of metabolic syndrome components, comorbidities and influence on certain biochemical markers. *Videosurgery Miniinvasive Tech*. 2020;15(1):136-147. doi:10.5114/wiitm.2019.84718

11. Patel JJ, Mundi MS, Hurt RT, Wolfe B, Martindale RG. Micronutrient deficiencies after bariatric surgery: an emphasis on vitamins and trace minerals. *Nutr Clin Pract Off Publ Am Soc Parenter Enter Nutr*. 2017;32(4):471-480. doi:10.1177/0884533617712226

12. Mohamed Elfadil O, Patel J, Patel I, Ewy MW, Hurt RT, Mundi MS. Processed foods—getting back to the basics. *Curr Gastroenterol Rep*. 2021;23(12):20. doi:10.1007/s11894-021-00828-z

13. Saltzman E, Karl JP. Nutrient deficiencies after gastric bypass surgery. *Annu Rev Nutr*. 2013;33(1):183-203. doi:10.1146/annurev-nutr-071812-161225

14. Academy of Nutrition and Dietetics. What is the effect of bariatric surgery on energy intake in adults? Evidence Analysis Library. Accessed November 4, 2022. www.andeal.org/topic.cfm?menu=5308&cat=5613

15. Schiavo L, Pilone V, Rossetti G, Iannelli A. The role of the nutritionist in a multidisciplinary bariatric surgery team. *Obes Surg*. 2019;29(3): 1028-1030. doi:10.1007/s11695-019-03706-w

16. Parrott JM, Craggs-Dino L, Faria SL, O'Kane M. The optimal nutritional programme for bariatric and metabolic surgery. *Curr Obes Rep*. 2020;9(3):326-338. doi:10.1007/s13679-020-00384-z

17. Velapati SR, Schroeder SE, Schroeder DR, et al. Use of home enteral nutrition in malnourished post-bariatric surgery patients. *JPEN J Parenter Enteral Nutr*. 2021;45(5):1023-1031. doi:10.1002/jpen.1973

18. Schiavo L, Scalera G, Pilone V, De Sena G, Capuozzo V, Barbarisi A. Micronutrient deficiencies in patients candidate for bariatric surgery: a prospective, preoperative trial of screening, diagnosis, and treatment. *Int J Vitam Nutr Res*. 2015;85(5-6):340-347. doi:10.1024/0300-9831/a000282

19.  Parrott J, Frank L, Rabena R, Craggs-Dino L, Isom KA, Greiman L. American Society for Metabolic and Bariatric Surgery integrated health nutritional guidelines for the surgical weight loss patient 2016 update: micronutrients. *Surg Obes Relat Dis.* 2017;13(5):727-741. doi:10.1016/j.soard.2016.12.018

20.  Frank LL. Thiamin in clinical practice. *J Parenter Enter Nutr.* 2015;39(5):503-520. doi:10.1177/0148607114565245

21.  Palmery M, Saraceno A, Vaiarelli A, Carlomagno G. Oral contraceptives and changes in nutritional requirements. *Eur Rev Med Pharmacol Sci.* 2013;17(13):1804-1813.

22.  Mohn ES, Kern HJ, Saltzman E, Mitmesser SH, McKay DL. Evidence of drug-nutrient interactions with chronic use of commonly prescribed medications: an update. *Pharmaceutics.* 2018;10(1):e36. doi:10.3390/pharmaceutics10010036

23.  Prescott JD, Drake VJ, Stevens JF. Medications and micronutrients: identifying clinically relevant interactions and addressing nutritional needs. *J Pharm Technol.* 2018;34(5):216-230. doi:10.1177/8755122518780742

24.  O'Kane M, Parretti HM, Pinkney J, et al. British Obesity and Metabolic Surgery Society guidelines on perioperative and postoperative biochemical monitoring and micronutrient replacement for patients undergoing bariatric surgery—2020 update. *Obes Rev.* 2020;21(11):e13087. doi:10.1111/obr.13087

25.  Bal BS, Finelli FC, Shope TR, Koch TR. Nutritional deficiencies after bariatric surgery. *Nat Rev Endocrinol.* 2012;8(9):544-556. doi:10.1038/nrendo.2012.48

26.  Lupoli R, Lembo E, Saldalamacchia G, Avola CK, Angrisani L, Capaldo B. Bariatric surgery and long-term nutritional issues. *World J Diabetes.* 2017;8(11):464-474. doi:10.4239/wjd.v8.i11.464

27.  Krzizek EC, Brix JM, Stöckl A, Parzer V, Ludvik B. Prevalence of micronutrient deficiency after bariatric surgery. *Obes Facts.* 2021;14(2):197-204. doi:10.1159/000514847

28.  Blaauw R, Osland E, Sriram K, et al. Parenteral provision of micronutrients to adult patients: an expert consensus paper. *JPEN J Parenter Enteral Nutr.* 2019;43 suppl 1:S5-S23. doi:10.1002/jpen.1525

29.  Cuesta M, Pelaz L, Pérez C, et al. Fat-soluble vitamin deficiencies after bariatric surgery could be misleading if they are not appropriately adjusted. *Nutr Hosp.* 2014;30(1):118-123. doi:10.3305/nh.2014.30.1.7471

30.  Gomes de Lima KV, de Carvalho Costa MJ, da Conceição Rodrigues Gonçalves M, Sousa BS. Micronutrient deficiencies in the pre-bariatric surgery. *Arq Bras Cir Dig.* 2013;26(suppl 1):63-66. doi:10.1590/s0102-67202013000600014

31. Slater GH, Ren CJ, Siegel N, et al. Serum fat-soluble vitamin deficiency and abnormal calcium metabolism after malabsorptive bariatric surgery. *J Gastrointest Surg*. 2004;8(1):48-55. doi:10.1016/j.gassur.2003.09.020

32. Mechanick JI, Youdim A, Jones DB, et al. Clinical practice guidelines for the perioperative nutritional, metabolic, and nonsurgical support of the bariatric surgery patient—2013 update: cosponsored by American Association of Clinical Endocrinologists, The Obesity Society, and American Society for Metabolic and Bariatric Surgery: AACE/TOS/ASMBS guidelines. *Obesity*. 2013;21(S1):S1-S27. doi:10.1002/oby.20461

33. Kennel KA, Drake MT, Hurley DL. Vitamin D deficiency in adults: when to test and how to treat. *Mayo Clin Proc*. 2010;85(8):752-758. doi:10.4065/mcp.2010.0138

34. Holick MF, Binkley NC, Bischoff-Ferrari HA, et al. Evaluation, treatment, and prevention of vitamin D deficiency: an Endocrine Society clinical practice guideline. *J Clin Endocrinol Metab*. 2011;96(7):1911-1930. doi:10.1210/jc.2011-0385

35. Montastier E, Chalret du Rieu M, Tuyeras G, Ritz P. Long-term nutritional follow-up post bariatric surgery. *Curr Opin Clin Nutr Metab Care*. 2018;21(5):388-393. doi:10.1097/MCO.0000000000000490

36. Sherf-Dagan S, Buch A, Ben-Porat T, Sakran N, Sinai T. Vitamin E status among bariatric surgery patients: a systematic review. *Surg Obes Relat Dis*. 2021;17(4):816-830. doi:10.1016/j.soard.2020.10.029

37. Mechanick JI, Kushner RF, Sugerman HJ, et al. American Association of Clinical Endocrinologists, The Obesity Society, and American Society for Metabolic and Bariatric Surgery Medical guidelines for clinical practice for the perioperative nutritional, metabolic, and nonsurgical support of the bariatric surgery patient. *Surg Obes Relat Dis*. 2008;4 (5 suppl):S109-S184. doi:10.1016/j.soard.2008.08.009

38. Rindi G. Thiamin absorption by small intestine. *Acta Vitaminol Enzymol*. 1984;6(1):47-55.

39. Shah HN, Bal BS, Finelli FC, Koch TR. Constipation in patients with thiamine deficiency after Roux-en-Y gastric bypass surgery. *Digestion*. 2013;88(2):119-124. doi:10.1159/000353245

40. Nordentoft M, Timm S, Hasselbalch E, Roesen A, Gammeltoft S, Hemmingsen R. Thiamine pyrophosphate effect and erythrocyte transketolase activity during severe alcohol withdrawal syndrome. *Acta Psychiatr Scand*. 1993;88(2):80-84. doi:10.1111/j.1600-0447.1993.tb03418.x

41. Schjønsby H. Vitamin B12 absorption and malabsorption. *Gut*. 1989;30(12):1686-1691.

42. Stabler SP. Vitamin B12 deficiency. *N Engl J Med*. 2013;368(21):2041-2042. doi:10.1056/NEJMcl304350

43. Saltzman E, Karl JP. Nutrient deficiencies after gastric bypass surgery. *Annu Rev Nutr.* 2013;33:183-203. doi:10.1146/annurev-nutr-071812-161225

44. Toninello P, Montanari A, Bassetto F, Vindigni V, Paoli A. Nutritional support for bariatric surgery patients: the skin beyond the fat. *Nutrients.* 2021;13(5):1565. doi:10.3390/nu13051565

45. Steenackers N, Van der Schueren B, Mertens A, et al. Iron deficiency after bariatric surgery: what is the real problem? *Proc Nutr Soc.* 2018;77(4): 445-455. doi:10.1017/S0029665118000149

46. Mahawar KK, Bhasker AG, Bindal V, et al. Zinc deficiency after gastric bypass for morbid obesity: a systematic review. *Obes Surg.* 2017;27(2): 522-529. doi:10.1007/s11695-016-2474-8

47. Bloomberg RD, Fleishman A, Nalle JE, Herron DM, Kini S. Nutritional deficiencies following bariatric surgery: what have we learned? *Obes Surg.* 2005;15(2):145-154. doi:10.1381/0960892053268264

48. Gletsu-Miller N, Broderius M, Frediani JK, et al. Incidence and prevalence of copper deficiency following Roux-en-Y gastric bypass surgery. *Int J Obes.* 2012;36(3):328-335. doi:10.1038/ijo.2011.159

49. Kumar P, Hamza N, Madhok B, et al. Copper deficiency after gastric bypass for morbid obesity: a systematic review. *Obes Surg.* 2016;26(6):1335-1342. doi:10.1007/s11695-016-2162-8

50. Majumdar MC, Reardon C, Isom KA, Robinson MK. Comparison of bariatric branded chewable multivitamin/multimineral formulations to the 2016 American Society for Metabolic and Bariatric Surgery Integrated Health Nutritional Guidelines. *Obes Surg.* 2020;30(4): 1560-1563. doi:10.1007/s11695-019-04169-9

51. Marques da Silva M, Waitzberg DL, Dipppolito RMS, et al. Nutritional guidance, monitoring, and supplementation before and after bariatric surgery—are we doing this correctly? *Nutr Hosp.* 2021;38(3):478-487. doi:10.20960/nh.03221

52. Ha J, Kwon Y, Kwon JW, et al. Micronutrient status in bariatric surgery patients receiving postoperative supplementation per guidelines: insights from a systematic review and meta-analysis of longitudinal studies. *Obes Rev.* 2021;22(7):e13249. doi:10.1111/obr.13249

53. Mahawar KK, Clare K, O'Kane M, Graham Y, Callejas-Diaz L, Carr WRJ. Patient perspectives on adherence with micronutrient supplementation after bariatric surgery. *Obes Surg.* 2019;29(5):1551-1556. doi:10.1007/s11695-019-03711-z

Metabolic & Bariatric Surgery

CHAPTER 15

# Burns

Beth A. Shields, MS, RDN, CNSC; Megan Nordlund, MS, RD, CSG; Kaitlin A. Pruskowski, PharmD, BCPS, BCCCP, FCCM; and Leopoldo C. Cancio, MD, FACS, FCCM

## Introduction

Severe burns, defined as those encompassing more than 20% of the total body surface area (TBSA), generate an extreme and prolonged hypermetabolic and catabolic response.[1,2] This response leads to increased utilization of micronutrients by the body and micronutrient losses across the burn wound and in the urine.[3] Meeting energy and protein requirements is fundamental to the care of patients with burns, as severe wasting may occur when these requirements are not met.[1] In addition to elevated energy and protein requirements, certain micronutrient requirements are also elevated.[3] Micronutrient deficiencies in patients with burns are caused by inadequate intakes and increased losses via wounds, urine, and feces; and they have effects on oxidative stress, immune function, and wound healing.[2,3]

   The assessment of micronutrient status and time needed for supplementation in patients with severe burns is unclear in the available guidelines. Laboratory values are not always indicative of nutriture, and those measuring micronutrients can be falsely low due to hemodilution from fluid resuscitation that occurs early in burn care as well as redistribution of nutrients from the plasma to other organs.[3] Decreases in carrier proteins result in lower total laboratory measurements of the micronutrients they carry. Inflammation can result in lower levels of vitamins A, C, and D, as well as iron, selenium, and zinc; and it can result in higher levels of vitamin B12 and copper.

The current evidence for vitamin and mineral supplementation in patients with severe burns is as follows (also summarized in Box 15.1)[1,2,4-9]:

- The 2016 guidelines from the Society of Critical Care Medicine and the American Society for Parenteral and Enteral Nutrition recommend supplementation of vitamin E, vitamin C, selenium, zinc, and copper for patients with severe burns.[4]

- The 2013 guidelines from the European Society for Clinical Nutrition and Metabolism also recommend supplementation of copper, selenium, and zinc, in addition to thiamin and vitamins C, D, and E.[1]

- In a 2009 survey of burn centers, all 65 participating centers reported giving patients a multivitamin; 62% gave additional vitamin C; and 80% gave additional zinc supplements.[5]

- A 2014 through 2015 international survey of 14 burn centers listed practices as being carried out during the first 12 days in the intensive care unit which included vitamin C given during 62% of patient-days, zinc given during 44% of patient-days, and selenium given during 25% of patient-days.[6]

- A 2018 cohort study evaluated the effectiveness of different vitamin and mineral combinations in patients with severe burns and found decreased hypermetabolic response and decreased inflammatory markers after supplementation with an intravenous cocktail of 6,600 IU vitamin A, 6 mg thiamin, 800 mcg folate, 10 mcg vitamin B12, 200 mg vitamin C, 400 IU vitamin D, 20 IU vitamin E, 30 mg zinc, 4 mg copper, 2 mg chromium, and 1,000 mcg selenium for 14 days, as well as 1,200 mg acetylcysteine and 400 IU vitamin E enterally twice a day for the first 7 days.[2]

**BOX 15.1  Summary of Evidence for Use of Vitamin and Mineral Treatments After Severe Burn Injury[a,1,2,4-9]**

### McClave 2016, American Society for Parenteral and Enteral Nutrition (ASPEN)/Society of Critical Care Medicine (SCCM) guidelines[4]

Supplementation suggested with low quality of evidence: copper, selenium, zinc, vitamin C, vitamin E

### Rousseau 2013, European Society for Clinical Nutrition and Metabolism (ESPEN guidelines)[1]

Strongly suggest supplementation with copper (intravenous [IV]), selenium (IV), zinc (IV), thiamin, vitamin C, vitamin D, vitamin E

### Graves 2009[5]

Survey of reported practices of 65 burn units:

- 92% of burn units reported routine use of micronutrient supplementation.
- 80% supplemented zinc
- 62% supplemented vitamin C
- 100% supplemented a multivitamin

### Chourdakis 2020[6]

Survey of actual practices of 14 burn units:

- Patients supplemented with selenium on 25% of admission days
- Patients supplemented with zinc on 44% of admission days
- Patients supplemented with vitamin C on 62% of admission days

### Berger 2006 and 2007[7,8]

Studies on copper, selenium, and zinc:

- Copper 2.5 to 3.7 mg daily (IV) for 7 to 21 days
- Selenium 230 to 280 mcg daily (IV) for 7 to 21 days
- Zinc 35 to 49 mg daily (IV) for 7 to 21 days

Outcomes:

- Decreased intensive care unit length of stay
- Fewer pulmonary infections
- Improved wound healing

*Continued on next page*

> **BOX 15.1  Summary of Evidence for Use of Vitamin and Mineral Treatments After Severe Burn Injury**[a,1,2,4-9] **(cont.)**

## *Barbosa 2009*[9]

Randomized controlled trial, pediatrics

Zinc twice the Recommended Dietary Allowance (enteral)

Vitamin C 1.5 times the upper limit (enteral)

Vitamin E 1.35 times the upper limit (enteral)

Outcomes: improved wound healing

## *Rehou 2018*[2]

Cohort study

Lactated ringers (1 L/d for 14 days), which contains:

- Copper 4 mg
- Selenium 1,000 mcg
- Zinc 30 mg
- Chromium 40 mcg
- Manganese 2 mg
- Vitamin A 6,600 IU (1,980 mcg RAE)
- Thiamin 6 mg
- Folic acid 800 mcg
- Vitamin B12 10 mcg
- Vitamin C 200 mg
- Vitamin D 10 mcg (400 IU)
- Vitamin E 20 IU
- Riboflavin 7.2 mg
- Niacinamide 80 mg
- D-panthenol 30 mg
- Pyridoxine 8 mg
- Biotin 120 mcg

Outcomes:

- Decreased inflammatory markers
- Decreased hypermetabolic response

[a] Stratified by guideline and original research.

- A 2006 study found fewer pulmonary infections in patients with burns encompassing 21% to 40% of their TBSA after they were given an intravenous cocktail consisting of approximately 3 mg copper, 350 mcg selenium, and 30 mg zinc for 2 weeks. The same occurred after 3 weeks for patients with burns covering more than 40% of their TBSA.[8]

- A randomized controlled trial found improved wound healing when pediatric patients with severe burns were given enteral vitamin C (1.5 times the upper limit), vitamin E (1.35 times the upper limit), and zinc (2 times the recommend dietary allowance).[9]

This chapter provides an overview of specific micronutrients and their role in metabolism, methods for evaluating deficiency status, and suggestions for repletion in adult patients with severe burns. Recommendations made at the end of each section are based on the available evidence.

# Copper

Copper plays a role in the cross-linking of collagen and elastin; deficiency can result in impaired wound healing, anemia, and neutropenia.[10,11] Studies have found decreased copper levels after severe burns. These decreases stem from both cutaneous and urinary losses, as well as from a decrease in copper's carrier protein (ceruloplasmin).[11,12] In addition, copper is sequestered in the liver, where it is incorporated into enzymes that fight oxidative stress (catalase and zinc-copper superoxide dismutase).[12,13] The decrease in copper levels is inversely correlated with the percentage of TBSA affected by burns and may resolve as the wounds heal; however, it does not always resolve quickly without supplementation.[11,14]

Zinc is often supplemented in patients with severe burns but can cause copper deficiency as copper and zinc compete for absorption. Clinicians should carefully monitor the copper status of patients who are receiving continuous renal replacement therapy (CRRT), as additional losses can occur with CRRT. Note that excessive copper supplementation can lead to hepatic damage and dementia.[10]

The clinician can consider giving 3 mg copper intravenously for the first 1 to 2 weeks of care, based on burn size regardless of copper status.[7,8] Otherwise, when copper deficiency is suspected or confirmed, intravenous copper supplementation should be given or enteral zinc supplementation should be discontinued, when applicable.

# Electrolytes: Calcium, Magnesium, Phosphorus, and Potassium

Low electrolyte levels are common after severe thermal injury, and the effects of these deficiencies can be substantial:

- Hypocalcemia can result in hypotension, decreased myocardial activity, and tetany.[15]

- Hypomagnesemia can result in arrhythmias, seizures, coma, and death.[15]

- Severe hypophosphatemia is common early in the hospitalization of patients with severe burns (peaking 3–5 days postburn) and can result in skeletal muscle and cardiac myopathy, impaired response to vasopressor agents, neurological dysfunction, paralysis, seizures, acute respiratory failure from impaired diaphragmatic contractility, and death.[15,16] Hypophosphatemia in burned patients, who sustain a rapid postburn increase in metabolic rate, is analogous to that seen in patients with refeeding syndrome.[15] Administering 30 mmol sodium phosphate intravenously every 6 hours, starting approximately 24 hours after thermal injury, has been found to result in fewer cardiac events and infections.[17] However, hypophosphatemia may persist, requiring additional phosphorus repletion and frequent testing of phosphorus levels.

- Hypokalemia can lead to vomiting, constipation, impaired respiratory function, paralysis, arrhythmias, and death.[15,18] It can be caused by medications commonly given to patients with burns, including β-agonists (such as albuterol), insulin, and loop diuretics.[15] Although kidney injury may impede the clearing of electrolytes from the body, patients receiving CRRT may experience additional electrolyte losses depending on the composition and dose of the replacement fluid.

Intravenous supplementation of calcium, phosphorus, and magnesium is preferred to enteral supplementation, as these micronutrients can be poorly absorbed when supplemented enterally. Enteral magnesium and phosphorus may also cause diarrhea.[15]

Decreases in carrier proteins can lead to lower electrolyte levels. For example, a decrease in albumin, a calcium carrier, can result in lower total calcium levels (but not in lower ionized calcium levels). Magnesium levels must be corrected before correcting potassium and calcium levels.[15]

The use of standardized replacement protocols for calcium, magnesium, phosphorus, and potassium is recommended. Also recommended is the initiation of 30 mmol sodium phosphate, administered intravenously every 6 hours, simultaneously with the initiation of enteral nutrition in patients with normal kidney function. This dose should then be adjusted based on the patient's phosphorus levels. In rare cases, enteral nutrition may need to be decreased temporarily or held when phosphorus levels cannot be controlled in order to avoid the aforementioned clinical manifestations of hypophosphatemia.[17]

# Iron

Iron plays a role in wound healing as a cofactor in collagen synthesis, but its role has not been thoroughly studied in patients with burns.[19] Iron levels decrease after severe thermal injury but return to normal without supplementation; they can even become elevated with numerous blood transfusions.[19,20] Low laboratory values are not always indicative of nutriture; an early decrease in iron level corresponds to an early increase in ferritin level.[20] Chapter 7 provides more details on iron deficiency.

Iron is not typically supplemented in patients with burns, because they often receive many blood transfusions that contain iron. Supplementation should be considered on an individual basis after evaluating a full iron panel to avoid iron overload. Obtaining an iron panel, including ferritin, is recommended for patients with microcytic anemia in order to evaluate for deficiency.

# Selenium

Selenium primarily functions as an antioxidant following severe thermal injury. Selenium levels decrease after burns, corresponding to increased losses through the urine and wounds.[21,22] Plasma selenium levels have been shown to inversely correlate with infection rates. Selenium deficiency is characterized by oxidative injury, altered thyroid hormone metabolism, increased plasma glutathione levels, muscle weakness, and cardiomyopathy.[10,21,22]

Clinicians can consider giving 400 mg selenium intravenously for the first 1 to 2 weeks after injury, based on burn size.[7,8] If intravenous selenium cannot be provided, enteral selenium supplementation, 400 mcg/d, can be considered; it should be discontinued when the open wound size reaches less than 10% TBSA but continued for patients receiving CRRT, as additional losses can occur with CCRT.

# Vitamin A

Whole-body vitamin A deficiency is rare, as the liver has stores that can last several months. Vitamin A deficiency can impair collagen synthesis and interfere with wound healing.[10,23] Experts recommend supplementing 3,000 to 15,000 IU/d (900 to 4,500 mcg RAE/d) in patients receiving corticosteroids (such as hydrocortisone). Vitamin A is thought to counteract the effects of corticosteroids, which may impair wound healing. However, these data are based on studies conducted in rats.[10,24]

Vitamin A levels decrease in the early days after severe burn.[20] In one study conducted in human subjects, vitamin A laboratory values were low for the first 3 weeks after severe burn unless vitamin A was supplemented[25]; yet another study in humans found that values normalized without supplementation by week 2.[26] The production of retinol-binding protein (which carries vitamin A) slows during the inflammatory response, contributing to decreased vitamin A levels that would not warrant supplementation.[10] Zinc plays a role in the production of retinol-binding protein; therefore, zinc deficiency can also cause decreased vitamin A values. In a 2009 survey, only 17% of burn centers reported routinely supplementing vitamin A as a separate micronutrient.[5]

Vitamin A toxicity has been reported in two patients with burns who received no supplementation other than a multivitamin.[27] Vitamin A levels can become elevated with acute kidney injury, which is a common complication of severe thermal injury,[10] and clinicians should bear this in mind when assessing patients with kidney disease.

Routine supplementation of vitamin A is not recommended. Supplementing 10,000 to 15,000 IU (3,000 to 4,500 mcg RAE) vitamin A enterally per day for a maximum of 10 days can be considered for patients taking corticosteroids whose wounds fail to heal. When supplementation is implemented, the clinician should monitor vitamin A and retinol-binding protein levels.

# Thiamin, Folate, and Vitamin B12

The B vitamins play a role in collagen formation but do not play a direct role in wound healing.[28] Folate assists in protein synthesis,[29] and pediatric patients with burns have been found to have increased losses of folate through the urine and low folate levels.[30] Alcohol abuse can decrease the intake and absorption of folate and thiamin.[10]

Vitamin B12 and folate do not decrease in the early days after severe thermal injury.[20] Folate supplementation is not commonly provided in burn centers (as reported by a 2009 survey).[5] Toxicity has only been noted at intakes of 100 times the Recommended Dietary Allowance (RDA).[10] Thiamin supplementation is associated with decreased lactate levels in patients with burns.[31]

Clinicians should consider enteral supplementation of 100 mg thiamin per day and 1 mg folate per day in critically ill patients with severe burns until the size of their open wounds reaches less than 10% TBSA. Note that patients with a high risk for deficiency (eg, older adults, patients who abuse alcohol, patients at risk for refeeding syndrome, and patients receiving CRRT) can have additional losses. Vitamin B12, folate, methylmalonic acid, and homocysteine levels should be checked in patients with macrocytic anemia in order to evaluate them for vitamin B12 and folate deficiencies.

# Vitamin C

Vitamin C plays a role in collagen synthesis, capillary strength, and wound healing.[10,23] Vitamin C levels decrease substantially in the early days after severe thermal injury.[20] One study found that levels increased to normal 3 weeks after severe burns without additional supplementation other than enteral nutrition (which did provide 8.5 to 11.4 times the RDA).[25] Deficiency of vitamin C can occur with alcohol use, decreased vitamin C intake, and increased excretion. It also occurs with smoking, which increases oxidative stress and vitamin C turnover.[28,32,33] Burn injuries caused by smoking while on home oxygen therapy are common, and individuals presenting with such injuries often have a positive blood alcohol level on admission.[34,35] Some studies have found improvements in wound healing with vitamin C supplementation, whereas others have not. In a 2009 survey, 87% of burn centers reported providing routine supplementation of vitamin C.[5]

Enteral supplementation with 1,000 to 1,500 mg vitamin C per day should be considered for patients with severe burns. This can be incrementally lowered to 500 mg/d once the open wound size reaches less than 10% TBSA. Higher doses should be continued for patients receiving CRRT, as additional losses can occur with CRRT. Monitoring of vitamin C levels is recommended to appropriately titrate doses and avoid over-supplementation.

# Vitamin D

Vitamin D plays a role in immunity, calcium metabolism, glucose metabolism, and muscle function,[10,36] and deficiency is a risk factor for infection and mortality.[36] Low vitamin D levels are prevalent in patients with burns in the early days of hospitalization, as a consequence of decreased levels of carrier proteins and hemodilution.[37] Limited sunlight exposure due to prolonged hospitalization, pressure garment use, and sunscreen use after hospital discharge can lead to decreased vitamin D production.[38] Both burn scars and adjacent nonburned skin produce less vitamin D than usual for more than 1 year after injury, and low serum levels can continue for 7 years after injury.[39]

Pruritus is a common concern among patients with burns and can be relieved with the correction of vitamin D deficiency.[38,40] Vitamin D deficiency following a burn injury has negative impacts on bone health, and there is an association between vitamin D status, bone mineral density, and long-bone fractures.[41] Deficiency also correlates with low scar elasticity and decreased skin barrier function.[42]

When researchers compared the administration of 100 IU vitamin D2 per kilogram of body weight per day vs the same amount of vitamin D3 vs placebo in pediatric patients throughout an initial hospitalization for burns, they found that subsequently, as outpatients, 31% of patients in the placebo group experienced fractures, 15% in the vitamin D2 group experienced fractures, and 0% in the vitamin D3 group experienced fractures ($P$ = .13).[41] In another study, patients had increased muscle strength after receiving both vitamin D3, at a dose of 200,000 IU intramuscularly every 3 months, and a daily oral calcium supplement for 1 year.[43] Clinicians should be aware that excessive vitamin D supplementation can result in hypercalcemia.

Consideration of enteral vitamin D3 supplementation is recommended for patients with severe burns. If implemented, the dose should be adjusted over the course of hospitalization according to the patient's 25-hydroxyvitamin D levels, and supplementation should be suspended when calcium levels are elevated.

# Vitamin E

Plasma and tissue vitamin E levels do not immediately decrease after severe thermal injury but do decrease throughout the first month after injury.[20,44] In one study, vitamin E levels returned to normal after 3 weeks without any supplementation other than enteral nutrition (which did provide 2.6 to 3.4 times the RDA for vitamin E).[25] Another study found lower levels of vitamin E in nonsurvivors of thermal injury compared to survivors.[45] In animal models, vitamin E supplementation has led to a decrease in the formation of pressure injuries, improved wound healing, amelioration of acute lung injury after inhalation injury, and worsening wound tensile strength.[46-50] Other benefits found in animal-burn models include decreased oxidative stress, improved anemia, and improved neutrophil function.[51-54] Excessive vitamin E supplementation can decrease neutrophil function and increase bleeding complications.[10]

Consideration of enteral vitamin E supplementation, 400 IU/d, is recommended for patients with severe burns. If implemented, the dose should be titrated throughout the hospital stay according to the patient's vitamin E levels, and supplementation should be discontinued when the open wound size reaches less than 10% TBSA.

# Zinc

Zinc is an antioxidant and plays a role in protein synthesis and immune function.[10,19,23] Zinc levels decrease after severe burns because of zinc sequestration to the liver, fewer zinc carrier proteins, hemodilution, and increased zinc losses through the urine and the skin.[12,14,20] Deficiency results in impaired wound healing.[10]

Daily doses of 40 mg elemental zinc can result in copper deficiency,[10] and zinc supplementation can increase urinary zinc losses.[55] Most burn centers do supplement zinc.[5] In one study, patients in burn units received 50 mg elemental zinc by mouth daily, which normalized zinc levels in 83% of the patients by the time of hospital discharge; furthermore, it did not interfere with copper absorption and caused no gastrointestinal side effects.[56] In another study, daily supplementation with 49 mg elemental zinc given intravenously normalized levels by day 20 of hospitalization.[57]

Clinicians can consider giving patients 40 mg zinc per day intravenously for the first 1 to 2 weeks after burn injury, based on burn size.[7,8,57] Patients with more severe burns should be given enteral supplementation of 50 mg elemental zinc (220 mg zinc sulfate) per day, which should be discontinued when the open wound size reaches less than 10% TBSA or when serum values normalize. Practitioners can consider switching to intravenous supplementation if enteral zinc supplementation results in low copper levels.

# Summary of Recommendations

The recommendations for micronutrient supplementation and monitoring in patients with burn injuries are summarized in Box 15.2.

---

**BOX 15.2   Recommendations for Micronutrient Supplementation and Monitoring in Patients With Burns**

### Copper

| | |
|---|---|
| Supplementation | 3 mg copper, intravenous (IV), for 1 to 2 weeks; or supplement when deficiency is suspected or confirmed. |
| Monitoring | Monitor copper and zinc levels, especially in patients receiving continuous renal replacement therapy (CRRT); replete intravenously (suspend enteral zinc if copper levels decline). |

### Selenium

| | |
|---|---|
| Supplementation | 400 mcg selenium, IV, for 1 to 2 weeks; or 400 mcg selenium enterally per day |
| Monitoring | Discontinue when open wound size reaches less than 10% total body surface area (TBSA) and patient is no longer receiving CRRT; monitor levels. |

### Zinc

| | |
|---|---|
| Supplementation | 40 mg zinc, IV, daily for 1 to 2 weeks; or 50 mg elemental zinc (220 mg zinc sulfate) enterally per day |
| Monitoring | Discontinue when open wound size reaches less than 10% TBSA or when serum values normalize; IV supplementation may be required if enteral zinc supplementation results in low copper levels. |

*Continued on next page*

---

**BOX 15.2  Recommendations for Micronutrient Supplementation and Monitoring in Patients With Burns** (cont.)

## Iron

Supplementation | Not typically supplemented

Monitoring | Check iron panel, including ferritin, in patients with microcytic anemia to evaluate for deficiency.

## Vitamin A

Supplementation | Not typically supplemented

Consider vitamin A supplementation, 10,000 to 15,000 IU (3,000–4,500 mcg RAE) enterally per day for a maximum of 10 days, in patients taking corticosteroids whose wounds fail to heal.

Monitoring | Check vitamin A levels along with retinol-binding protein.

## Thiamin

Supplementation | 100 mg thiamin enterally per day

Monitoring | Discontinue when open wound size reaches less than 10% TBSA and the patient is no longer receiving CRRT.

## Folate

Supplementation | 1 mg folate enterally per day

Monitoring | Discontinue when open wound size reaches less than 10% TBSA and the patient is no longer receiving CRRT.

## Vitamin B12

Supplementation | No dosing recommendations available

Monitoring | Check vitamin B12, folate, methylmalonic acid, and homocysteine levels in patients with macrocytic anemia.

> **BOX 15.2** Recommendations for Micronutrient Supplementation and Monitoring in Patients With Burns (cont.)

### Vitamin C

| | |
|---|---|
| Supplementation | 1,000 to 1,500 mg vitamin C enterally per day |
| Monitoring | Wean down to 500 mg/d when open wound size reaches less than 10% TBSA and the patient is no longer receiving CRRT. |

### Vitamin D

| | |
|---|---|
| Supplementation | Cholecalciferol (vitamin D3) is preferred; no dosing recommendations are available. |
| Monitoring | Adjust the dose of vitamin D throughout hospitalization according to the patient's 25-hydroxyvitamin D levels and suspend supplementation if calcium levels increase. |

### Vitamin E

| | |
|---|---|
| Supplementation | 400 IU vitamin E enterally per day |
| Monitoring | Discontinue when open wound size reaches less than 10% TBSA; titrate the dose based on the patient's vitamin E levels. |

# References

1. Rousseau AF, Losser MR, Ichai C, Berger MM. ESPEN endorsed recommendations: nutritional therapy in major burns. *Clin Nutr.* 2013;32(4):497-502. doi:10.1016/j.clnu.2013.02.012

2. Rehou S, Shahrokhi S, Natanson R, Stanojcic M, Jeschke MG. Antioxidant and trace element supplementation reduce the inflammatory response in critically ill burn patients. *J Burn Care Res.* 2018;39(1):1-9. doi:10.1097/BCR.0000000000000607

3. Berger MM. Antioxidant micronutrients in major trauma and burns: evidence and practice. *Nutr Clin Pract.* 2006;21(5):438-449. doi:10.1177/0115426506021005438

4.  McClave SA, Taylor BE, Martindale RG, et al. Guidelines for the provision and assessment of nutrition support therapy in the adult critically ill patient: Society of Critical Care Medicine (SCCM) and American Society for Parenteral and Enteral Nutrition (A.S.P.E.N.). *JPEN J Parenter Enteral Nutr.* 2016;40(2):159-211. doi:10.1177/0148607115621863

5.  Graves C, Saffle J, Cochran A. Actual burn nutrition care practices: an update. *J Burn Care Res.* 2009;30(1):77-82. doi:10.1097/BCR.0b013e3181921f0d

6.  Chourdakis M, Bouras E, Shields BA, Stoppe C, Rousseau AF, Heyland DK. Nutritional therapy among burn injured patients in the critical care setting: an international multicenter observational study on "best achievable" practices. *Clin Nutr.* 2020;39(12):3813-3820. doi:10.1016/j.clnu.2020.04.023

7.  Berger MM, Baines M, Raffoul W, et al. Trace element supplementation after major burns modulates antioxidant status and clinical course by way of increased tissue trace element concentrations. *Am J Clin Nutr.* 2007;85(5):1293-1300. doi:10.1093/ajcn/85.5.1293

8.  Berger MM, Eggimann P, Heyland DK, et al. Reduction of nosocomial pneumonia after major burns by trace element supplementation: aggregation of two randomised trials. *Crit Care.* 2006;10(6):R153. doi:10.1186/cc5084

9.  Barbosa E, Faintuch J, Machado Moreira EA, et al. Supplementation of vitamin E, vitamin C, and zinc attenuates oxidative stress in burned children: a randomized, double-blind, placebo-controlled pilot study. *J Burn Care Res.* 2009;30(5):859-866. doi:10.1097/BCR.0b013e3181b487a8

10. McKeever L. Vitamins and trace elements. In: Mueller CM, ed. *The ASPEN Adult Nutrition Support Core Curriculum eBook.* 3rd ed. American Society for Parenteral and Enteral Nutrition; 2017:18.

11. Voruganti VS, Klein GL, Lu HX, Thomas S, Freeland-Graves JH, Herndon DN. Impaired zinc and copper status in children with burn injuries: need to reassess nutritional requirements. *Burns.* 2005;31(6):711-716. doi:10.1016/j.burns.2005.04.026

12. Berger MM, Cavadini C, Bart A, et al. Cutaneous copper and zinc losses in burns. *Burns.* 1992;18(5):373-380. doi:10.1016/0305-4179(92)90035-s

13. Shewmake KB, Talbert GE, Bowser-Wallace BH, Caldwell FT Jr, Cone JB. Alterations in plasma copper, zinc, and ceruloplasmin levels in patients with thermal trauma. *J Burn Care Rehabil.* 1988;9(1):13-17. doi:10.1097/00004630-198801000-00005

14. Gosling P, Rothe HM, Sheehan TM, Hubbard LD. Serum copper and zinc concentrations in patients with burns in relation to burn surface area. *J Burn Care Rehabil.* 1995;16(5):481-486. doi:10.1097/00004630-199509000-00004

15. McKeever L. Fluids, electrolytes, and acid-base disorders. In: Mueller CM, ed. *The ASPEN Adult Nutrition Support Core Curriculum eBook*. 3rd ed. American Society for Parenteral and Enteral Nutrition; 2017:17.

16. Bollaert PE, Levy B, Nace L, Laterre PF, Larcan A. Hemodynamic and metabolic effects of rapid correction of hypophosphatemia in patients with septic shock. *Chest*. 1995;107(6):1698-1701. doi:10.1378/chest.107.6.1698

17. Kahn SA, Bell DE, Stassen NA, Lentz CW. Prevention of hypophosphatemia after burn injury with a protocol for continuous, preemptive repletion. *J Burn Care Res*. 2015;36(3):e220-e225. doi:10.1097/BCR.0000000000000114

18. Kraft MD, Btaiche IF, Sacks GS, Kudsk KA. Treatment of electrolyte disorders in adult patients in the intensive care unit. *Am J Health Syst Pharm*. 2005;62(16):1663-1682. doi:10.2146/ajhp040300

19. Żwierełło W, Styburski D, Maruszewska A, et al. Bioelements in the treatment of burn injuries—the complex review of metabolism and supplementation (copper, selenium, zinc, iron, manganese, chromium and magnesium). *J Trace Elem Med Biol*. 2020;62:126616. doi:10.1016/j.jtemb.2020.126616

20. Vinha PP, Martinez EZ, Vannucchi H, et al. Effect of acute thermal injury in status of serum vitamins, inflammatory markers, and oxidative stress markers: preliminary data. *J Burn Care Res*. 2013;34(2):e87-e91. doi:10.1097/BCR.0b013e31826fc506

21. Berger MM, Cavadini C, Bart A, et al. Selenium losses in 10 burned patients. *Clin Nutr*. 1992;11(2):75-82. doi:10.1016/0261-5614(92)90014-h

22. Dylewski ML, Bender JC, Smith AM, et al. The selenium status of pediatric patients with burn injuries. *J Trauma*. 2010;69(3):584-588. doi:10.1097/TA.0b013e3181e74c54

23. McKeever L. Wound healing. In: Mueller CM, ed. *The ASPEN Adult Nutrition Support Core Curriculum eBook*. 3rd ed. American Society for Parenteral and Enteral Nutrition; 2017:33.

24. Wicke C, Halliday B, Allen D, et al. Effects of steroids and retinoids on wound healing. *Arch Surg*. 2000;135(11):1265-1270. doi:10.1001/archsurg.135.11.1265

25. Rock CL, Dechert RE, Khilnani R, Parker RS, Rodriguez JL. Carotenoids and antioxidant vitamins in patients after burn injury. *J Burn Care Rehabil*. 1997;18(3):269-278. doi:10.1097/00004630-199705000-00018

26. Rai K, Courtemanche AD. Vitamin A assay in burned patients. *J Trauma*. 1975;15(5):419-424. doi:10.1097/00005373-197505000-00008

27. Bremner NA, Mills LA, Durrani AJ, Watson JD. Vitamin A toxicity in burns patients on long-term enteral feed. *Burns*. 2007;33(2):266-267. doi:10.1016/j.burns.2006.06.007

28. Alvarez OM, Gilbreath RL. Thiamine influence on collagen during the granulation of skin wounds. *J Surg Res.* 1982;32(1):24-31. doi:10.1016/0022-4804(82)90180-9

29. Zhang XJ, Chinkes DL, Herndon DN. Folate stimulation of wound DNA synthesis. *J Surg Res.* 2008;147(1):15-22. doi:10.1016/j.jss.2007.07.012

30. Barlow GB, Wilkinson AW. 4-amino-imidazole-5-carboxamide excretion and folate status in children with burns and scalds. *Clin Chim Acta.* 1970;29(3):355-359. doi:10.1016/0009-8981(70)90002-1

31. Falder S, Silla R, Phillips M, et al. Thiamine supplementation increases serum thiamine and reduces pyruvate and lactate levels in burn patients. *Burns.* 2010;36(2):261-269. doi:10.1016/j.burns.2009.04.012

32. Lim DJ, Sharma Y, Thompson CH. Vitamin C and alcohol: a call to action. *BMJ Nutr Prev Health.* 2018;1(1):17-22. doi:10.1136/bmjnph-2018-000010

33. Lykkesfeldt J, Loft S, Nielsen JB, Poulsen HE. Ascorbic acid and dehydroascorbic acid as biomarkers of oxidative stress caused by smoking. *Am J Clin Nutr.* 1997;65(4):959-963. doi:10.1093/ajcn/65.4.959

34. Holmes WJ, Hold P, James MI. The increasing trend in alcohol-related burns: it's [*sic*] impact on a tertiary burn centre. *Burns.* 2010;36(6):938-943. doi:10.1016/j.burns.2009.12.008

35. Edelman DA, Maleyko-Jacobs S, White MT, Lucas CE, Ledgerwood AM. Smoking and home oxygen therapy—a preventable public health hazard. *J Burn Care Res.* 2008;29(1):119-122. doi:10.1097/BCR.0b013e31815f5a3a

36. Braun A, Chang D, Mahadevappa K, et al. Association of low serum 25-hydroxyvitamin D levels and mortality in the critically ill. *Crit Care Med.* 2011;39(4):671-677. doi:10.1097/CCM.0b013e318206ccdf

37. Krishnan A, Ochola J, Mundy J, et al. Acute fluid shifts influence the assessment of serum vitamin D status in critically ill patients. *Crit Care.* 2010;14(6):R216. doi:10.1186/cc9341

38. Schumann AD, Paxton RL, Solanki NS, et al. Vitamin D deficiency in burn patients. *J Burn Care Res.* 2012;33(6):731-735. doi:10.1097/BCR.0b013e31824d1c2c

39. Klein GL, Chen TC, Holick MF, et al. Synthesis of vitamin D in skin after burns. *Lancet.* 2004;363(9405):291-292. doi:10.1016/S0140-6736(03)15388-3

40. Goetz DW. Idiopathic itch, rash, and urticaria/angioedema merit serum vitamin D evaluation: a descriptive case series. *W V Med J.* 2011;107(1):14-20.

41. Mayes T, Gottschlich MM, Khoury J, Kagan RJ. Investigation of bone health subsequent to vitamin D supplementation in children following burn injury. *Nutr Clin Pract*. 2015;30(6):830-837. doi:10.1177/0884533615587720

42. Cho YS, Seo CH, Joo SY, Song J, Cha E, Ohn SH. The association between postburn vitamin D deficiency and the biomechanical properties of hypertrophic scars. *J Burn Care Res*. 2019;40(3):274-280. doi:10.1093/jbcr/irz028

43. Rousseau AF, Foidart-Desalle M, Ledoux D, et al. Effects of cholecalciferol supplementation and optimized calcium intakes on vitamin D status, muscle strength and bone health: a one-year pilot randomized controlled trial in adults with severe burns. *Burns*. 2015;41(2):317-325. doi:10.1016/j.burns.2014.07.005

44. Shimoda K, Nakazawa H, Traber MG, Traber DL, Nozaki M. Plasma and tissue vitamin E depletion in sheep with burn and smoke inhalation injury. *Burns*. 2008;34(8):1137-1141. doi:10.1016/j.burns.2008.01.015

45. Nguyen TT, Cox CS, Traber DL, et al. Free radical activity and loss of plasma antioxidants, vitamin E, and sulfhydryl groups in patients with burns: the 1993 Moyer Award. *J Burn Care Rehabil*. 1993;14(6):602-609. doi:10.1097/00004630-199311000-00004

46. Houwing R, Overgoor M, Kon M, Jansen G, van Asbeck BS, Haalboom JR. Pressure-induced skin lesions in pigs: reperfusion injury and the effects of vitamin E. *J Wound Care*. 2000;9(1):36-40. doi:10.12968/jowc.2000.9.1.25939

47. Musalmah M, Fairuz AH, Gapor MT, Ngah WZ. Effect of vitamin E on plasma malondialdehyde, antioxidant enzyme levels and the rates of wound closures during wound healing in normal and diabetic rats. *Asia Pac J Clin Nutr*. 2002;11 (suppl 7):S448-S451. doi:10.1046/j.1440-6047.11.s.7.6.x

48. Taren DL, Chvapil M, Weber CW. Increasing the breaking strength of wounds exposed to preoperative irradiation using vitamin E supplementation. *Int J Vitam Nutr Res*. 1987;57(2):133-137.

49. Ehrlich HP, Tarver H, Hunt TK. Inhibitory effects of vitamin E on collagen synthesis and wound repair. *Ann Surg*. 1972;175(2):235-240. doi:10.1097/00000658-197202000-00013

50. Morita N, Shimoda K, Traber MG, et al. Vitamin E attenuates acute lung injury in sheep with burn and smoke inhalation injury. *Redox Rep*. 2006;11(2):61-70. doi:10.1179/135100006X101020

51. Naziroğlu M, Kökçam I, Yilmaz S. Beneficial effects of intraperitoneally administered alpha-tocopheryl acetate on the levels of lipid peroxide and activity of glutathione peroxidase and superoxide dismutase in skin, blood and liver of thermally injured guinea pigs. *Skin Pharmacol Appl Skin Physiol*. 2003;16(1):36-45. doi:10.1159/000068286

52. Bekyarova G, Yankova T, Kozarev I, Yankov D. Reduced erythrocyte deformability related to activated lipid peroxidation during the early postburn period. *Burns*. 1996;22(4):291-294. doi:10.1016/0305 -4179(95)00131-x

53. Chai J, Guo Z, Sheng Z. Protective effects of vitamin E on impaired neutrophil phagocytic function in patients with severe burn. Article in Chinese. *Zhonghua Zheng Xing Shao Shang Wai Ke Za Zhi*. 1995;11(1):32-35.

54. Haberal M, Hamaloğlu E, Bora S, Oner G, Bilgin N. The effects of vitamin E on immune regulation after thermal injury. *Burns Incl Therm Inj*. 1988;14(5):388-393. doi:10.1016/0305-4179(88)90008-3

55. Boosalis MG, Solem LD, Cerra FB, et al. Increased urinary zinc excretion after thermal injury. *J Lab Clin Med*. 1991;118(6):538-545.

56. Caldis-Coutris N, Gawaziuk JP, Logsetty S. Zinc supplementation in burn patients. *J Burn Care Res*. 2012;33(5):678-682. doi:10.1097/BCR .0b013e31824799a3

57. Berger MM, Binnert C, Chiolero RL, et al. Trace element supplementation after major burns increases burned skin trace element concentrations and modulates local protein metabolism but not whole-body substrate metabolism. *Am J Clin Nutr*. 2007;85(5):1301-1306. doi:10 .1093/ajcn/85.5.1301

# APPENDIX

# Top Food Sources for Micronutrients

### TABLE A.1  Vitamin A

| Food | Standard portion | Amount (mcg RAE) |
| --- | --- | --- |
| Beef liver | 3 oz | 6,582 |
| Sweet potato, baked in skin | 1 medium | 1,403 |
| Spinach, cooked | 1 c | 573 |
| Carrot, raw | ½ c | 459 |
| Milk, nonfat, with vitamins A and D | 1 c | 149 |
| Cantaloupe | ½ c | 135 |
| Ricotta cheese | ½ c | 133 |
| Peppers, red, raw | ½ c | 117 |
| Mango | 1 each | 112 |
| Breakfast cereal, ready-to-eat, fortified | ¾-1 c | 90 |

Abbreviation: RAE, retinol activity equivalent.
Vitamin A and carotenoids: fact sheet for health professionals. Office of Dietary Supplements, National Institutes of Health. Updated December 15, 2023. Accessed August 26, 2024. https://ods.od.nih.gov/factsheets/VitaminA-HealthProfessional

### TABLE A.2  Vitamin D

| Food | Standard portion | Amount (IU)[a] |
|---|---|---|
| Mushrooms (various types), exposed to ultraviolet light, raw | 1 c | 732-1,110 |
| Trout, cooked | 3 oz | 645 |
| Salmon, cooked | 3 oz | 570 |
| Fish oil | 1 tsp | 450 |
| Milk, evaporated, with vitamins A and D | 1 c | 403 |
| Milk, fluid, various | 1 c | 124-128 |
| Soy or almond milk, with vitamin D | 1 c | 100-144 |
| Egg, scrambled | 1 egg | 44 |
| Tuna, canned in water, drained | 3 oz | 40 |

[a] 1 mcg cholecalciferol = 40 IU vitamin D
Vitamin D: fact sheet for health professionals. Office of Dietary Supplements, National Institutes of Health. Updated July 26, 2024. Accessed August 27, 2024. https://ods.od.nih.gov/factsheets/VitaminD-HealthProfessional

### TABLE A.3  Vitamin E

| Food | Standard portion | Amount (mg -tocopherol) |
|---|---|---|
| Sunflower seeds, roasted | 1 oz | 7.4 |
| Almonds, roasted | 1 oz | 6.8 |
| Sunflower oil | 1 tbsp | 5.6 |
| Hazelnuts, roasted | 1 oz | 4.3 |
| Peanut butter (smooth or chunky) | 2 tbsp | 2.9 |
| Spinach, cooked | ½ c | 1.9 |
| Broccoli, cooked | ½ c | 1.2 |
| Kiwifruit | 1 medium | 1.1 |

Vitamin E: fact sheet for health professionals. Office of Dietary Supplements, National Institutes of Health. Updated March 26, 2021. Accessed August 27, 2024. https://ods.od.nih.gov/factsheets/VitaminE-HealthProfessional

# Top Food Sources for Micronutrients

### TABLE A.4  Vitamin K

| Food | Standard portion | Amount (mcg phylloquinone) |
| --- | --- | --- |
| Collards, cooked | ½ c | 530 |
| Turnip greens, boiled | ½ c | 426 |
| Spinach, raw | 1 c | 145 |
| Kale, raw | 1 c | 113 |
| Broccoli, boiled | ½ c | 110 |
| Soybeans, roasted | ½ c | 43 |
| Soybean oil | 1 tbsp | 25 |
| Pumpkin, canned | ½ c | 20 |
| Blueberries, raw | ½ c | 14 |
| Iceberg lettuce, raw | 1 c | 14 |

Vitamin K: fact sheet for health professionals. Office of Dietary Supplements, National Institutes of Health. Updated March 29, 2021. Accessed August 27, 2024. https://ods.od .nih.gov/factsheets/VitaminK-HealthProfessional

### TABLE A.5  Thiamin (Vitamin B1)

| Food | Standard portion | Amount (mg) |
| --- | --- | --- |
| Breakfast cereal, ready-to-eat, fortified | ¾-1 c | 1.2 |
| Egg noodles, enriched, cooked | 1 c | 0.5 |
| English muffin, enriched | 1 each | 0.3 |
| Pork, cooked | 3 oz | 0.4 |
| Black beans, cooked | ½ c | 0.4 |
| Acorn squash, cooked | ½ c | 0.2 |
| Rice, enriched, cooked | ½ c | 0.1 |
| Bread, whole wheat | 1 slice | 0.1 |
| Orange juice, frozen concentrate | 1 c | 0.1 |
| Milk, reduced-fat | 1 c | 0.1 |

Thiamin: fact sheet for health professionals. Office of Dietary Supplements, National Institutes of Health. Updated February 9, 2023. Accessed August 27, 2024. https://ods.od.nih .gov/factsheets/thiamin-HealthProfessional

**TABLE A.6  Riboflavin (Vitamin B2)**

| Food | Standard portion | Amount (mg) |
|---|---|---|
| Beef liver, cooked | 3 oz | 2.9 |
| Breakfast cereal, ready-to-eat, fortified | ¾-1 c | 1.7-2.1 |
| Oats, cooked with water | 1 c | 1.1 |
| Milk, reduced-fat | 1 c | 0.5 |
| Beef, cooked | 3 oz | 0.4 |
| Clams, cooked | 3 oz | 0.4 |
| Almonds, roasted | 1 oz | 0.3 |
| Cheese, Swiss | 3 oz | 0.3 |
| Chicken or turkey, cooked | 3 oz | 0.2 |
| Egg, scrambled | 1 each | 0.2 |
| Bread, whole wheat | 1 slice | 0.1 |
| Tomatoes, canned | ½ c | 0.1 |

Riboflavin: fact sheet for health professionals. Office of Dietary Supplements, National Institutes of Health. Updated May 11, 2022. Accessed August 27, 2024. https://ods.od .nih.gov/factsheets/riboflavin-HealthProfessional

**TABLE A.7  Niacin (Vitamin B3)**

| Food | Standard portion | Amount (mg) |
|---|---|---|
| Beef liver, cooked | 3 oz | 14.9 |
| Chicken breast, cooked | 3 oz | 10.3 |
| Marinara (spaghetti) sauce, ready-to-serve | 1 c | 10.3 |
| Salmon, cooked | 3 oz | 8.6 |
| Tuna, canned in water, drained | 3 oz | 8.6 |
| Pork, cooked | 3 oz | 6.3 |
| Beef, ground, cooked | 3 oz | 5.8 |
| Brown rice, cooked | 1 c | 5.2 |
| Peanuts, roasted | 1 oz | 4.2 |
| Breakfast cereal, ready-to-eat, fortified | ¾-1 c | 4 |
| Potato, russet, baked | 1 medium | 2.3 |

Niacin: fact sheet for health professionals. Office of Dietary Supplements, National Institutes of Health. Updated November 18, 2022. Accessed August 27, 2024. https://ods.od .nih.gov/factsheets/niacin-HealthProfessional

## Top Food Sources for Micronutrients

### TABLE A.8  Vitamin B6 (Pyridoxine)

| Food | Standard portion | Amount (mg) |
| --- | --- | --- |
| Chickpeas, canned | 1 c | 1.1 |
| Tuna, cooked | 3 oz | 0.9 |
| Salmon, cooked | 3 oz | 0.6 |
| Chicken or turkey, cooked | 3 oz | 0.4-0.5 |
| Breakfast cereal, ready-to-eat, fortified | ¾-1 c | 0.4 |
| Potatoes, cooked | 1 c | 0.4 |
| Banana | 1 medium | 0.4 |
| Beef, ground, cooked | 3 oz | 0.3 |
| Cottage cheese | 1 c | 0.2 |
| Squash, winter, cooked | ½ c | 0.2 |
| Rice, cooked | 1 c | 0.1 |
| Raisins | ½ c | 0.1 |

Vitamin B6: fact sheet for health professionals. Office of Dietary Supplements, National Institutes of Health. Updated June 16, 2023. Accessed August 27, 2024. https://ods.od.nih.gov/factsheets/VitaminB6-HealthProfessional

### TABLE A.9  Folate (Vitamin B9)

| Food | Standard portion | Amount (mcg DFE) |
| --- | --- | --- |
| Beef liver, cooked | 3 oz | 215 |
| Pasta, enriched | 1 c | 148 |
| Spinach, cooked | ½ c | 131 |
| Breakfast cereal, ready-to-eat, fortified | ¾-1 c | 100 |
| Rice, cooked | ½ c | 90 |
| Asparagus, cooked | ½ c (4 spears) | 89 |
| Mixed greens, raw | 1 c | 55-65 |
| Broccoli, cooked | ½ c | 52 |
| Bread, white, enriched | 1 slice | 50 |
| Kidney beans, canned | ½ c | 46 |
| Orange juice | 1 c | 44 |

Abbreviations: DFE, dietary folate equivalent.
Folate: fact sheet for health professionals. Office of Dietary Supplements, National Institutes of Health. Updated November 30, 2022. Accessed August 27, 2024. https://ods.od.nih.gov/factsheets/folate-HealthProfessional

## TABLE A.10  Vitamin B12 (Cobalamin)

| Food | Standard portion | Amount (mcg) |
|------|------------------|--------------|
| Beef liver, cooked | 3 oz | 71 |
| Nutritional yeast, fortified | ¼ c | 8-24 |
| Salmon, cooked | 3 oz | 2.6 |
| Tuna, canned in water | 3 oz | 2.5 |
| Beef, ground, cooked | 3 oz | 2.4 |
| Yogurt | 6 oz | 1 |
| Breakfast cereal, ready-to-eat, fortified | ¾-1 c | 0.6 |
| Cheese, cheddar | 1.5 oz | 0.5 |
| Egg | 1 each | 0.5 |
| Turkey, cooked | 3 oz | 0.3 |
| Tempeh | ½ c | 0.1 |

Vitamin B12: fact sheet for health professionals. Office of Dietary Supplements, National Institutes of Health. Updated March 6, 2024. Accessed August 27, 2024. https://ods.od.nih.gov/factsheets/VitaminB12-HealthProfessional

## TABLE A.11  Vitamin C

| Food | Standard portion | Amount (mg) |
|------|------------------|-------------|
| Peppers, red, yellow, or green, raw | 1 c | 120-190 |
| Orange juice | 1 c | 116 |
| Strawberries, frozen and raw | 1 c | 98 |
| Grapefruit juice | 1 c | 87 |
| Kiwifruit | 1 medium | 64 |
| Orange, raw | 1 medium | 70 |
| Broccoli, cooked | ½ c | 51 |
| Brussels sprouts, cooked | ½ c | 48 |
| Tomato juice | 1 c | 41 |
| Cantaloupe | ½ c | 29 |

Vitamin C: fact sheet for health professionals. Office of Dietary Supplements, National Institutes of Health. Updated March 26, 2021. Accessed August 27, 2024. https://ods.od.nih.gov/factsheets/VitaminC-HealthProfessional

### TABLE A.12  Iron

| Food | Standard portion | Amount (mg) |
| --- | :---: | :---: |
| Breakfast cereal, ready-to-eat, fortified | ¾-1 c | 18 |
| White beans, canned | 1 c | 8 |
| Lentils, cooked | 1 c | 6 |
| Spinach, cooked | ½ c | 3 |
| Tofu, firm | ½ c | 3 |
| Chickpeas, cooked | ½ c | 2 |
| Tomatoes, canned | ½ c | 2 |
| Beef, cooked | 3 oz | 2 |
| Potato, baked | 1 medium | 2 |
| Bread, whole wheat | 1 slice | 1 |

Iron: fact sheet for health professionals. Office of Dietary Supplements, National Institutes of Health. Updated June 15, 2023. Accessed August 27, 2024. https://ods.od.nih.gov/factsheets/Iron-HealthProfessional

### TABLE A.13  Calcium

| Food | Standard portion | Amount (mg) |
| --- | :---: | :---: |
| Yogurt, plain | 1 c | 415 |
| Orange juice, fortified with calcium | 1 c | 349 |
| Cheese, mozzarella | 1.5 oz | 333 |
| Cheese, cheddar | 1.5 oz | 306 |
| Milk, nonfat | 1 c | 299 |
| Soy milk, fortified with calcium | 1 c | 299 |
| Tofu, firm, with calcium sulfate | ½ c | 253 |
| Salmon, canned with bones | 3 oz | 181 |
| Breakfast cereal, ready-to-eat, fortified | ¾-1 c | 130 |
| Spinach, cooked | 0.5 c | 123 |

Calcium: fact sheet for health professionals. Office of Dietary Supplements, National Institutes of Health. Updated July 24, 2024. Accessed August 27, 2024. https://ods.od.nih.gov/factsheets/calcium-HealthProfessional

### TABLE A.14  Copper

| Food | Standard portion | Amount (mcg) |
| --- | --- | --- |
| Beef liver, cooked | 3 oz | 12,400 |
| Oysters, cooked | 3 oz | 4,850 |
| Baking chocolate, unsweetened | 1 oz | 938 |
| Potato, cooked with skin | 1 medium | 675 |
| Cashews, roasted | 1 oz | 629 |
| Crab, Dungeness, cooked | 3 oz | 624 |
| Tofu, raw, firm | ½ c | 476 |
| Salmon, cooked | 3 oz | 273 |
| Pasta, whole wheat, cooked | 1 c | 263 |
| Avocado, raw | ½ c | 219 |

Copper: fact sheet for health professionals. Office of Dietary Supplements, National Institutes of Health. Updated October 18, 2022. Accessed August 27, 2024. https://ods.od.nih.gov/factsheets/copper-HealthProfessional

### TABLE A.15  Selenium

| Food | Standard portion | Amount (mcg) |
| --- | --- | --- |
| Brazil nuts | 1 oz | 544 |
| Tuna, yellowfin, cooked | 3 oz | 92 |
| Spaghetti, cooked | 1 c | 33 |
| Turkey, cooked | 3 oz | 26 |
| Ham, cooked | 3 oz | 24 |
| Chicken, cooked | 3 oz | 22 |
| Cottage cheese, low-fat | 1 c | 20 |
| Beef, ground, cooked | 3 oz | 18 |
| Brown rice, cooked | 1 c | 12 |
| Bread, whole wheat | 1 slice | 8 |

Selenium: fact sheet for health professionals. Office of Dietary Supplements, National Institutes of Health. Updated April 15, 2024. Accessed August 27, 2024. https://ods.od.nih.gov/factsheets/selenium-HealthProfessional

## Top Food Sources for Micronutrients

### TABLE A.16  Zinc

| Food | Standard portion | Amount (mg) |
|---|---|---|
| Oysters, cooked | 3 oz | 32 |
| Beef, sirloin, cooked | 3 oz | 3.8 |
| Breakfast cereal, ready-to-eat, fortified | ¾-1 c | 2.8 |
| Oatmeal, cooked with water | 1 c | 2.3 |
| Pork, cooked | 3 oz | 1.9 |
| Turkey breast, cooked | 3 oz | 1.5 |
| Cheese, cheddar | 1.5 oz | 1.5 |
| Yogurt, Greek | 6 oz | 1 |
| Peanuts, roasted | 1 oz | 0.8 |
| Egg | 1 each | 0.6 |
| Kidney beans, canned | ½ c | 0.6 |
| Bread, whole wheat | 1 slice | 0.6 |

Zinc: fact sheet for health professionals. Office of Dietary Supplements, National Institutes of Health. Updated September 28, 2022. Accessed August 27, 2024. https://ods.od.nih.gov/factsheets/zinc-HealthProfessional

Top Sources for Micronutrients

# Continuing Professional Education

This edition of *Academy of Nutrition and Dietetics Pocket Guide to Micronutrient Management* offers readers Continuing Professional Education (CPE) credit. Please check the expiration date and the number of hours offered at the link that follows or on the product page at www.eatrightSTORE.org. Readers may earn credit by completing the interactive online quiz at: https://publications .webauthor.com/PG_micronutrient_mgmt

The Academy of Nutrition and Dietetics Product Strategy & Development team can be reached at publications@eatright.org. Additional notes, errata, related products, and information on licensing and permissions can be found on the product page at www.eatrightSTORE.org or at the QR code below.

# Index

Letters *b*, *f*, and *t* after page number indicate box, figure, and table, respectively.